Handbook of Public Health: Advanced Research

Volume III

Handbook of Public Health: Advanced Research Volume III

Edited by **Felix Rohmer**

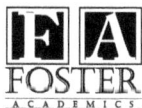

FA **FOSTER**
ACADEMICS

New Jersey

Published by Foster Academics,
61 Van Reypen Street,
Jersey City, NJ 07306, USA
www.fosteracademics.com

Handbook of Public Health: Advanced Research
Volume III
Edited by Felix Rohmer

International Standard Book Number: 978-1-63242-216-3 (Hardback)

Contents

Preface

This book explains the advanced research developments in Public health. Public health is considered as the cornerstone and basis of health, commonly and in medicine. It is described as the science and art of prolonging life, preventing disease and promoting health through the systematized efforts and smart choices of organizations, private and public, society, communities and individuals. This field has evolved by the incorporation of multiple factors, knowledge fields, professionals and it has also been promoted by various technologies, primarily – information technology. As a transforming field of knowledge, public health needs information based on evidence and timely updates. This book provides up-to-date information on several topics associated with actual fields of interest in this emerging and exciting medical science, with the philosophy and conception to enhance the health of the population. Rather than treating illnesses of specific patients, taking decisions regarding cumulative health care that are based on the best available, recent, authentic and significant evidence, are finally within the context of available resources. This book offers a broad geographical perspective since information in this book has been contributed by researchers and scientists from across the globe. It includes important sections on Non-Communicable Diseases in Public Health; Environmental Public Health; Pharmaco-epidemiology and Pharmaco-surveillance; and Research, Ethics, Social and Teaching Issues. All these aspects make this book a great update on several subjects of world public health.

This book unites the global concepts and researches in an organized manner for a comprehensive understanding of the subject. It is a ripe text for all researchers, students, scientists or anyone else who is interested in acquiring a better knowledge of this dynamic field.

I extend my sincere thanks to the contributors for such eloquent research chapters. Finally, I thank my family for being a source of support and help.

Editor

Non-Communicable Diseases in Public Health

Topics in Prevention of Diseases in Gastroenterology

Leonardo Sosa Valencia and Erika Rodriguez-Wulff

Additional information is available at the end of the chapter

1. Introduction

Cancer is a disease caused by an uncontrolled division of abnormal cells in a part of the body, in another words, is a malignant growth or tumor resulting from such a division of cells. Is the leading cause of death worldwide. Attributed 7.6 million deaths (approximately 13% of total) occurred worldwide in 2008. The most common types of cancer are shown in Figure 1 [1]

- Gastric (736,000 deaths);

- Liver (695,000 deaths);

- Colorectal (608,000 deaths);

- Pancreas (227,000 deaths).

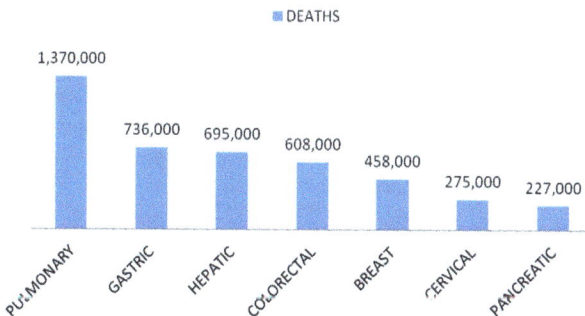

Figure 1. Cancer deaths in 2008

Cancers that cause more deaths per year are lung, stomach, liver, colon and breast.

In this problem, are involving genetic factors and lifestyle of the population, approximately 30% of cancer deaths are due to five behavioral risk factors and diet: high body mass index, reduced intake of fruits and vegetables, sedentary lifestyle, smoking and alcohol use.

More than 50% of cancer could be prevented if people implemented what is already known about cancer prevention, according to researchers at the Union for International Cancer Control (UICC) World Cancer Congress 2012 [2].

In this chapter, we summarize the relationship of some gastrointestinal cancer and factors that can be change in our population to decrease and prevent them in the future.

2. Helicobacter pylori and gastric cancer

Gastric cancer is the second leading cause of cancer death in the world [3,4,5]. A number of environmental factors such as Helicobacter pylori status, smoking, alcohol, decrease vitamin C intake, nitrosamines and nitrates, and salt intake are related to gastric cancer development. Also the presence of a family history of gastric cancer is significantly associated with increased risk of developing the disease [6] Figure 2. Gastric carcinogenesis is a multifactorial process, involving complex interactions between host and environmental factors [7]. It is known that gastric cancer involves the interaction of three major factors: the agent (in the great part of the cases, H. pylori) and its pathogenicity, the characteristics of the host, and the external environment [8].

Among these factors, have been associated with the development of gastric cancer, premalignant conditions within which include chronic atrophic gastritis, intestinal metaplasia, Helicobacter pylori infection and gastric adenoma [3,4,5,8]. Chronic inflammation plays an important role in the development of gastric cancer. Inflammation-induced injury may compromise tissue integrity and drive the multistage process of carcinogenesis by altering targets and pathways crucial to normal tissue homeostasis [7].

Helicobacter pylori (H. pylori), is a spiral, Gram-negative microaerophilic bacterial pathogen that is distributed worldwide and is in particular found in developing countries, infecting the stomach of about 50 % of the world's population [9]. H. pylori infection is closely related to the development of gastric cancer [10]. In 1994 the results of epidemiological studies carried, the World Health Organization's International Agency for Research on Cancer to concluded that H. pylori has a causal link with gastric carcinogenesis and was defined as a type I carcinogen, a definite human carcinogen [10,8]. The evidence in the population of whole world shows that H. pylori infection, has been known to induce chronic gastric inflammation that leads to atrophy, metaplasia, dysplasia, and gastric cancer [3,7]. All patients with H. pylori infection have histological gastritis, which corresponds to classical chronic gastritis and is characterized by the infiltration of neutrophils and other inflammatory cells. However, most patients are asymptomatic for life, while only some will come to develop a digestive disease [8]. The transmission route of H. pylori infection has been the topic of sev-

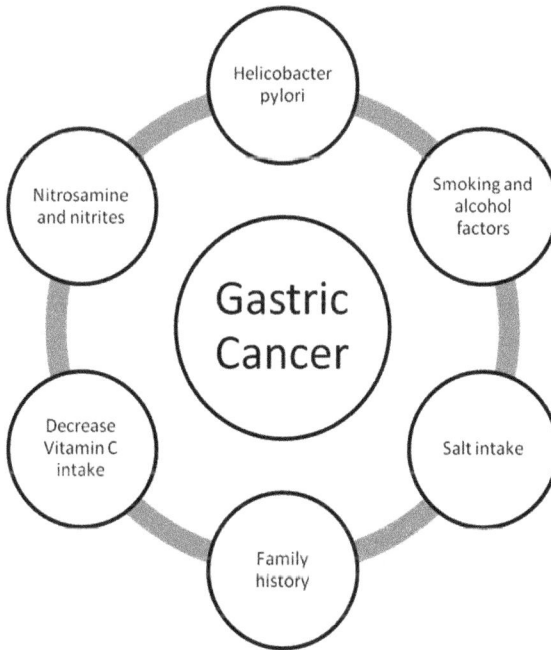

Figure 2. Associated factors in Gastric Cancer

eral studies. Most infections are probably acquired in childhood, mainly via oral-oral or fecal-oral routes; H. pylori has been found in saliva, dental plaques and feces, which shows that oral and fecal cavities are probably involved in H. pylori transmission, however, the exact mode of transmission is still unknown [11].

Gastric cancer can develop both in the proximal and the distal region. Dietary factors and H. pylori infection are major risk factors for the development of distal tumors; the major risk factors for proximal cancers are gastroesophageal reflux disease and obesity [5].

The gastric intestinal metaplasia is recognized as a premalignant condition that may be the result of adaptive response to environmental stimuli such as infection by H. pylori, smoking and high concentrations of salt intake. Patients with intestinal metaplasia are up to 10 times greater risk of developing gastric cancer, which may be higher in certain geographical areas and in patients infected with H. pylori [12]. Figure 3.

Despite advances in diagnosis, the disease is usually detected after invasion of the muscular propia, because most patients experience vague and nonspecific symptoms in the early stages and the classic triad of anemia, weight loss, and refusal of meat-based foods is seen only in advanced stages. Furthermore, surgery and chemotherapy have limited value in advanced disease and there is a paucity of molecular markers for targeted therapy. Since cancer of the stomach has a very poor prognosis and the 5-year survival rate is only around 20 per cent, a new look at the results of epidemiological and experimental studies is important to establish strategies for primary prevention [5]. As treatment of gastric cancer at the symptomatic stage represents a significant medical burden, clinicians have been encouraged to focus on designing preventive strategies instead of multimodal therapies [13].

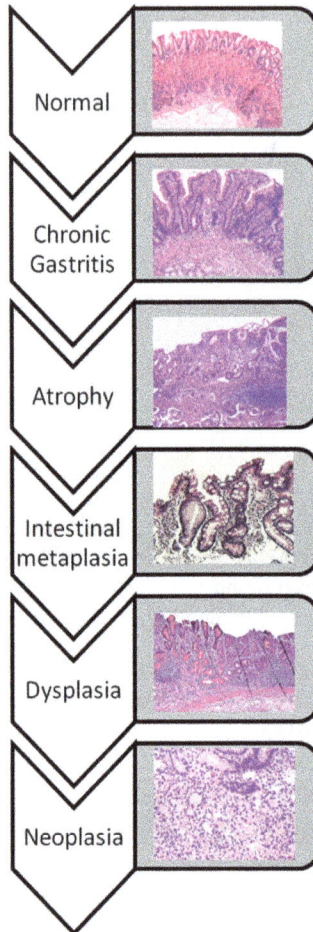

Figure 3. Gastric carcinogenesis: Histologyc changes from normal gastric mucosa to neoplasia.

As a primary prevention, some behavior modifications have been suggested, including reduction of salt intake with the diet, increase of vitamin C consumption, abolition of smoking and H. pylori eradication wich is recommended as it is able to reduce gastric cancer incidence up to 35% [14]. If infection with H. pylori is identified, eradication should be considered the same because it is considered a class I carcinogen [12]. After eradicating H. pylori, precancerous lesions may regress. Testing and treating for the H pylori infection earlier rather than later in life is suggested to be the more beneficial approach [7]. The eradication of H. pylori prophylactically pylori remains controversial in humans, has not shown a significant reduction in the risk of gastric cancer after eradication of H pylori [10], but in a recent population-based study, early H pylori eradication was found to be associated with decreased risk of gastric cancer [7]. There are some studies indicating that the eradication of the microorganisms in the system could reduce the incidence of gastric cancer in patients without precancerous lesions or, when lesions are presents, that the eradication may or may not reduce this incidence. Also, when the eradication is done after endoscopic mucosal resection in patients with early gastric adenocarcinoma, it could decrease the recurrence of metachronous gastric cancer in some patients [8].

3. Hepatitis virus and liver cancer

The hepatocellular carcinoma (HCC), is the most frequent form of primary liver cancer [15], it accounts for up to 90% [16], and is one of the most common malignancies in the world [17], is the third most common cause of cancer-related death worldwide [18,19], results in between 250.000 and one million deaths globally per annum, the increasing incidence rates are in many parts of the world, including the United States and Central Europe. The Incidence of HCC in the United States is expected to continue to rise as a consequence of high hepatitis C infection rates between 1960 and 1990 and the average 20 to 30 year lag time between virus acquisition and the development of cirrhosis and carcinoma.

Cancers caused by viral infections such as infections of hepatitis B virus (HBV), hepatitis C virus (HCV) and human papillomavirus (HPV), are responsible for up to 20% of cancer deaths in middle-income countries low and medium [1]. The major risk factors for the development of HCC include liver cirrhosis of any etiology [16]. Almost 80 percent of cases are due to underlying chronic hepatitis B and C virus infection [19]. Occur with particular frequency in patients with cirrhosis caused by hepatitis virus. HCC can develop in patients with chronic HBV, even in the absence of cirrhosis. However, 70 to 90 percent of patients with HBV who develop HCC will have cirrhosis [18]. The strong association between liver cancer and cirrhosis has been recognized in patients with HCV [17]. Chronic infection of HBV and hepatitis C virus are well-documented major etiologic factors for HCC [20,21].

The majority of HCC occur in patients with chronic liver disease or cirrhosis. Thus, older patients with longstanding liver disease are more likely to develop HCC, it develops commonly, but not exclusively, in a setting of chronic liver cell injury, inflammation which leads to, hepatocyte regeneration, liver matrix remodeling, fibrosis, and ultimately, cirrhosis. The major etiologies of liver cirrhosis are diverse and include chronic HBV and HCV, alcohol consumption, steatosis, diabetes, certain medications or toxic exposures, including dietary aflatoxins and genetic metabolic diseases [22,23]. In addition to cirrhosis, a number of other factors have been associated with the risk of developing HCC among patients with chronic HBV, including the viral load, the presence of hepatitis B e antigen (HBeAg), and the presence of hepatitis B surface antigen (HBsAg). The risk of HCC is much greater in patients with high serum levels of HBV DNA compared with those who have low levels (<10,000 copies/mL). Figure 4.

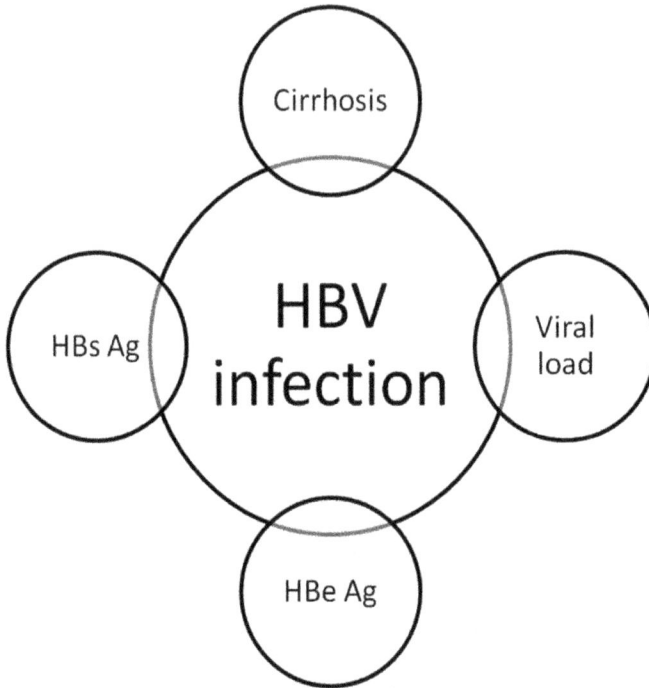

HCC: Hepatocellular Carcinoma. HBV: Virus Hepatitis B. HBs Ag: Hepatitis B surface antigen. HBe Ag: Hepatitis B e antigen

Figure 4. Factors associated with the risk of develop HCC in patients with chronic HBV

The mechanisms by which these varied etiologies lead to cirrhosis and HCC are not yet fully understood [21,22,23]. A common pathway from these varied etiologies to HCC may involve chronic inflammation, which is increasingly recognized as a procarcinogenic condition [21,22]. Both viruses have been classified as human carcinogens by the International Agency for Research on Cancer [20]. Malignant transformation that is induced by chronic HBV infection is a multistage pathogenic process and involves multiple risk predictors [20]. Other many factors determining the risk of developing an HCC are host dependent, some are genetic and not modifiable, other are linked to lifestyle and can be influenced [15]; age, gender, family history of HCC, alcohol consumption habits, serostatus of hepatitis B e antigen, HBV genotype and mutant types, as well as serum quantitative levels of ALT and HBV DNA are important long-term risk predictors of HCC [20]. Figure 5.

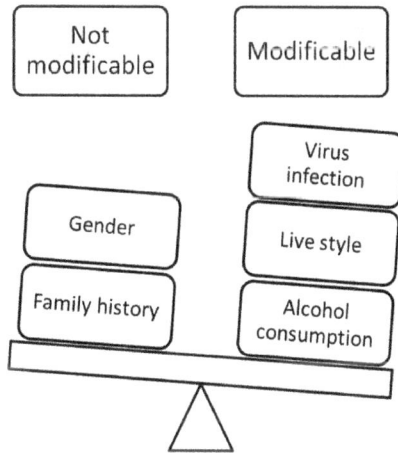

HCC: Hepatocellular Carcinoma.

Figure 5. Host dependant factors that determining risk of HCC

A variety of important risk factors for the development of HCC have been identified. These include viral infections, environmental toxins, comorbid conditions, inherited errors of metabolism, and autoimmune disorders [18]. At one major referral center in the United States, the most commonly seen risk factors for HCC were HCV infection, alcohol use, and nonalcoholic fatty liver disease. In a 5-year cumulative incidence, hepatocellular carcinoma in patients with HCV cirrhosis is about 15%, the risk is increased 2-6 fold in the presence of other risk factors such as alcohol, obesity, diabetes mellitus and HBV [24]. HBeAg positivity, which indicates active viral replication, is also associated with the development of HCC. The risk of HCC is also elevated in patients who are HBsAg positive but HBeAg negative (inactive carriers) compared with the general population.

Because of the association of HBV with HCC, screening for HCC is recommended for many patients with hepatitis B. Currently, it is recommended that patients with high HBV DNA levels and signs of active inflammation (elevated ALT) for several years undergo surveillance for HCC.

Coinfection with HCV has also been associated with an increased risk of HCC. Some studies suggest that patients with dual HBV and HCV infection may have a higher rate of HCC compared with patients infected by either virus alone, particularly those who are anti-HCV and HBeAg positive. Coinfection with hepatitis D virus (HDV) also appears to increase the risk of HCC among patients with HBV. Hepatitis C accounts for at least one-third of the cases of HCC in the United States. An important clinical observation is that HCC in patients with HCV occurs almost exclusively in patients with advanced stages of hepatic fibrosis or cirrhosis.

Symptoms attributable to HCC are usually absent, when symptomatic, is often associated with nonspecific complaints, including right upper abdominal or epigastric pain, early satiety, weight loss, and malaise. Rather, patients typically manifest symptoms related to underlying cirrhosis, a condition present in 80%–90% of patients with HCC. Consequently, the majority of patients are diagnosed with advanced disease, often precluding potentially curative therapies. HCC is associated with a number of paraneoplastic syndromes resulting in hypoglycemia, erythrocytosis, hypercholesterolemia, hypercalcemia, severe watery diarrhea, and cutaneous manifestations. Extrahepatic spread at presentation is relatively uncommon, ranging between 10% and 30% [18].

Eradicating the main viruses associated with cancer worldwide by implementing widespread infant and childhood immunization programs targeting 3 viruses — human papillomavirus and hepatitis B and C — could lead to a 100% reduction in viral-related cancer incidence in 20 to 40 years [2].

4. Colonoscopy and colon cancer

The colonoscopy consists in visualizing the entire large bowel mucosa and the terminal ileum, is widely used for diagnosis and treatment of diseases of the colon; performed properly, is safe, accurate and well tolerated by most patients [25]. Is used for primary colorectal cancer screening, monitoring of patients with colon cancer and for diagnosis in patients with lower gastrointestinal tract symptoms, also used to evaluate patients with screening tests for colorectal cancer such as occult blood positive stool, sigmoidoscopy, fecal DNA, or images studies [26,27,28], having shown in ramdom studies that has been effective in reducing deaths from colorectal cancer [28,29,30].

Colorectal cancer is a leading cause of cancer worldwide [29,31,32,33] increased in both sexes with an increase in incidence and mortality, which is why we have emphasized the need to improve prevention and control in order to modify the course of the disease and improve prognosis [29,31,34]. The rate of colorectal cancer mortality has declined substantially in part by the increase in the performance of studies including screening colonoscopy, which aims to reduce mortality based on a reduction in the incidence of advanced disease [34,35].

There is evidence that most colon cancers develop from adenomatous polyps (adenoma-carcinoma sequence) [36,37] and takes about 10 years when a polyp of 1 cm from becoming invasive colorectal cancer [38], the risk is higher in advanced adenomas, greater than or equal to 1 cm and / or villous component and / or high grade dysplasia [37]. Being a long term process which involves multiple steps, the disease is preventable, on the other hand, if the disease is detected in a first step, the curative is possible [26].

Many colorectal cancer studies focus on symptomatic populations, however, the majority of colorectal adenomas are asymptomatic and are detected by chance during colonoscopy [39].

This finding that adenomatous polyps are precursors to cancer and these are usually asymptomatic, has gained strength in the screening asymptomatic individuals for early cancer detection and prevention [38].

Colonoscopy is considered the preferred tool for colorectal cancer screening [25,29,31,32,33,38,40,41] because it allows us both to make detection and sampling of the lesions and to detect and remove polypoid lesions [25,26,34,35,38,42]. Colonoscopy with removal of adenomas is a useful tool to reduce the incidence and mortality of colorectal cancer, and is recommended as the first choice for screening in patients with intermediate risk of colorectal cancer [36,37,43,44,45].

In individuals with average risk, the U.S. Multi-Society Task Force on Colorectal Cancer and the American Cancer Society recommend screening should begin at age 50 regardless of sex and race [38,46], however, the American College of Gastroenterology suggests to consider these two factors and to be started earlier in blacks because they have a higher incidence and age of onset of colorectal cancer earlier [46]. Other authors suggest could benefit from colorectal cancer screening people with abdominal obesity or metabolic syndrome from 45 years of age reported having these risk factors are independent [45]. In patients at high familial risk, screening is different.

The ASGE publish this guideline for colorectal cancer screening and surveillance [38]:

1. Individuals at Risk for FAP Flexible sigmoidoscopy screening should undergo yearly starting at age 10 to 12 years. The Development of multiple, diffuse adenomas in the colon is an indication for colectomy Total.

2. Individuals at Risk for HNPCC should undergo colonoscopy every 1 to 2 years starting at age 20 to 25 years or 10 years younger than the age of the earliest diagnosis of cancer in the family, whichever is earlier.

3. Individuals with a family history of 1 or more first degree relatives with sporadic CRC regardless of age, should have a colonoscopy beginning at age 40 years or 10 years younger than the affected relative, whichever is earlier. If the index has regular colonoscopy results, repeat colonoscopy should be performed on the basis of the relative age of the affected.

4. Individuals with a first-degree relative age 60 years with adenomatous polyps should undergo colonoscopy at age 40 years or 10 years younger than the affected relative, whichever is earlier. If the index examination is normal, recommend repeat colonoscopy every 5 years.

5. In patients with a first-degree relative more than 60 years old at diagnosis of adenomatous polyps, the timing of screening colonoscopy should be individualized. The timing interval follow-up examinations between should be the same as for average-risk patients.

6. In individuals with UC and Crohn's extensive colitis. Surveillance colonoscopy with multiple biopsy specimens should be performed every 1 to 2 years after beginning 8 to 10 years of disease.

7. A complete colonoscopy should be performed in all patients diagnosed with CRC to rule out synchronous or adenomatous lesions cancers. If a complete examination can not be performed at the time of CRC diagnosis, a colonoscopy should be performed within 6 months after surgical resection.

8. Surveillance colonoscopy after surgical resection of CRC should be performed 1 year after surgery and, if results are normal, every 3 to 5 years thereafter.

Adenomatous polyps are the most frequent neoplasm found during colorectal screening and removal of these lesions have been shown to reduce the risk for future colorectal cancer or advanced adenomas (gastrointestinal). One of the parameters critical to the viability and profitability of colonoscopy for colorectal cancer screening is the time interval for surveillance colonoscopy after resection of an adenoma, surveillance intervals are based primarily on the recurrence of adenoma and not in the incidence of colorectal cancer [43]. In 2006, the U.S. Multi-Society Task Force on Colorectal Cancer joint the American Cancer Society to Provide a broader consensus and thereby increase the use of the recomendations by endoscopists, publishing guidelines for colonoscopy surveillance These after polypectomy:

1. Patients with small rectal polyps should be considered to have normal colonoscopies and therefore, the interval for subsequent colonoscopy should be 10 years. An exception is patients with hyperplastic polyposis syndrome, they are at an increased risk of colorectal adenomas and cancer and need to be identified for more intensive monitoring.

2. Patients with only 1 or 2 small tubular adenomas (less than 1 cm) with only low-grade dysplasia should have their next colonoscopy control in 5 to 10 years, the precise time within this range should be based on other clinical factors such as a result of previous colonoscopy, family history and patient preference and physician's discretion.

3. Patients with 3 or more adenomas, adenomas larger than 1 cm or villous features or adenoma with high grade dysplasia should have their next colonoscopy in control 3 years after complete resection of the adenoma. If the colonoscopy is normal or shows up in 1 or 2 small tubular adenomas or low-grade dysplasia, the interval for further study should be 5 years.

4. Patients who have 10 or more adenomas in an examination, should be reevaluated in a shorter period as 3 years, interval established by clinical judgment, it being necessary to consider an underlying familial syndrome.

5. Patients with sessile adenomas that are removed by picemeal monitoring should be considered for short intervals between 2-6 months to verify complete removal, which, once established, subsequent surveillance should be individualized based on the judgment of the endoscopist, the integrity of elimination by both endoscopy and biopsy evaluations.

6. More intensive monitoring is indicated when the family history may indicate HNPCC.

Subsequent studies suggest that it may be considered to extend surveillance intervals even in people 5 years after detection and elimination of high-risk polyps [43].

It has been reported that colonoscopy could prevent approximately 85% of cases of distal colorectal cancer while the risk reduction for proximal colon is significantly lower ranging from 0-55% [42], but colonoscopy is not perfect have been diagnosed with cancer between the intervals of follow-up examinations, reporting an incidence rate ranging from 1.7 to 2.4 cancers per 1,000 persons / year of observation [44]. The effectiveness of colonoscopy in reducing colon cancer incidence depends on adequate visualization of the mucosa, diligence in examining the mucosa and patient acceptance of the procedure [25]. That is why for the reporting of colonoscopies are suggested previously structured reports that include quality indicators such as colonoscopies specific point as far as progress, quality of bowel preparation, cecal intubation, polyp detection [27], since it has been shown that the quality of colonoscopy is also important in screening, low quality colonoscopies reduce the effectiveness especially in the proximal colon [29]. It has been reported that conventional colonoscopy some lesions may be missed even with adequate colonic preparation, this may be partly because flat lesions which makes them difficult to recognize or be injuries that are located behind the colonic haustral; it is proposes that autofluorescence imaging are better for the detection of colorectal neoplasia than conventional colonoscopy [33]. With the increase of colonoscopy in the general population over 50 years, has contributed to the decreased incidence of colorectal cancer observed since the mid-year 1980 [40].

Should bear in mind the risk cost benefit of screening colonoscopy for colorectal cancer in elderly patients, remains controversial at this stage because the net benefit of screening reduces the risk of mortality from other diseases, reporting especially in octogenarians, a increased risk of complications during and after colonoscopy [32], the benefits of screening are significantly limited due to their short life expectancy [47].

A recent study showed that after a median follow-up of 11.9 years, there was a 21% relative risk reduction in the incidence of colorectal cancer and a 26% reduction in mortality in adults screened with flexible sigmoidoscopy, with a repeat screening at 3 or 5 years, compared with those treated with the usual care [2].

5. Obesity and pancreatic cancer

Pancreatic cancer is the eighth leading cause of cancer-related death [48], is one of the most lethal malignant diseases due to the high rate of advanced stage disease at diagnosis, and the lack of any affective medical therapy [49]. Currently, there are no methods of screening established for early detection; thus, at present, primary prevention by altering modifiable risk factors will probably be the most effective way of reducing the burden pancreatic cancer [50]. The etiology of pancreatic cancer is complex and poorly understood, therefore the indentification of risk factors, specially those which are modifiable through medication or behavioral change, is important for the development and progression preventing of pancreatic cancer. The risk factors for pancreatic cancer include family history, smoking, obesity, diabetes mellitus and chronic pancreatitis [49,51,52,53] Figure 6.

Family history	Smoking	Obesity

Diabetes mellitus	Chronic pancreatitis

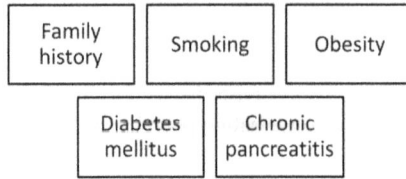

Figure 6. Risk factors for pancreatic cancer

Obesity is defined as abnormal or excessive accumulation of fat that can be harmful to health [48]. A World Health Organization (WHO) report demonstrates that more than 400 million people are obese in the world, with a predicted increase to 700 million by 2015 [52]. Since 1990, the prevalence of obesity has doubled in the United States [12]. Statistics from 2007 to 2008 indicate that 33.8% of american adults are obese [51]. According to WHO/Food and Agriculture Organization (FAO), obesity and overweight conditions can be diagnosed by measuring the body mass index (BMI) of the individual [52]. The BMI is the ratio of calculated with weight in kilograms divided by the square of height in meters kg/m2. The current standard categories of BMI are as follows: underweight <18.5, normal weight 18.5-24.9, overweight 25.0-29.9, obese 30.0-34.9, and severely obese > or = 35.0 [52,54,55].

Many studies based on large population have shown that obesity and insulin resistance are independent risk factors may types of cancer [50,52,55,56], reporting that the strength of the association varies with the organ and histologic type; this evidence supports the notion that controlling obesity can be an important tool for a number of preventing cancers among the populations of modern societies [57].

A number of recent studies indicate that obesity may be an important risk factor for pancreatic diseases including pancreatitis and pancreatic cancer and is associated with a lower age of onset [54,58]. Between the positive association with BMI and high risk of pancreatic cancer has been in at least observed 19 of 29 prospective studies and three meta-analyzes. The magnitude of the association varied from 10 to 45% increased risk for every 5 kg/m2 increase in BMI. It has been reported that people with a BMI greater than 40 kg/m2 in both sexes have higher cancer mortality rate when compared with normal weight [59], associated with a 50-60% death rate from cancer increased of pancreas [49]. Among the many possible mechanisms involved, hyperinsulinemia, diet and nutritional factors, and other hormone abnormalities have been suggested as causal factors [49]. There are sparse data on the association whether between BMI and pancreatic cancer risk is modified by age, sex, smoking, physical activity and history of diabetes [51,60]. Study showed that increased risk of pancreatic cancer was more strongly associated with obesity at younger adulthood (30-40years) than was weight gain at older age (older than 40years) [51].

In the obese patient, becomes important both visceral fat and ectopic fat, as well as waist circumference and the waist-to-hip ratio in relation to pancreatic cancer risk [50]. It has been described that may centralized increased fat distribution pancreatic cancer risk, especially in women [53]. In these patients and have fat deposits in hepatocytes do in pancreatic cells, resulting in an entity called pancreatic steatosis, it has been hypothesized that pancreatic steatosis could promote the development of chronic pancreatitis and pancreatic cancer [61].

Obesity has also been associated with major metabolic abnormalities including insulin resistance and diabetes, and therefore may be associated with the risk of pancreatic cancer.

It has also demonstrated strong association between pancreatic cancer and two medical conditions chronic pancreatitis and diabetes mellitus. Since these conditions are often present many years before the diagnosis of cancer, they should be considered etiologically relevant [58].

Epidemiological studies have demonstrated that diabetes is a risk factor for multiple forms of malignancy including the pancreatic cancer. Previous studies have implicated long-term diabetes as a modifiable risk factor for pancreatic cancer [51]. Roughly half of all the patients with pancreatic cancer are found to have diabetes at the time of diagnosis, and roughly half of the diabetic patients present which is at the time of pancreatic cancer diagnosis is of new onset having developed over the preceding 2-3 years the diagnosis of pancreatic cancer [49]. There has been a long debate about whether diabetes mellitus is a risk factor for, or a consequence of cancer, pancreatic cancer, but there are findings that suggest that diabetic individuals with a history of 5 or more years and have a 2-fold increase risk of pancreatic cancer compared with those with no history of diabetes or with less than 5 years [58], reporting that the long-standing diabetes increases the risk of pancreatic cancer [54]. The association between pancreatic cancer and diabetes has been investigated extensively, but the causal relationships have yet to be fully elucidated [49].

The association between type 2 diabetes and pancreatic cancer risk can be the result of high concentrations of glucose in the after load and gradual alterations glucose tolerance for years. It supports the hypothesis that glucose tolerance and diabetes play a role in carcinogenesis of pancreatic cancer.

Obesity has been associated with a negative prognostic factor, higher BMI is associated with decreased survival and increased mortality in pancreatic cancer [54,62,63]. Furthermore, in pancreatic cancer, increased BMI has been reported to be an adverse prognostic factor for survival after surgery in two surgical series [63].

A majority of prospective epidemiological studies have found that a high body mass index and/or a lack of physical activity are associated with an increased risk of pancreatic cancer incidence or mortality, independently of prior history of diabetes [53]. Physical activity and reduced caloric intake have to been shown to reduce the risk of pancreatic cancer especially in those who are overweight [49,54]. The successful treatment of obesity and diabetes has been shown to reduce the risk of pancreatic cancer, but the treatment with insulin, insulin analogs, and insulin secretagogues maintains or increases the risk. Metformin as well as livestyle alterations has been shown to reduce the risk of pancreatic cancer [49].

It is estimated that being overweight or obese causes approximately 20% of cancer today. If people could maintain a healthy body mass index (BMI), the incidence of cancer could be reduced by approximately 50% in 2 to 20 years [2].

6. Conclusion

Having the knowledge of the cancer associated factors, interventions could be implemented to prevent and treat it, in order to reduce and control the disease. We should apply science-based strategies for the prevention of disease as well as early detection and treatment of these patients.

A percentage of all cancer deaths could be prevented by modifying or avoiding key risk factors, such as: smoke, overweight or obese, unhealthy diets with a low consumption of fruit and vegetables, physical inactivity, consumption of alcoholic beverages, HPV infection and HBV, air pollution in cities.

It is critical the knowledge of the risk factors to apply prevention strategies in the future to modify the morbidity of this disease.

Author details

Leonardo Sosa Valencia and Erika Rodriguez-Wulff

CITE (National Center of Ecoendoscopia), Caracas, Venezuela

References

[1] Organización Mundial de La SaludNota descriptiva N°297, Febrero de (2012).

[2] Pam HarrisonLifestyle Changes Could Prevent 50% of Common Cancers . Medscape Medical News, September 5, 2012. Union for International Cancer Control (UICC) World Cancer Congress 2012 August (2012). Montreal, Canada, 27-30.

[3] Kenichi SaitoMD, PhD, Kazuko Arai, MD, Masatomo Mori, MD, PhD, Ryouta Kobayashi, MD, Ichiro Ohki, MD, PhD. Effect of Helicobacter pylori eradication on malignant transformation of gastric adenoma. *Gastrointestinal Endoscopy*; (2000).

[4] Anna, D. Wagner, Wilfried Grothe, Johannes Haerting, et al. Chemotherapy in Advanced Gastric Cancer: A Systematic Review and Meta-Analysis Based on Aggregate Data. *Journal Of Clinical Oncology*. 24 (18): 2903-2909, (2006).

[5] Siddavaram NaginiCarcinoma of the stomach: A review of epidemiology, pathogenesis, molecular genetics and chemoprevention. World J Gastrointest Oncol. 4(7): 156-169, (2012).

[6] Mi Ah HanMyueng Guen Oh, Il Ju Choi, et al. Association of Family History With Cancer Recurrence and Survival in Patients With Gastric Cancer. *Journal Of Clinical Oncology*. 30 (7): 701-708, (2012).

[7] Chun-Ying WuMing-Shiang Wu, Ken N. Kuo, et al. Effective Reduction of Gastric Cancer Risk With Regular Use of Nonsteroidal Anti-Inflammatory Drugs in Helicobacter Pylori-Infected Patients. *Journal Of Clinical Oncology.* , 28(18), 2952-2957.

[8] BrunaMaria RoeslerSandra Cecilia Botelho Costa and Jose Murilo Robilotta Zeitune. Eradication Treatment of Helicobacter pylori Infection: Its Importance and Possible Relationship in Preventing the Development of Gastric Cancer. ISRN Gastroenterol. (2012).

[9] Aneta TargoszTomasz Brzozowski, Piotr Pierzchalski et al. Helicobacter pylori promotes apoptosis, activates cyclooxygenase (COX)-2 and inhibits heat shock protein HSP70 in gastric cancer epithelial cells. Inflamm. Res. 61:955-966, (2012).

[10] Yuji MaehataShotaro Nakamura, Kiyoshi Fujisawa, Motohiro Esaki, Tomohiko Moriyama, Kouichi Asano, Yuta Fuyuno et al. Long-term effect of Helicobacter pylori eradication on the development of metachronous gastric cancer after endoscopic resection of early gastric cancer. *Gastrointestinal Endoscopy;* (2012).

[11] Hassan MomtazNegar Souod, Hossein Dabiri et al. Study of Helicobacter pylori genotype status in saliva, dental plaques, stool and gastric biopsy samples. World J Gastroenterol. 18(17): 2105-2111, (2012).

[12] ASGE guideline: the role of endoscopy in the surveillance of premalignant conditions of the upper GI tract*Gastrointestinal Endoscopy;* (2006).

[13] Yi-Chia LeeTony Hsiu-Hsi Chen, Han-Mo Chiu, Chia-Tung Shun, et al. The benefit of mass eradication of Helicobacter pylori infection: a community-based study of gastric cancer prevention. Gut doi:10.1136/gutjnl-, 2012-302240.

[14] Angelo ZulloCesare Hassan, Adriana Romiti et al. Follow-up of intestinal metaplasia in the stomach: When, how and why. World J Gastrointest Oncol. 4(3): 30-36, (2012).

[15] Lorenz KuskeArmand Mensen, Beat Müllhaupt et al. Characteristics of patients with chronic hepatitis C who develop hepatocellular carcinoma. Swiss Med Wkly. 142: 1-9, (2012).

[16] Chung-Hwa ParkSeung-Hee Jeong, Hyeon-Woo Yim et al. Family history influences the early onset of hepatocellular carcinoma. World J Gastroenterol. 18 (21): 2661-2667, (2012).

[17] Katsuya ShirakiAtsuya Shimizu, Koujiro Takase, Atsushi Suzuki, Yukihiko Tameda, Takeshi Nakano. Prospective study of laparoscopic findings with regard to the development of hepatocellular carcinoma in patients with hepatitis C virus-associated cirrhosis. *Gastrointestinal Endoscopy;* (2001).

[18] Christopher L Tinkle and Daphne Haas-KoganHepatocellular carcinoma: natural history, current management, and emerging tools. Biologics: Targets and Therapy. 6: 207-219, (2012).

[19] So Young BaeMoon Seok Choi, Geum-Youn Gwak et al. Comparison of usefulness of clinical diagnostic criteria for hepatocellular carcinoma in a hepatitis B endemic area. Clinical and Molecular Hepatology. 18: 185-194, (2012).

[20] Chien-Jen Chen and Mei-Hsuan LeeEarly Diagnosis of Hepatocellular Carcinoma by Multiple microRNAs: Validity, Efficacy, and Cost-Effectiveness. J Clin Oncol. 29 (36): 4745-4747, (2011).

[21] Hany ElewaManal Abd-Elmeneem, Ahmed Murad Hashem et al. Study of interleukin 8 (IL8) serum level in patients with chronic liver disease due to hepatitis C virus (HCV) with and without hepatocellular carcinoma (HCC). International Journal of Hepatology.

[22] Melanie, B. Thomas and James L. Abbruzzese. Opportunities for Targeted Therapies in Hepatocellular Carcinoma. Journal of Clinical Oncology. 23 (31): 8093-8108, (2005).

[23] Jing GaoLi Xie, Wan-Shui Yang et al. Risk Factors of Hepatocellular Carcinoma- Current Status and Perspectives. Asian Pacific J Cancer Prev. 13: 743-752, (2012).

[24] Thuluvath Paul JEUS-guided FNA could be another important tool for the early diagnosis of hepatocellular carcinoma. *Gastrointestinal Endoscopy* ; (2007).

[25] Douglas, K. Rex, John L. Petrini, Todd H. Baron et al. Quality indicators for colonoscopy. Gastrointest Endosc. 63 (4): SS28, (2006). , 16.

[26] Christian StockUlrike Haug and Hermann Brenner. Population-based prevalence estimates of history of colonoscopy or sigmoidoscopy: review and analysis of recent trends. Gastrointest Endosc. 71 (2): 366-381, (2010).

[27] David, A. Lieberman, Douglas O. Faigel, Judith R. Logan et al. Assessment of the quality of colonoscopy reports: results from a multicenter consortium. Gastrointest Endosc. 69 (3): 645-653, (2009).

[28] Andrew, N. Freedman, Martha L. Slattery, Rachel Ballard-Barbash et al. Colorectal Cancer Risk Prediction Tool for White Men and Women Without Known Susceptibility. Journal of Clinical Oncology. 27 (5): 686-693, (2009).

[29] Nancy, N. Baxter, Joan L. Warren, Michael J. Barrett et al. Association Between Colonoscopy and Colorectal Cancer Mortality in a US Cohort According to Site of Cancer and Colonoscopist Specialty. Journal of Clinical Oncology. 30 (21): 2664-2669, (2012).

[30] Hye Won ParkSeungbong Han, Jong-Soo Lee et al. Risk stratification for advanced proximal colon neoplasm and individualized endoscopic screening for colorectal cancer by a risk-scoring model. Gastrointest Endosc (2012). in press

[31] Wei-Chih LiaoHan-Mo Chiu, Chien-Chuan Chen et al. A prospective evaluation of the feasibility of primary screening with unsedated colonoscopy. Gastrointest Endosc. 70 (4):724-731, (2009).

[32] Lukejohn, W. Day, Annette Kwon, John M. Inadomi et al. Adverse events in older patients undergoing colonoscopy: a systematic review and meta-analysis. Gastrointest Endosc. 74 (4): 885-896, (2011).

[33] Yoji TakeuchiTakuya Inoue, Noboru Hanaoka et al. Autofluorescence imaging with a transparent hood for detection of colorectal neoplasms: a prospective, randomized trial. Gastrointest Endosc 72 (5): 1006-1013, (2010).

[34] Binu, J. Jacob, Rahim Moineddin, Rinku Sutradhar et al. Effect of colonoscopy on colorectal cancer incidence and mortality: an instrumental variable analysis. Gastrointest Endosc. 76 (2): 355-364, (2012).

[35] Christian StockAmy B. Knudsen, Iris Lansdorp-Vogelaar et al. Colorectal cancer mortality prevented by use and attributable to nonuse of colonoscopy. Gastrointest Endosc. 73 (3): 435-443, (2011).

[36] Christine, N. Manser, Lucas M. Bachmann, Jakob Brunner et al. Colonoscopy screening markedly reduces the occurrence of colon carcinomas and carcinoma-related death: a closed cohort study. Gastrointest Endosc. 76 (1): 110-117, (2012).

[37] Franco ArmelaoCorrado Paternolli, Gaia Franceschini et al. Colonoscopic findings in first-degree relatives of patients with colorectal cancer: a population-based screening program. Gastrointest Endosc. 73 (3): 527-34, (2011).

[38] ASGE guideline: colorectal cancer screening and surveillanceGastrointestinal Endoscopy; (2006).

[39] Wai, K. Leung, Khek Yu Ho, Won-ho Kim et al. Colorectal neoplasia in Asia: a multicenter colonoscopy survey in symptomatic patients. Gastrointest Endosc. 64 (5): 751-759, (2006).

[40] Christian StockDianne Pulte, Ulrike Haug et al. Subsite-specific colorectal cancer risk in the colorectal endoscopy era. Gastrointest Endosc. (2012). , 75(3), 621-630.

[41] Hermann BrennerJenny Chang-Claude, Christoph M. Seiler et al. Long-Term Risk of Colorectal Cancer After Negative Colonoscopy. Journal of Clinical Oncology. 29 (28): 3761-3767, (2011).

[42] Eveline, J. A. Rondagh, Mariëlle W.E. Bouwens, Robert G. Riedl et al. Endoscopic appearance of proximal colorectal neoplasms and potential implications for colonoscopy in cancer prevention. Gastrointest Endosc. 75 (6): 1218-1225, (2012).

[43] Hermann BrennerJenny Chang-Claude, Alexander Rickert et al. Risk of Colorectal Cancer After Detection and Removal of Adenomas at Colonoscopy: Population-Based Case-Control Study. Journal of Clinical Oncology. 30 (24): 2969- 2976, (2012).

[44] Keith LeungPaul Pinsky, Adeyinka O. Laiyemo et al. Ongoing colorectal cancer risk despite surveillance colonoscopy: the Polyp Prevention Trial Continued Follow-up Study. Gastrointest Endosc. 71 (1): 111-117, (2010).

[45] Sung Noh HongJeong Hwan Kim, Won Hyeok Choe et al. Prevalence and risk of colorectal neoplasms in asymptomatic, average-risk screenees 40 to 49 years of age. Gastrointest Endosc. 72 (3): 480-489, (2010).

[46] Iris Lansdorp-VogelaarMarjolein van Ballegooijen, Ann G. Zauber et al. Individualizing colonoscopy screening by sex and race. Gastrointest Endosc. 70 (1): 96-108, (2009).

[47] Charles, J. Kahi, Faouzi Azzouz, Beth E. Juliar et al. Survival of elderly persons undergoing colonoscopy: implications for colorectal cancer screening and surveillance. Gastrointest Endosc. 66 (3): 544-550, (2007).

[48] Organización Mundial de La SaludNota descriptiva N°311, Mayo de (2012).

[49] YunFeng Cui and Dana KAndersen. Diabetes and Pancreatic Cancer. Endocr Relat Cancer. (2012). doi:ERC-, 12-0105.

[50] Aune, D, Greenwood, D. C, & Chan, D. S. M. et al. Body mass index, abdominal fatness and pancreatic cancer risk: a systematic review and non-linear dose-response meta-analysis of prospective studies. Annals of Oncology. 23: 843-852, (2012).

[51] Hongwei TangXiaoqun Dong, Manal Hassan et al. Body Mass Index and Obesity- and Diabetes-Associated Genotypes and Risk for Pancreatic Cancer. Cancer Epidemiol Biomarkers Prev. 20(5):779-792, (2011).

[52] Bin BaoZhiwei Wang, Yiwei Li et al. The complexities of obesity, diabetes, and the development and progression of pancreatic cancer. Biochim Biophys Acta. 1815(2): 135-146, (2011).

[53] Alan, A. Arslan, Kathy J. Helzlsouer, Charles Kooperberg et al. Anthropometric Measures, Body Mass Index and Pancreatic Cancer: a Pooled Analysis from the Pancreatic Cancer Cohort Consortium (PanScan). Arch Intern Med. 170(9): 791-802, (2010).

[54] Ho Gak Kim and Jimin HanObesity and Pancreatic Diseases. Korean J Gastroenterol. 59 (1): 35-39, (2012).

[55] Carolyn, C. Gotay. Behavior and Cancer Prevention. *Journal Of Clinical Oncology*. 23 (2): 301-310, (2005).

[56] Sang Min ParkMin Kyung Lim, Kyu Won Jung et al. Prediagnosis Smoking, Obesity, Insulin Resistance, and Second Primary Cancer Risk in Male Cancer Survivors: National Health Insurance Corporation Study. *Journal Of Clinical Oncology*. 25 (30): 4835-4843, (2007).

[57] Sang Woo OhYeong Sook Yoon, and Soon-Ae Shin. Effects of Excess Weight on Cancer Incidences Depending on Cancer Sites and Histologic Findings Among Men: Korea National Health Insurance Corporation Study. *Journal Of Clinical Oncology*. 23 (21): 4742-4754, (2005).

[58] Michaud Dominique SThe epidemiology of pancreatic, gallbladder, and other biliary tract cancers. *Gastrointestinal Endoscopy*; (2002). S6)

[59] Lauren, B. Gerson. Impact of obesity on endoscopy. *Gastrointestinal Endoscopy*; (2009).

[60] Body mass indexeffect modifiers, and risk of pancreatic cancer: a pooled study of seven prospective cohorts. Li Jiao, Amy Berrington de Gonzalez, Patricia Hartge et al. Cancer Causes Control. 21(8): 1305-1314, (2010).

[61] Paul, S. Sepe, Ashray Ohri, Sirish Sanaka, Tyler M. Berzin, Sandeep Sekhon, Gayle Bennett, et al. A prospective evaluation of fatty pancreas by using *Eus. Gastrointestinal Endoscopy*; (2011).

[62] Wen-Ko ChiouJawl-Shan Hwang, Kuang-Hung Hsu et al. DiabetesMellitus IncreasedMortality RatesMore in Gender-Specific than in Nongender-Specific Cancer Patients: A Retrospective Study of 149,491 Patients. Exp Diabetes Res. (2012). doi:

[63] Robert, R. McWilliams, Martha E. Matsumoto, Patrick A. Burch et al. Obesity Adversely Affects Survival in Pancreatic Cancer Patients. Cancer. 116 (21): 5054-5062, (2010).

Chapter 2

Burden of Cardiovascular Disease in Colombia

Adrián Bolívar-Mejía and Boris E. Vesga-Angarita

Additional information is available at the end of the chapter

1. Introduction

Cardiovascular Diseases (CVD) is the first cause of mortality in the world. According to the World Health Statistics issued by the World Health Organization (WHO) in 2012, noncommunicable diseases (NCDs) caused 63% (36 millions) of 57 million of deaths that occurred in the world during 2008 [1]. Also, in the same period of time, CVD were the first cause of death by NCDs with 17 million of deaths (48% of the total deaths caused by NCDs). In 2010, this number reached to 18.1 million and it is estimated that will rise to 25 million by 2030. [1,2]. Likewise, it is calculated in That year, the number of deaths caused by NCDs in the world will reach to 55 million [1].

The outlook previously exposed at beginning worsen when it is consider that 80% of the deaths caused by NCDs have place in low and medium income countries, where the percentage of deaths in people under 70 years (48%) is greater than high income countries (26%). In fact, reports indicate that each year eight million people die prematurely in low and medium income countries due to NCDs, situation that produces a greater impact in terms of healthy life years lost and greater economic lose caused by no productivity in populations, that due to deficitary socioeconomic conditions are less able to face the burden that generates this growing public health problem [1,3]. In Latin America, according to the report about the health situation in the Americas issued by the Pan American Health Organization in 2011, between 2007 - 2009 the NCDs caused 76% of deaths reported, and 69% took place in medium and low income countries [4].

In Colombia similar to world statistics, NCDs are the main cause of death. According to the paper "Noncommunicable diseases country profiles 2011", issued by WHO, it is estimated that during 2008, NCDs caused 66% of total deaths, and CVD were the first cause of death from NCDs, causing 28% of all deaths, with a mortality rate of 205.9 and 166.7 by each 100,000 inhabitants in men and women, respectively (Figure 1) [5].

Colombia

2010 total population: 46 294 841
Income group: Upper middle

NCD mortality

2008 estimates	males	females
Total NCD deaths (000s)	66.3	68.2
NCD deaths under age 60 (percent of all NCD deaths)	30.7	26.8
Age-standardized death rate per 100 000		
All NCDs	437.6	351.3
Cancers	112.9	92.1
Chronic respiratory diseases	43.0	29.9
Cardiovascular diseases and diabetes	205.9	166.7

Behavioural risk factors

2008 estimated prevalence (%)	males	females	total
Current daily tobacco smoking	...	...	...
Physical inactivity	38.1	47.1	42.7

Metabolic risk factors

2008 estimated prevalence (%)	males	females	total
Raised blood pressure	40.4	33.8	37.0
Raised blood glucose	6.0	5.7	5.9
Overweight	43.5	52.7	48.3
Obesity	11.3	22.9	17.3
Raised cholesterol	40.8	41.8	41.4

Proportional mortality (% of total deaths, all ages)

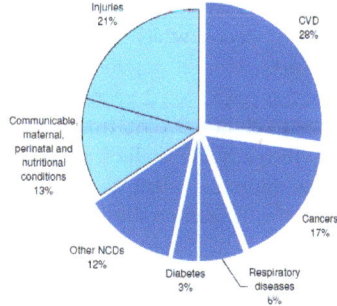

Injuries 21%
CVD 28%
Cancers 17%
Respiratory diseases 5%
Diabetes 3%
Other NCDs 12%
Communicable, maternal, perinatal and nutritional conditions 13%

NCDs are estimated to account for 66% of all deaths.

Metabolic risk factor trends

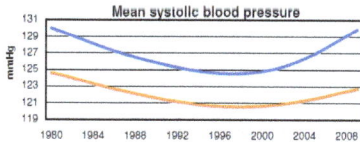

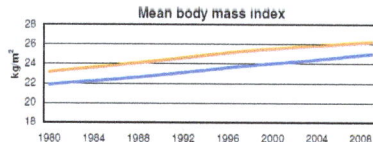

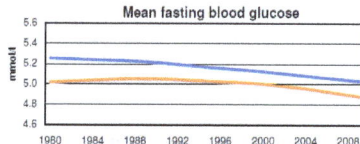

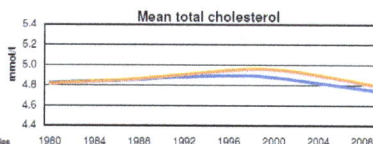

Mean systolic blood pressure
Mean body mass index
Mean fasting blood glucose
Mean total cholesterol

■ Males
■ Females

Country capacity to address and respond to NCDs

Has a Unit / Branch / Dept in MOH with responsibility for NCDs	ND
There is funding available for:	
NCD treatment and control	ND
NCD prevention and health promotion	ND
NCD surveillance, monitoring and evaluation	ND
National health reporting system includes:	
NCD cause-specific mortality	ND
NCD morbidity	ND
NCD risk factors	ND
Has a national, population-based cancer registry	ND

Has an integrated or topic-specific policy / programme / action plan which is currently operational for:	
Cardiovascular diseases	ND
Cancer	ND
Chronic respiratory diseases	ND
Diabetes	ND
Alcohol	ND
Unhealthy diet / Overweight / Obesity	ND
Physical inactivity	ND
Tobacco	ND
Number of tobacco (m)POWER measures implemented at the highest level of achievement	2/5

... = no data available
ND = Country did not respond to country capacity survey

Figure 1. Noncommunicable diseases: epidemiological profile for Colombia, according to World Health Organization, 2011 [5].

Historically, coronary atherosclerotic disease represented a great burden in terms of mortality, which rises significantly after sixth decade of life. In Colombia, reports from late twentieth century, between 1998 and 2000, the mortality rate of coronary disease in men and
women was 93.4 and 60.9 by each 100.000 inhabitants, respectively [6], nevertheless, between 2007 and 2009, the mortality rate was 124.7 for males and 88.3 for females by each
100.000 inhabitants, with a global rate of 104.5 by each 100,000 inhabitants [4]. This increase
in mortality is probably associated to the demographic changes that have been taking place
during the last decades, which are characterized by an increase in life expectancy at birth
and a continued ageing of population. In Colombia, in the last 50 years, life expectancy at
birth increased from 50 to 72 years-old, added to an increase in population older than 60
years from six to eight per cent, from 600,000 in 1950 to three million in 2001, and it is estimated that will reach 15.5 million in 2050 [7,8]. Such changes increased the population in
which CVD are more prevalent, so it is expected that as the population continues ageing, the
burden of CVD will continue showing a steady increase.

Stroke represents also a great social and economic burden, it is the second cause of death in
the world, and the first cause of acquired disability in whole population [2]. Several reports
show that the cerebrovascular disease is responsible of 55% of the total disability-adjusted
life years (DALYs) produced by the neurological diseases in the world, estimating that in
2005 produced a total of 788.4 years of DALYs by each 100,000 inhabitants, representing
3.45% of the total DALYs worldwide [9]. It is estimated that in 2005, stroke caused a 9.9% of
total deaths worldwide, according to estimations, it will rise up to 10.19% in 2015 and up to
10.63% in 2030 [9].

In Colombia, a study performed in 1997 in a northwestern town called Sabaneta (Figure 2),
the annual incidence of cerebrovascular disease was calculated in 88.9 by each 100,000 inhabitants, with a greater incidence in men (118.7/100,000 inhabitants) versus women
(61.8/100,000 inhabitants) [10]. Nevertheless, there are not national data available about the
incidence of stroke.

Neuroepidemiological studies performed in different areas of Colombia, reported different
prevalence of sequels of cerebrovascular disease according to the study area, data varied between 1.42 to 19.9 by each 1,000 inhabitants. Nevertheless, the results of these studies vary
significantly due to some differences between the study populations, cultural habits, implementation of promotion and prevention strategies and ethnic factors. The most recent study,
conducted in 2002 in Piedecuesta, Santander, northeastern Colombia, reported a prevalence
of 5.7 by each 1,000 inhabitants [11-14].

In the State of Santander, Colombia, the analysis of mortality causes during 2007, reported
that CVD were responsible of 32.07% of all deaths, with a mortality rate of 159.7 by each
100,000 inhabitants [15]. In the group of CVD, the ischemic heart disease produced 47.9% of
deaths, followed by stroke (23.3%) and heart failure (9.6%) [15].

It is evident the growing problem that exists in the national and international context, where
NCDs and specially CVD have become a great burden for populations, producing a great
amount of deaths, that in low and medium income countries (included Colombia) occurred

in an early way, affecting the life of their inhabitants at the time they are more productive economically. Therefore, the study of the CVD burden, as well as the design of intersectoral strategies to reduce the impact related to this burden, should be taken as a national and international priority, looking for mitigate and control this epidemic disease.

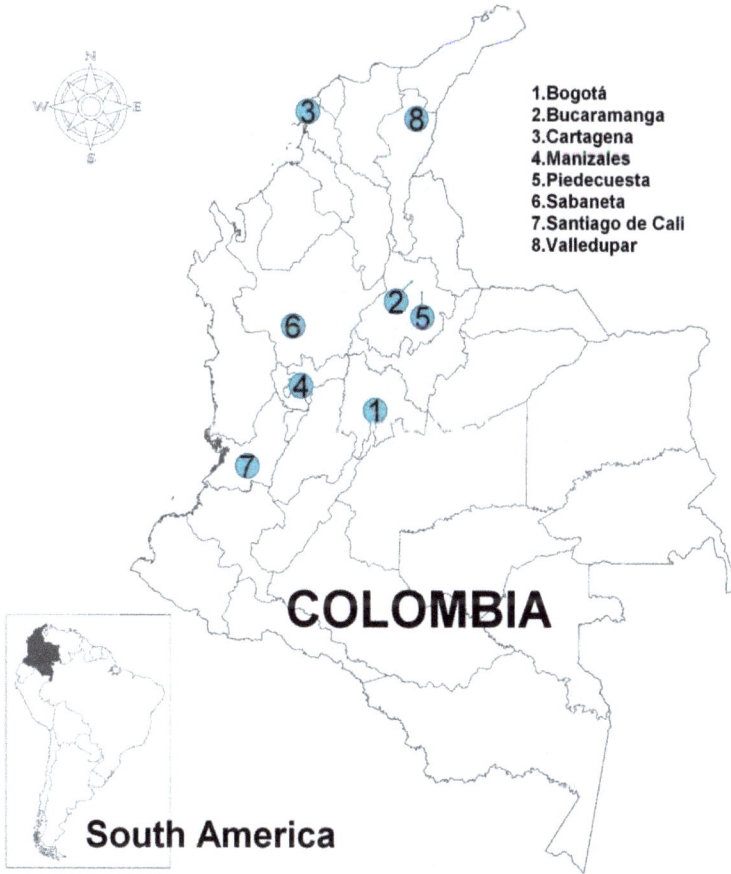

1.Bogotá
2.Bucaramanga
3.Cartagena
4.Manizales
5.Piedecuesta
6.Sabaneta
7.Santiago de Cali
8.Valledupar

Figure 2. Geographic location of the Colombian cities mentioned on this paper.

2. Burden of CVD in Colombia according to DALYs

The DALYs are used as an indicator that estimates the global burden of a disease and the effectiveness of the health interventions aimed to diminish this burden, considering both,

the years lived with disability and those lost by premature death [16,17]. Thus, when determining the burden of a disease through this indicator, we can observe the gap that exists
between the real conditions of morbidity and mortality of a population and the ideals that
this could reach if it was free from a particular disease [17].

According to the last study about Burden of Disease in Colombia, published in the 2005, the
CVD (hypertensive heart disease, ischemic heart disease and cerebrovascular disease) are
found to be in the first 10 causes of DALYs for both, disability and mortality in the adult
population [17].

The hypertensive heart disease is the main cause of DALYs by disability in both gender, in
the age groups of 30-44 years old (55.2 DALYs/1,000 inhabitants), 45-59 years old (78.5 DA-
LYs/1,000 inhabitants) and 60-69 years old (75.6 DALYs/1,000 inhabitants). So, in a concerning way was observed that this disease was the second cause of DALYs by disability in both
gender in the age group of 15-29 years-old (104.5 DALYs/1.000 inhabitants) and the fifth
cause of DALYs in the age group of 5-14 years-old (2,9 DALYs/1,000 inhabitants) [17].

Meanwhile, ischemic heart disease is the main cause of DALYs by disability in people older
than 70 years-old, with a total of 48.2 by each 1,000 inhabitants in the age group 70-79 years-
old and 42.9 by each 1,000 inhabitants in the age group of 80 years-old or more. In the same
way, this disease is the third cause of DALYs by disability in both gender in the age group
60-69 years old (31.8/1,000 inhabitants) and the sixth cause of DALYs by disability in the age
group of 45-59 years old (12.9/1,000 inhabitants) [17].

When assessing the number of DALYs produced by mortality in both gender, it was found
that ischemic heart disease was the first cause in group of 45-59 years-old (12.2/1,000 inhabitants), 60-69 years-old (29.5/1,000 inhabitants), 70-79 years (45.9/1,000 inhabitants) and 80
years-old or more (41.3/1,000 inhabitants). Stroke was the second cause of DALYs for mortality in both gender, in groups of 60-69 years old (11.8/1,000 inhabitants), 70-79 years old
(21.8/1,000 inhabitants) and 80 years old or more (19.2/1,000 inhabitants) [17].

Finally, hypertensive heart disease was found as disease that more DALYs produces in the
Colombian population, with a total of 52.5 DALYs by each 1,000 inhabitants when adding
those produced by disability and mortality, accounting for 19% of the total DALYs [17].

The above results reveal that the CVD are the main cause of death in Colombia, but also represent a great burden for the population in what concerns to DALYs. It is surprisingly how
CVD, besides producing a great proportion of the DALYs in the older population, also produce a great burden disease in the young adult population. These data are consistent with
recent informs in where there is estimated that in lower and medium income countries the
29% of deaths by NCDs are produced in the population under 60 years-old. In contrast, the
high-income countries only the 26% and 13% of deaths by NCDs are produce in the population under 70 and 60 years-old, respectively [1,18]. Additionally, it has been estimated that
CVD are the main cause of death by NCDs in people under 70 years-old because, they produce the 39% of the total death in group, followed by cancer (27%) and chronic respiratory
diseases [18].

Therefore, an important amount of the promotion and prevention strategies that emerge with the purpose of fighting the continuous increase of the CVD should be directed to sensitize the young people about the importance of adopting healthy life habits, in order to diminish the negative impact that CVD produce in the Colombian population.

3. The burden of the risk factors for CVD in Colombia

The risk factors more highly related with CVD include physical inactivity, smoking, alcohol drinking, unhealthy diet, overweight, obesity, hypertension, and high blood levels of cholesterol and glucose [2,19]. It is estimated that implementing effective prevention strategies based on the knowledge about the control of these risk factors, could prevent up to 70% of ischemic heart disease events and stroke and increase the life expectancy of the population in at least five years [2.20], in addition to reducing the risk for other diseases that share some risk factors with CVD such as cancer, respiratory chronic disease and diabetes [19]. Hence the importance of coordinating the implementation of promotion and prevention strategies in which it is linked the general population and the health personnel, in order to improve the risk profile for CVD of a particular community.

Even though, CVD continue being the main cause of mortality in the world, it has been documented in high-income countries that during the last two decades the mortality rates by CVD have diminished in a significant. While part of this decline is product of the improvements that have been presented during the treatment of the acute cardiovascular events, there is evidence that supports that the primary prevention strategies directed to the control of the main risk factors have contributed significantly to this decline [19,21]. In England and Gales, it is estimated that the mortality rate by coronary disease diminish from 1981 - 2000 to 65% in men and 45% in women between 25 - 84 years-old, which resulted in a decrease of approximately 68,230 deaths by the 2000 year, become interesting that such reduction in mortality was attributed in 58% to population control of risk factors for CVD, which empathizes the importance of knowing and identifying the more prevalent risk factors, in order to implement promotion strategies aimed to diminish their impact [21].

4. Tobacco consumption

It is estimated that tobacco consumption is responsible of 10% of the CVD deaths worldwide [19,20]. Despite the current knowledge about the consequences that tobacco produces in the human health and educational campaigns directed to the population in order to reduce its consumption, it is estimated that tobacco consumption causes approximately six million death each year, being responsible of six per cent of all deaths in women and 12% in men [19,20].

WHO considers tobacco consumption as a completely avoidable risk factor. Its association with CVD has been ratified in different studies, as also has been the benefits of its interruption. The INTERHEART study, in which Colombia participated, showed an odds ratio for acute myocardial infarction of 2.87 in smokers [22]. In a cohort of British doctors followed during 50 years was observed when comparing the mortality during the following in smokers versus nonsmokers and the ones who stop smoking, it was observed that those that stop smoking before the fourth decade can reach a similar life expectancy to those that have been never smoked [23]. Nevertheless, even after this age, the interruption of tobacco consumption brings significant benefits, so, life expectancy can be increase in 9 years if interruption of tobacco consumption is done around the age of 40, in 6 years if interruption is done at the age of 50 and still it can be increase in 3 years if interruption of tobacco consumption is done by the age of 60, when comparing with those that keep smoking. Therefore, it is emphasizing the tobacco interruption is justified almost in any moment of life [23].

In Latin America, the CARMELA study conducted between 2003 and 2005 in seven cities (Barquisimeto, Venezuela; Bogota, capital of Colombia; Buenos Aires, Argentina; Lima, Peru; Mexico City, Mexico; Quito, Ecuador; and Santiago de Chile), which sought to evaluate the prevalence of tobacco consumption in adult between 25 and 64 years old, the study found a prevalence between 21.8% and 45.4%. The ages where the consumption was highest were between 25 and 44 years old. In this study, Bogota showed a global prevalence of 22.2% with a confidence interval of 95% (CI 95%) of 19.1-25.2, being the consumption more prevalent in men (31.3, CI 95%: 27.1-35.5) than in women (15.0 CI 95% 11.1-18.9) [24].

In Colombia, as part of the *Tobacco-Free Initiative* developed in association with the WHO, the United Nations Children's Fund (UNICEF), the Center for Disease Control (CDC), and the Office on Smoking and Health (OSH) with the purpose of giving the countries the knowledge about the burden of tobacco consumption, the Global Youth Tobacco Survey (GYTS) was applied in Bogota city in 3,599 youths between 11 and 17 years old belonging to 231 official schools [25, 26]. In a concerning way, this study reported that the 62% of students have tasted at least once the tobacco, without finding significant differences between men and women [26]. From the total, 29.8% have consumed some tobacco derivatives in the last month, being the cigarette the most frequent (94.4%), without findings significant differences between gender. Nevertheless, the results also evidenced that seven of each 10 students considered the tobacco smoke as harmful for their health, seven of each 10 desire to drop the tobacco consumption and in fact seven of each 10 have tried [26]. Not being enough with the exposure to tobacco smoke by direct consumption, it was found that nonsmokers are exposed in a 40% to the tobacco smoke in public places and in a 28% in their homes, fact that urge the need of a legislation that prompts the creation of free smoke places in order to protect those nonsmokers from the exposition equally harmful to the tobacco smoke. In consideration to that, it was found that 63.8% of students (including smokers and nonsmokers) considered that tobacco consumption in public places must be forbidden [26].

Other studies done in Colombia in which the prevalence of tobacco consumption has been determined, have found similar data to CARMELA study. In this way, a paper done in university students in Cartagena de Indias city (a touristic city located in northern Colombia on the Caribbean Coast) and Santiago de Cali (the third city more populated of Colombia, located in the western country) reported prevalence of 23.9% and 23.2%, respectively [27,28]. Another study done in five cities (Bogota, Santiago de Cali, Bucaramanga, Manizales y Valledupar) (Figure 2) reported a prevalence that changes between 7.4% and 34.1% [29]; in this study the onset of tobacco consumption was 11.9 years old. This, added to results that indicate that in Colombia 57.5% of smokers between 11 and 17 years old had acquired cigarette in stores, reflects a poor authority control on the tobacco sale to minors.

As a result of knowledge about the negative impact that tobacco produces on the health of the smoker and nonsmoker population, as well as the failings in relation to the sell control of these products in minors, in Colombia, the authorities tend for optimizing the laws that regulate the policies about tobacco consumption prevention. Thus, on July 21st of 2009, the Colombian Republic Congress issued the law number 1335, law that seeks to regulate the consumption, selling, advertising and promotion of tobacco and its derivatives, as well as the creation and implementation of promotion programs directed to minimize the consumption and promoting the dropping of tobacco [30].

Some measures contained in the 1335 law include the ratification of the ban on the sale of tobacco products to the population under 18 years old, as well as the ban of tobacco products unit sales. It is forbidden that packaging expresses attractive advertising to minor as well as messages suggesting a soft, light or low nicotine product. The law provides that 30% of the packing area must contain clear, explicit and striking messages that warm with images or texts in Spanish about the damage produced by tobacco to the human health. It is forbidden the advertising of tobacco derivatives products on radio, television, film or other media directed to the general public as well as the sponsorship of these products to sporting or cultural events. On the other hand, the law encourages the creation of promotion strategies directed specially to the minor population, where this, may receive quality education about the negative effects of tobacco consumption [30].

Similarly, considering the rights of the nonsmokers are the possibility to breath smoke-free air, the 1335 law forbidden the tobacco consumption in public places like malls, parks, nightclubs, casinos, waiting rooms, among others where nonsmokers people may result affected by the tobacco smoke [30].

Thus, from knowledge about the prevalence of tobacco consumption, the health problems arising from this consumption and the burden of disease generated by this, is duty of the health personnel the promotion of non-consumption of tobacco-based products, in order to reduce the risk that this causes on the Colombians' health.

5. Physical inactivity

Adequate physical activity had been defined as at list 30 minutes of moderate physical activity during five days per week or 20 minutes of vigorous physical activity during three days per week [19]. The physical inactivity is considered as one of the most related factors with inadequate maintenance of the cardiovascular health [3]. It had been calculated that in the world, the physical inactivity produces around 3.2 million of deaths (six per cent of the deaths produced worldwide) and 32.1 million of DALYs (2.1% of the total DALYs in the world) by year, estimating that it causes the 30% of the cases of coronary disease, this fact, added to its association with another chronic diseases like cancer and diabetes mellitus, has placed it as the fourth risk factor of mortality in the world [19].

One of the most relevant aspects about the importance of an adequate physical activity promotion, sedentary is not only an independent risk factor for developing CVD, also is related with the development of another risk factors for CVD as overweight, obesity and high blood levels of glucose and cholesterol.

When evaluating the prevalence of the fulfillment of the recommendations for realization of an adequate physical activity, the National Survey of the Nutritional Situation in Colombia (Encuesta Nacional sobre la Situación Nutricional en Colombia, ENSIN) performed in 2010, reported that when adding the physical activity as a way of transportation and development during the free time [31], the national prevalence was 53.3%, prevalence increased when comparing with the results obtained in the ENSIN done in 2005 with a prevalence of 46.5%; the prevalence of physical inactivity, was found to be associated with female gender, low socioeconomic level and low scholarity [31,32].

Other Colombian studies determined the prevalence of physical inactivity in children, adolescents and adults founding numbers that varies from 26% to 85% [27.33-36]. Nevertheless, such studies can not be compared between them, due that definition of physical activity varies between them. It is noteworthy that as well as reported by the ENSIN, women has the highest prevalence of physical inactivity, in scholars between 7 and 14 years, the same trend is observed with a prevalence in girls of 83.8% and boys of 44.2%.

In Bogota, a study from 2003 evaluated the burden of mortality associated to physical inactivity and found a physical inactivity prevalence of 53.2%, data associated with a population attributable risk of 19.3% for mortality by coronary disease, 24.2% for mortality by stroke and a 13.8% for mortality by arterial hypertension [36]. Additionally, the mortality by NCDs in adults older than 45 years could be reduced between 1.9% and 5.1% if the prevalence of physical inactivity is reduced in a 37.2%. In that way, it must be considered as a priority the implementation of strategies that promote the realization of physical activity in the Colombian population.

In Bogota, during the last years some changes in the policies about transportation and recreation had been implemented, policies that have seek for the generation of spaces for physical activity promotion [36]. As a part of this initiative, the use of the bicycle as an alternative mean of transportation has been promoted with the building of bike paths. Also, some city streets have been intended as bikeways during holidays to promote the recreation and the physical activity as a frequent habit. These and other similar policies, have been extended to another cities of the country with the purpose of improving the population health conditions and reducing the impact of CVD and others non-communicable diseases on Colombians mortality [36]. Nevertheless, studies that allow the evaluation of the effectiveness of these measures must be done, in order to determine if these measures have been enough to reduce in a significant way the prevalence of physical inactivity in Colombian people.

6. Alcohol consumption

Alcohol consumption can be seen as a major public health problem since the consequences of abuse are reflected not only in an increased risk for many types of diseases, but also are related with high violence indexes, sexual abuse, suicide and traffic accidents; events that together affect millions of teenagers and young adults in the world.

It is estimated that during the 2004 the alcohol consumption was responsible of 3.8 %(2.5 million) of the deaths in the world, from which over 50% were due to CVD, liver cirrhosis and cancer [19]. According to the report done by the WHO in the 2009 where, based on the DALYs, the burden of the risk factors over mortality in the world was estimated; the alcohol consumption produced the 4.5% of total DALYs worldwide, being surpassed only by child malnutrition (5.9%) and risk sexual practices, nevertheless, this burden is greater in men, in which the alcohol produces the 6.0% of deaths and the 7.4% of the DALYs, while in women it produces the 1.1% of deaths and the 1.4% of the DALYs, aspects that are related with the study's results in which a higher prevalence of alcohol consumption in men than in women is reported [20].

Multiple diseases have been associated with excessive alcohol consumption, among these are included the CVD like coronary disease, arterial hypertension, cardiac arrhythmias and the cerebrovascular disease, nevertheless, the relation between alcohol consumption and CVD is complex due to there is evidence that supports that a moderate alcohol consumption could reduce the risk of dying by CVD, especially if it is red wine and in quantities not exceeding the 5-30 gr/day. In contrary, high quantities of alcohol consumption have shown a clear association with the risk of developing CVD [19,37].

In Colombia, according to diverse studies done mainly between teenagers and young adults, the lifetime prevalence of alcohol consumption ranges between 63% and 89%, with a past month consumption prevalence that ranges between 33 and 51% [38-42]. In a concerning way, the results of these studies have shown that in most cases, the onset age for alcohol consumption is between 13 and 16 years old [38-42]. Such is the case of a study conducted in Cartagena city, where after studying 1,031 university students, whose ages ranged between 15 and 38 years old, it was found that the 97.6% of those that have consumed alcohol for at least once in their life, have started the consumption before the 19 years old [41], which reflects an exposition to the harmful alcohol effects since very early stages of life and a greater risk for becoming a chronic consumer, since, according to a study done by the Epidemiologic Observatory of Cardiovascular Diseases of the Industrial University of Santander (Bucaramanga, Colombia) (Figure 2), during the years 2005 and 2006 in Bucaramanga city, the probability of being an alcohol consumer increases in a 17% in the individuals whose onset consumption was before the 16 years old and in an 11% in those who get drunk for the first time before this age [43].

Thus, it is clear that in Colombia a greater control on the alcohol drinks consumption in the adolescent population must be applied. Strategies directed to educate this population group about the harmful effects of alcohol consumption have been proposed by the Ministry of Social Protection as part of a policy that aims to reduce the negative impact of the alcoholic beverages consumption on the premature death in the Colombian population [44]. It is expected that these measures are implemented as proposed, and with this, reduce the alcohol beverages consumption in the Colombian territory, as well as the detrimental effects this produces in their inhabitants' health.

7. Unhealthy diet

It is estimated that in the world are produced approximately 16 million DALYs and 1.7 million of deaths related directly with a low fruits and vegetables consumption, which represents 1% of the total DALYs and 2.8% of the total deaths worldwide [19]. The impact of diet over cardiovascular death has been widely studied during the last years, resulting in an important quantity of evidence that shows a relation between the bad dietary habits and an increase of the risk for CVD [19,45,46]. Thus, it has been described that high-calorie diet, rich in trans-fat and with high salt levels is associated with an increase of cardiovascular risk, while a diet rich in vegetables, fruits and unsaturated fatty acids is associated with a decrease of cardiovascular risk.

In the 2010, the results of the ENSIN revealed the dietary habits of the Colombian population evidencing that vegetables and fruits consumption is well below the recommendations that have been considered to prevent the CVD (Figure 3) [31]. Thus, it was found that 66.8% of the population consumes some kind of fruit at least once a day, describing that such consumption has its maximum prevalence during the childhood and decreases steadily as the age advances. Moreover, the daily vegetables consumption was only 25.7%. In contrast, high values for the daily use of sweeteners (94.6%), fried foods (32%), soda drinks (22.1%), packaged food (15.2%) and candies (36.6%) were reported, values that were the highest in the 9 to 18 years old population [31].

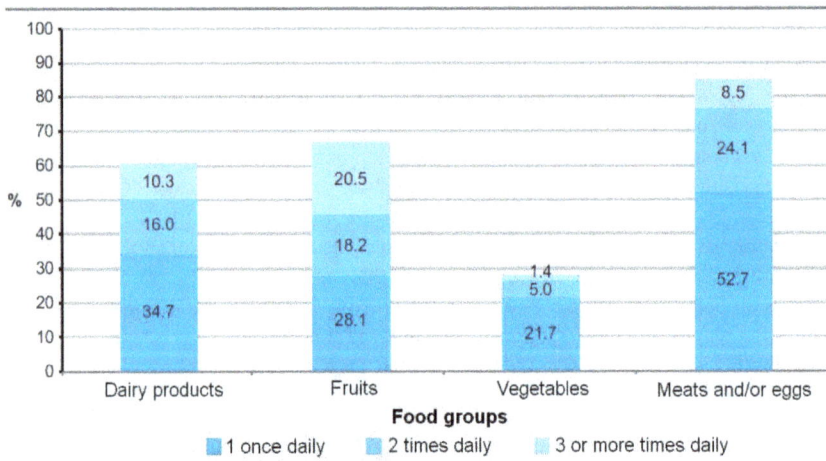

Figure 3. National proportions (5 to 64 years) of the daily frequencies of consumption by food groups in Colombia (Modified from ENSIN 2010) [31].

The previously exposed results, explain why despite existing in Colombia a high malnutrition prevalence, which in the 2010 year was of 13.2% for children between 0 and 4 years old, recently, in a simultaneous way the overweight and obesity are beginning to become a great public health problem because dietary habits as described previously, predispose the population to an alteration in their corporal mass index, with an increase in the cardiovascular risk as a consequence, which will eventually begin to appear in more earlier ages, as it is evidenced by the results in which it is observed that the overweight and obesity prevalence in the children population of 0 to 4 years old, went from 4.9% in the 2005 to 5.2% in the 2010, and is expected to continue rising in the next years as a result of the constant urbanization that exists nationally, and the changes in the lifestyles that this process entails [31].

8. Overweight and obesity

Overweight and obesity represent a great burden concerning the risk of developing CVD because, not only are independent risk factors for the development of these diseases, but also are directly related with an increase of other risk factors as the metabolic syndrome, hyperglycemia, hypertension and hyperlipidemia [22,47]. It is estimated that annually 2.8 million deaths are produced and 35.8 million of DALYs (2.3%) in the world due to overweight and obesity, expecting that this burden keeps increasing through the years as it is estimated that overweight and obesity prevalence will continue rising, affecting people at earlier ages [19,31].

In Colombia, during the last decades a steadily increase in the mass corporal index has been experimented in men as well as in women (Figure 1). The ENSIN, showed the numbers of prevalence of excess weight in the Colombian population, evidencing a continuous increase of such prevalence as the age advances(Table 1), which, associated to the aging population and the increase of others cardiovascular risks factors in the adult population, brings a great burden on the health system [31].

Age (years)	Prevalence %
0 - 4	5.2
5 - 17	17.5
18 - 22	21.4
23 - 27	35.0
28 - 32	48.1
33 - 37	54.9
38 - 42	60.5
43 - 47	63.3
48 - 52	66.4
53 - 57	67.1
58 - 64	65.7

Table 1. Prevalence of excessive weight in Colombian population by age groups [31].

Therefore, strategies through which the population could be educated about the importance of maintaining their weight in normal values must be created, and the consequences that the obesity and overweight bring to their health. Similarly, is the duty of the health personnel to inform the users about the normal values in which their weight should be kept, because, according to the ENSIN, when assessing the self-perception of body weight, the 23.6% of the youths (under 18 years old) and the 32.3% of the adults underestimated their corporal mass index, which may bring as a consequence a lack of motivation for weight losing in those individuals that, even though they have an excess weight, consider this as normal [31].

9. Raised blood pressure

Arterial hypertension is perhaps one of the risk factors for cardiovascular diseases most studied, estimating that it produces 12.8% (7.5 million) of the total deaths in the world and 3.7% (57 million) of the total DALYs [19]. Its prevalence increases with age producing a great impact in the mortality of adult people, estimating that it is present in the 35% of the total cardiovascular events secondary to atherosclerosis and in the 49% of heart failure cases [48].

Multiple studies have assessed the prevalence of arterial hypertension in different Colombian regions. Nationally, the Second National Study of Risk Factors for Chronic Diseases (SNSRFCD II) published in 1999 [49], reported a prevalence of arterial hypertension of 12.3%. Nevertheless, recent publications, evidenced an increase in the prevalence, thus, the report about the Americas Health Situation issued in 2011 by the Pan American Health Organization, showed a prevalence of arterial hypertension in Colombia of 27.8% and 19.1% in men and in women respectively, data that agree with other regional reports like the Study of the Prevalence of Risk Factors for Chronic Diseases done in Santander Department, in which a prevalence of arterial hypertension of 22.9% was reported in men and 17% in women [38]. Besides, is concerning that in this last report, despite the great amount of advances that have been made for the treatment and control of blood pressure, the 58.1% of hypertensive patients was not receiving any kind of antihypertensive treatment and the 18% was receiving a treatment but their blood pressure was not controlled at the time the study was conducted. Thus, the health authorities in Colombia, must implement strategies that seek to ensure that all the hypertensive people receive an adequate antihypertensive treatment, looking forward to reduce the impact that arterial hypertension represents in terms of morbidity and mortality over the Colombian population [38].

10. Raised blood cholesterol

It is estimated that high blood levels of total cholesterol (TC) produce the 4.5% (2.6 million) of the total deaths in the world and the 2 % of the total DALYs (29.7 million) [19]. The high levels of cholesterol represent a factor clearly implicated in the pathophysiology underneath the vascular processes related with the development of cardiovascular diseases like the coronary disease and the cerebrovascular disease. High levels of low density lipoprotein (LDL) (traditionally called 'bad cholesterol') have been related with the CVD due to the atherogenic effect they produce in the blood vessels, while high levels of high density lipoproteins (HDL) (traditionally called 'good cholesterol') represent a protector factor due to their anti-oxidant, anti-inflammatory, antiproliferative and antithrombotic functions [50].

In Colombia, multiple studies have been conducted with the purpose of assessing the prevalence of cardiovascular risk factors, among which are included the blood measurement of TC, HDL and LDL [38, 51-53]. In studies where those biological indicators have been evaluated, numbers of high TC prevalence have been found in the population over 15 years old, which varies between the 6 and 39%, evidencing an increase of the same with the age [51]. Thus, the study about Prevalence of Risk Factors for Chronic Diseases in Santander showed a prevalence of 14.2%, 36.2% and 32.0% in the age groups of 15 to 24 years old, 25 to 44 years old and 45 to 64 years old respectively [38]. In relation to the high levels of LDL, numbers of prevalence in the population older than 15 years old which varies between the 24% and 39% have been found, showing, as with TC an increase in these values as the age advances. Finally, when assessing the prevalence of low levels of HDL, values between 13% and 22% were found [51,53].

On the other hand, in a concerning way, a study done in children and adolescents between the 6 and 18 years old, found a prevalence of high TC and LDL of 13.5% and 17% respectively, with a prevalence of low HDL levels of 19.1%, evidencing an early presentation of the dyslipidemias as biological factors related to a premature increase of the risk for developing CVD [54].

Considering the facts previously exposed, it is clearly that the alterations in cholesterol blood values represent a risk factor highly prevalent in the Colombian population, which is found even since early ages. It is necessary to intervene early on the factors that may potentially modify these numbers, like consumption of a healthy diet and a regular physical activity, in order to stop the increase that has been showing the prevalence of dyslipidemias in younger population.

11. Raised blood glucose (Diabetes Mellitus)

Diabetes Mellitus is without any doubt one of the main risk factors for CVD. The increase of the cardiovascular risk associated to Diabetes Mellitus is due in part to the coexistence of other risk factors like obesity, hypertension, dyslipidemia and physical inactivity, nevertheless, the increase of blood glucose represents by itself a risk factor for the development of CVD [55], noting for example that glucose blood values at the admission moment of a patient with acute myocardial infarction, behave as an independent predictor of in-hospital mortality [55,56].

It has been estimated that the diabetic population has an increase in the risk for developing a cardiovascular disease that is 2 to 4 times greater, when compared to the rest of the population, because approximately the 80% of the deaths associated to diabetes are related in a direct way to the CVD [19].

In Colombia, the prevalence of Diabetes Mellitus varies between 4.0% and 8.9% in urban areas, and it's around the 1.4% in rural areas, according to the reported by different studies in which the behavior of this risk factor in different cities of the country has been studied [38,51,55]. Such prevalence has shown to vary significantly with age, being higher during the seventh decade of life, where it can reach up to 18.6% [38,51].

The Diabetes Mellitus represents a great economic burden for Colombian society due to the costs generated by the treatment of the disease, as well as by the complications produced, being the CVD the group of complications that more costs generates. Thus, it is estimated that during the 2007, the costs generated by the Colombian population with Diabetes Mellitus reached the 2,708 million dollars, from which, 1,404 million (51.8%) were secondary to coronary disease, cardiac disease and cerebrovascular disease [57]. In turn, the 74.4% (1044 million dollars) of the costs generated by cardiovascular complications previously mentioned, corresponded to direct medical costs (drugs, laboratories, hospitalizations, professional care) while the 25.6% (360 million dollars) were secondary to indirect costs (losses by non-productivity secondary to acquired disability in population under 65 years old and losses by non-productivity secondary to deaths in the population under 65 years old) [57].

Thus, it becomes clearly the need to control the impact that Diabetes Mellitus produces over the Colombian population. It is essential that, the health authorities and also the medical-assistance personnel, consider a priority the early detection of patients with diabetes mellitus through screening strategies, from which an early treatment could be done, looking for to reduce the number of short term, medium term and long term complications, with the purpose of improving life quality in the diabetics and reduce the direct and indirect economic costs secondary to this disease.

12. Conclusion

The NCD and specially the CVD are nowadays the main cause of mortality in Colombia, being these consequence of a high prevalence of the major risk factors that have been related to their development, within the tobacco consumption, alcohol consumption, physical inactivity, unhealthy diet, overweight and obesity, arterial hypertension and high blood cholesterol and glucose levels are the leading ones, which constitute also important risk factors for the development of other NCD.

Thus, as part of a search of cost-effective strategies, that allow to potentially reduce the burden of CVD in Colombia, programs directed specifically to the prevention of each one of the modifiable risk factors identified in the present chapter must be implemented, in order to impact significantly in the reduction of the prevalence of the CVD. Such strategies, must be based in educational programs directed to the general population, making emphasis on children because as seen before, is on this age in which in most cases bad habits that will define the future behavior of this population group are adopted. Besides, is responsibility of authorities to guarantee the fulfillment of the laws by which the alcohol and tobacco products consumption are regulated, looking for to avoid an early onset of tobacco consumption among children and the exposition of non-smokers to the harmful effects of the tobacco smoke, considering the morbidity and mortality associated to these two risk factors.

Finally, is duty of the medical personnel to participate in an active way in the promotion of healthy lifestyles, constantly looking for an excellent adherence of the patients to the indications related to the frequent fruits and vegetables intake and the regular physical activity, educating them about the importance of following these recommendations, in order to guarantee a reduction in their risk profile for the development of NCD and through this reduce the constant increase in the prevalence of this group of diseases in the Colombian population.

Author details

Adrián Bolívar-Mejía[1] and Boris E. Vesga-Angarita[2]

1 Medical School, Faculty of Health, Universidad Industrial de Santander, Bucaramanga, Santander, Colombia

2 Instituto del Corazón de Bucaramanga, Internal Medicine Department, Universidad Industrial de Santander, Bucaramanga, Santander, Colombia

References

[1] World Health Organization. World Health Statistics 2012. http://www.who.int/healthinfo/EN_WHS2012_Full.pdf. (accessed 20 July 2012).

[2] Pan American Health Organization. Regional Consultation: Priorities for Cardiovascular Health in the Americas. Key Messages for Policymakers. http://www.cardiosource.org/acc/international-center/~/media/Files/ACC/International/Priorities.ashx (accessed 20 July 2012).

[3] World Health Organization. State of the Heart: Cardiovascular Disease Report. http://www.world-heart-federation.org/fileadmin/user_upload/documents/WHD2010/FINALStateoftheHeartCVDReport121010.pdf (accessed 20 July 2012).

[4] Pan American Health Organization. Health Situation in the Americas. Basic Indicators 2011. http://ais.paho.org/chi/brochures/2011/BI_2011_ENG.pdf (accessed 20 July 2012).

[5]   World Health Organization. Noncommunicable diseases country profiles 2011. http://whqlibdoc.who.int/publications/2011/9789241502283_eng.pdf (accessed 20 July 2012).

[6]   Beltrán-Bohórquez JR., García-Ramírez M., Beltrán-Pineda R., Gómez-López E., Bohórquez-Rodríguez R. et al. Guías Colombianas de Cardiología: Síndrome coronario agudo con elevación del ST. Rev Col Cardiol 2010; 17(suppl 3): 121-275

[7]   Gómez LA. Las enfermedades cardiovasculares: un problema de salud pública y un reto global. Biomedica 2011;31(4):469-73.

[8]   Abegunde DO., Mathers CD., Adam T., Ortegon M., Strong K. The burden and costs of chronic diseases in low-income and middle-income countries. Lancet. 2007; 370(9603):1929-1938.

[9]   Dua T., Garrido-Cumbrera M., Mathers C., Saxena S. Global Burden of Neurological Disorders: Estimates and Projections. In Campanini B. (ed.) Neurological Disorders: Public Health Challenges. Geneva: WHO Press; 2006. P27-39.

[10] Uribe CS., Jimenez I., Mora MO., Arana A., Sánchez JL. et al. Epidemiología de las enfermedades cerebrovasculares en Sabaneta, Colombia (1992 1993). Rev Neurol 1997;25(143):1008-1012.

[11] Pradilla G., Vesga BE., Diaz LA., Pinto NX., Sanabria CL. et al. Estudio neuroepidemiológico en comunidad urbana de Piedecuesta Santander. Acta Med Colomb 2002;27(6):407-420.

[12] Pradilla G., Vesga B., Leon FE and GENECO group. ational neuroepidemiological study in Colombia (EPINEURO). Pan Am J Public Health 2003;14(2): 104-111.

[13] Pradilla G., Vesga BE., Leon-Sarmiento FE., Bautista LE., Núñez LC. Neuroepidemiology in the eastern region of Colombia. Rev Neurol 2002;34(11):1035-43.

[14] Silva F., Quintero C., Zarruk JG. Guía Neurológica 8: Enfermedad Cerebrovascular. In Pérez G. (Ed.) Comportamiento Epidemiológico de la Enfermedad Cerebrovascular en la población colombiana. Bogotá: Mavarac LTDA; 2008. p23-29

[15] Ochoa-Vera ME., Otero-Wandarruga JA., Hormiga-Sánchez CM., López-Moreno L. Perfil de morbilidad y mortalidad de Santander. Revista del Observatorio de Salud Pública de Santander 2010;5(2):3-30.

[16] World Bank. Investing in Health. World Development Report, 1993. http://wdronline.worldbank.org/worldbank/a/c.html/world_development_report_1993/back_matter/WB.0-1952-0890-0.back (accessed 20 July 2012).

[17] Acosta-Ramírez N., Peñaloza RE., Rodríguez-García J. Carga de la Enfermedad Colombia 2005: Resultados Alcanzados. http://www.cendex.org.co/GPES/informes/PresentacionCarga_Informe.pdf (accessed 20 July 2012).

[18] World Health Organization. Global status report on noncommunicable diseases 2010. http://www.who.int/nmh/publications/ncd_report_full_en.pdf (accessed 20 July 2012).

[19] World Health Organization. Global Atlas on cardiovascular disease prevention and control. http://www.world-heart-federation.org/fileadmin/user_upload/documents/ Publications/Global_CVD_Atlas.pdf (accessed 20 July 2012).

[20] World Health Organization. Global Health Risks Mortality and burden of disease attributable to selected major risks (OMS) http://www.who.int/healthinfo/global_burden_disease/GlobalHealthRisks_report_full.pdf (accessed 20 July 2012).

[21] Unal B., Critchley JA., Capewell S. Explaining the decline in coronary heart disease mortality in England and Wales between 1981 and 2000. Circulation 2004;109(9): 1101-1107.

[22] Yusuf S., Hawken S., Ounpuu S., Dans T., Avezum A. Effect of potentially modifiable risk factors associated with myocardial infarction in 52 countries (the INTERHEART study): case-control study. Lancet 2004;364(9438):937-952.

[23] Doll R., Peto R., Boreham J., Sutherland I. Mortality in relation to smoking: 50 years' observations on male British doctors. BMJ 2004;328(7455): 1519 -1528.

[24] Champagne BM., Sebrié EM., Schargrodsky H., Pramparo P., Boissonnet C. et al. Tobacco smoking in seven Latin American cities: the CARMELA study. Tob Control 2010;19(6):457-462.

[25] World Health Organization. Tobacco Free Initiative (TFI). http://www.who.int/tobacco/surveillance/gyts/en/ (accessed 20 July 2012).

[26] Wiesner C., Peñaranda D. Encuesta mundial de tabaquismo en jóvenes, reporte de Bogotá, Colombia. Rev Col Cancerol 2002;6(4): 5-14.

[27] Hernández-Escolar J., Herazo-Beltrán Y., Valero MV. The frequency of cardiovascular disease-associated risk factors in a university student population. Rev Salud Publica 2010;12(5): 852-864.

[28] Tafur LA., Ordóñez G., Millán JC., Varela JM., Rebellón P. Prevalencia de tabaquismo en estudiantes recién ingresados a la Universidad Santiago de Cali. Colomb Med 2006; 37(2): 126-132.

[29] Pardo C., Piñeros M. Teenage tobacco consumption in five Colombian cities. Biomedica 2010;30(4): 509-518.

[30] Congreso de la República de Colombia. Ley 1335 de 2009. http://www.secretariasenado.gov.co/senado/basedoc/ley/2009/ley_1335_2009.html ((accessed 20 July 2012).

[31] Instituto Colombiano de Bienestar Familiar. Encuesta Nacional de la Situacion Nutricional en Colombia 2010. https://www.icbf.gov.co/icbf/directorio/portel/libreria/pdf/ LibroENSIN2010.pdf (accessed 20 July 2012).

[32] Instituto Colombiano de Bienestar Familiar. Encuesta Nacional de la Situacion Nutricional en Colombia 2005. https://www.icbf.gov.co/icbf/directorio/portel/libreria/pdf/1ENSINLIBROCOMPLETO.pdf (accessed 20 July 2012).

[33] Mantilla-Toloza SC., Gómez-Conesa A., Hidalgo-Montesinos. Physical activity and tobacco and alcohol use in a group of university students. Rev Salud Publica 2011;13(5): 748-58.

[34] Alayón AN., Castro-Orozco R., Gaviria-Esquivia L., Fernández-Franco M., Benítez-Peña L. Cardiovascular risk factors among 7-and 14-year old schoolchildren in Cartagena, Colombia, 2009. Rev Salud Publica 2011;13(2): 196-206.

[35] Patiño-Villada FA., Arango-Vélez EF., Quintero-Velásquez MA., Arenas-Sosa MM. Cardiovascular risk factors in an urban Colombia population. Rev Salud Publica 2011;13(3): 433-45.

[36] Lobelo F., Pate R., Parra D., Duperly J., Pratt M. Burden of mortality associated to physical inactivity in Bogota, Colombia. Rev Salud Publica 2006;8(Suppl 2): 28-41.

[37] Böhm M., Rosenkranz S., Laufs U. Alcohol and red wine: impact on cardiovascular risk. Nephrol Dial Transplant 2004;19(1): 11-16.

[38] Hormiga-Sánchez CM., Otero-Wandarraga JA., Rodríguez Villamizar LA., León-Franco MH. Prevalencia de factores de riesgo para enfermedades crónicas en Santander, 2010. Revista del Observatorio de Salud Pública de Santander 2010;5(3): 2-24.

[39] Manrique-Abril FG., Ospina JM., Garcia-Ubaque JC. Children and adolescents' alcohol and tobacco consumption in Tunja, Colombia, 2009. Rev Salud Publica 2011;13(1): 89-101.

[40] López-Maldonado MC., Luis MA., Gherardi-Donato EC. Licit drugs consumption among nursing students at a private university in Bogotá, Colombia. Rev Lat Am Enfermagem 2011;19: 707-13.

[41] Arrieta-Vergara KM. Pathological alcohol consumption amongst students from the University of Cartagena, 2008. Rev Salud Publica 2009;11(6): 878-86.

[42] Observatorio de Drogas de Colombia. Estudio Nacional de Consumo de Sustancias Psicoactivas en Poblacion Escolar Colombia - 2011. http://odc.dne.gov.co/docs/publicaciones_nacionales/Estudio%20Sustancias%20Psicoactivas%20en%20Escolares%202011.pdf (accessed 20 July 2012).

[43] Ardila MF., Herrán OF. Expectancies towards alcohol consumption in Bucaramanga, Colombia. Rev Med Chil 2008;136(1): 73-82.

[44] Ministry of Social Protection. Decreto número 120 de 2010. http://web.presidencia.gov.co/decretoslinea/2010/enero/21/dec12021012010.pdf (accessed 20 July 2012).

[45] Belin RJ., Greenland P., Allison M., Martin L., Shikany JM. et al. Diet quality and the risk of cardiovascular disease: the Women's Health Initiative (WHI). Am J Clin Nutr 2011;94(1): 49-57.

[46] Socarrás-Suárez MM., Bolet-Astoviza M. Healthy feeding and nutrition in cardiovascular diseases. Rev Cubana Invest Bioméd 2010; 29(3): 353-363.

[47] Webber L., Kilpi F., Marsh T., Rtveladze K., Brown M. et al. High Rates of Obesity and Non-Communicable Diseases Predicted across Latin America. PLoS One 2012;7(8): 1-6

[48] Báez L., Blanco MI., Bohórquez R., Botero R., Cuenca G. et al. Guías colombianas para el diagnóstico y tratamiento de la hipertensión arterial. Rev Col Cardiol 2007;13(suppl 1): 187-313

[49] Ministerio de Salud. II Estudio Nacional de Factores de Riesgo de Enfermedades Crónicas - Enfrec II. http://www.col.ops-oms.org/sivigila/IndiceBoletines1999.asp (accessed 20 July 2012).

[50] National Institute of Health. Detection,Evaluation,and Treatmentof High BloodCholesterolin Adults(Adult TreatmentPanel III). http://www.nhlbi.nih.gov/guidelines/ cholesterol/atp3full.pdf (accessed 20 July 2012).

[51] Bautista LE., Oróstegui M., Vera LM., Prada GE., Orozco LC. et al. Prevalence and impact of cardiovascular risk factors in Bucaramanga, Colombia: results from the Countrywide Integrated Noncommunicable Disease Intervention Programme (CINDI/CARMEN) baseline survey. Eur J Cardiovasc Prev Rehabil 2006;13(5): 769-75.

[52] Feliciano-Alfonso JE., Mendivil CO., Ariza ID., Pérez CE. Cardiovascular risk factors and metabolic syndrome in a population of young students from the National University of Colombia. Rev Assoc Med Bras 2010;56(3): 293-8.

[53] Alayón AN., Ariza S., Baena K., Lambis L., Martínez L. et al. Active search and assessment of cardiovascular risk factors in young adults, Cartagena de Indias, 2007. Biomedica 2010;30(2): 238-44.

[54] Uscátegui-Peñuela RM., Alvarez-Uribe MC., Laguado-Salinas I., Soler-Terranova W., Martínez-Maluendas L. et al. Cardiovascular risk factors in children and teenagers aged 6-18 years old from Medellin (Colombia). An Pediatr (Barc) 2003;58(5): 411-417.

[55] Aschner P. Epidemiology of diabetes in Colombia. Av Diabetol 2010;26(2): 95-100.

[56] Takada JY., Ramos RB., Avakian SD., dos Santos SM., Ramires JA. et al. BNP and admission glucose as in-hospital mortality predictors in non-ST elevation myocardial infarction. ScientificWorldJournal. 2012;2012: 1-7.

[57] Gozáles JC., Walter JH., Einarson TR. Cost-of-illness study of type 2 diabetes mellitus in Colombia. Rev Panam Salud Publica 2009;26(1): 55-63.

Environmental Public Health

Biological Responses of in vivo Studies to Contaminants: A Contribution to Improve Public Health Knowledge

Maria de Lourdes Pereira,
Irvathur Krishnananda Pai and
Fernando Garcia e Costa

Additional information is available at the end of the chapter

1. Introduction

Global climate changes and ecosystems deterioration due to several human activities in-volving environmental hazards have a great impact on human welfare [1]. These factors added to many other stressors are responsible for emerging diseases worldwide, which represent an important endeavour. For this reason the risk of contaminants on human health is an expanding area of environmental epidemiology. This sub-field of epidemiol-ogy addresses, not only the environmental factors affecting the health and illness of pop-ulations but also offers public education on environmental issues. Matters such as sources of environmental contaminants, assessment of how exposure to a hazardous chemical may occur, measurement of health effects, and applying appropriate controls are relevant issues of this branh [2]. Surveillance platforms for hazardous environmental factors involving data collection and analyses, and public health promotion through evi-dence-based approaches are also within the scope of this growing field. Nowadays, at-tention to chemical and physical factors have gained special care within the scope of environmental epidemiology due to the myriad of pollutants persisting in water bodies, air, crop lands, and other environmental settings.

The example of the adverse effects on humans and other species induced by heavy metals, and metalloids spread within environment [3-12] illustrates the intersection between the en-vironmental and human health issues. Another example, based on epidemiological studies has revealed that pesticides may cause birth deficiencies, and cancer [13].

Latest advances in scientific research and new developments on important environmental
and human health topics such as the potential risk to humans from toxic chemicals in the
environment were recently communicated [14]. In this matter, research elucidating the cellular and molecular mechanisms by which these environmental agents induce toxicity, muta-
genesis, and carcinogenesis, among others were underlined.

Human exposure to environmental contaminants and their potentially harmful impacts
on public health was more recently discussed by a panel of international experts on the
conference "Human Biomonitoring: Political benefits – scientific challenges", held in Berlin 2010 [15]. In fact, health measures surveys have been implemented worldwide, and
the role of human biomonitoring data has been underlined due to important risk assessment, and risk management procedures. Quantitative measure of exposure to environmental chemicals by measuring them or their metabolites in tissues (eg. hair, nails),
fluids (e.g., saliva, breast milk, blood, and urine) or exhaled air are indicators of the degree of human exposure to potentially hazardous chemicals. Some widespread health impacts like diabetes, obesity, attention deficit, or hyperactivity are related to chemical
exposure, as evidenced by linking human biomonitoring and epidemiological data to
health effects [16].

Additionally to this topic, the importance of sentinel animal species for evaluating the potential human health impacts of chemical stressors was previously debated and the possible
use of animal data into the human risk assessment process was emphasized [17]. In fact, the
scientific literature evidences reports on a wide range of animal sentinels and their relevance
as models for epidemiologic studies of human diseases and environmental exposures. For
example, domestic and wild animals may be sensitive indicators of environmental hazards
and provide an early warning system for public health, corroborating or informing epidemiologic studies in humans [18]. For example, the suitability of pet dogs was focussed since
they share the same environment as humans. Additionally, large mammals were pointed in
these studies due to the role as top predator species.

Advances in the development of environmental epidemiology are then illustrated by the
interrelationships between humans and other forms of life sharing the same environment. In this context, several effects occurring in organisms (eg. mortality, reproductive
dysfunction) in a particular ecological niche may alert to potential harmful effects on human health.

Comparison between human and wildlife exposure models revealed similarities in exposure
endpoints, chemical stressors (i.e., pesticides and metals), and extent of model validation
(for review see) [19].

More recently the topic "Contaminant and Pollutant effects" was discussed in a workshop
organised by the Society of Environmental Toxicology and Chemistry (SETAC e Italian
Branch), and newly reported [20]. Under this concern, this working group underlined that
almost all the contaminants thought to be of concern in large marine vertebrates (eg. pelagic
fish, whales) is of great relevance to contaminant-related human diseases. In addition, concerns over newly emerging threats such as perfluorinated compounds and nanomaterials

were debated. Workshop participants also highlighted the role of biomarkers to accomplish this study. To reinforce this idea the relevance of biological responses of some species was mentioned to clarify questions concerning the behaviour of persistent organic pollutants, and emerging contaminants and their impact on humans and the environment [21].This report focussed on the importance of archiving biological and environmental samples (eg. plankton, fish, marine mammals, water, sediment) for monitoring anthropogenic contaminants and a global coordination need in environmental research.

The measurement of the health consequences due to contaminants exposure is a very hard task, since different actors play in this scenario. Factors such as complexes mixtures within the environment (including chemical and biological agents), added to physical parameters (eg. see level rise, heat), and individual factors (eg. species, gender, age, nutritional, and immunological status) take an important part in this evaluation.

Apart from field studies, the use of laboratory animals in biomedical research for the benefit of human health conducted in accordance with ethical procedures, and based on the 3Rs (replacement, reduction, and refinement) remain vital. These reports emphasize the crucial value of research findings on animal species for understanding the extent and burden of health-related problems induced by xenobiotics. In fact, decisions in public health based on these findings contribute for a better formulation of health policy planning and intervention.

Although substantial progress has been devoted to the production, management, and disposal of chemicals, added to the Directives and other regulations aiming to minimise threats, past and present experiences revealed that, it is still a very multifaceted process due to several interacting factors among genetic features and environmental exposures, which deserve much attention.

This chapter is a contribution for the *in vivo* data knowledge on the relevance of both experimental laboratory mice and field studies including wildlife species in which concern to contaminants. Although some exposure models for either wildlife or humans are available following regulatory guidelines focussing on relevant endpoints, some examples, offered as a case study, include, among others, those based on our experiments. For example, the disease potential of some copepods due to their role as vectors of waterborne pathogens of humans is focussed; some fish species used as pollutants indicators are mentioned; finally, some experimental studies conducted on laboratory mice exposed to some contaminants are analysed. Those reports based on interdisciplinary techniques including histopathological, ultrastructural, biochemical, molecular and/or analytical approaches aims to characterize the biological responses to several contaminants within target organs. The last goal intends to integrate these experimental findings for environmental monitoring, and is a contribution for the understanding of human health impacts.

Finally, some issues for a more robust public health-based interdisciplinary research are recommended.

2. Relevance of animal studies for human health

A growing body of research focuses on the impact of chemical contamination on a wide range of animal species among different phyla and habitats. Adverse effects have been described alerting for the risk to humans. In this part, some representative examples are given with special emphasis for zooplankton, and fish. In addition, studies on the toxicity of contaminants on laboratory mice are presented.

Birds have been used to evaluate the presence of heavy metals in some habitats [22]. Some marine gastropod molluscs such as *Nucella lapillus* (L.) are used as bioindicators of tributyltin pollution in the North Atlantic coastlines through an important imposex assessment index [23]. Amphibians can serve as crucial and valuable research models for understanding the ecological effects of persistent contaminants such as mercury amplifying the risk of transfer of accumulated contaminants to higher trophic levels [24]. Amphibians living near uranium mines were used to assess the impacts of the locally produced acidic and metal-rich materials [25]. Copepods have broad geographic ranges, and sustain the world fisheries that nourish and support human populations [26]. They are key sensitive indicators of local and global climate change, and potential vectors of waterborne diseases. Mussels such as *Mytilus galloprovincialis,* and *Mytilus edulis* are key bivalves widely used as sentinel species [27, 28]. Mussels are suitable test species for monitoring persistent pollutants because they are sessile, filter feeders with low rates of metabolic transformation [29].

The biological signals of exposure in the above mentioned species include suitable biomarkers (eg. subcellular, cellular, functional levels) added to pollutant analysis in species. Of course, parameters such as biological cycles must be regarded as for a proper interpretation of data. Another factor to consider when dealing with wild animals is the availability of food once it may have a great influence on the immune system condition of animals [25].

2.1. Role of zooplankton with special reference to copepods in human health

The name plankton is derived from the Greek adjective - *planktos,* meaning "errant", and by extension "wanderer" or "drifter". This is in contrast to nekton organisms that can swim against the ambient flow and control their position (e.g. squid, fish, and marine mammals). Though many planktic or planktonic species are microscopic in size, plankton includes organisms covering a wide range of sizes, including large organisms such as jellyfish.

Plankton are any drifting organisms (animals, plants, or bacteria) that, inhabit the pelagic zone of oceans, seas, or bodies of freshwater. That is, plankton are defined by their ecological niche rather than phylogenetic or taxonomic classification. They provide a crucial source of food to larger, more familiar aquatic organisms such as fish and whales. Freshly hatched fish larvae are also plankton for a few days as long as they cannot swim against currents. Their density and distribution pattern varies horizontally, vertically and seasonally. This variability is mainly due to the availability of light, availability of nutrient. Besides from representing the bottom few levels of a food chain that supports commercially important fisheries, plankton ecosystems play a role in the biogeochemical cycles of many important chemical elements, including the ocean's carbon cycle. In addition, plankton species play important role in the disposal of sewage and in the natural purification of polluted water. But, some of them like dinoflagellates, their harmful bloom causes high mortality in the aquatic environment. They also act as indicator of petroleum too [30]. They are responsible for causing various diseases to animals and human beings.

Plankton are primarily divided into broad functional (or trophic level) groups: Phytoplankton (from Greek *phyton*, or plant), autotrophic, prokaryotic or eukaryotic algae that live near the water surface, where there is sufficient light to support photosynthesis. E.g. diatoms, cyanobacteria, dinoflagellates and coccolithophores; Zooplankton (from Greek *zoon*, or animal), small protozoans or metazoans (e.g. crustaceans and other animals) that feed on other plankton; Bacterioplankton, bacteria and archaea, which play an important role in remineralising organic material down the water column.

Plankton are further classified into holoplankton, which spend their entire life cycle as plankton (e.g. most algae, copepods, salps, and some jellyfish) and meroplankton, which lead a planktonic life only for a part of their lives (usually the larval stage), and then develop in to a nektic or sea floor living benthic form (eg: larvae of sea urchins, starfish, crustaceans, marine worms, and most fish).

Plankton are also classified into the following groups, based on the size of these organisms (Table 1).

Plankton inhabits in ponds, lakes, seas and oceans too and their density and distribution pattern varies horizontally, vertically and seasonally. This variability is mainly due to the availability of light, availability of nutrient.

Zooplankton can also act as a disease reservoir. They have been found to house the bacterium *Vibrio cholerae*, which causes cholera, by allowing the cholera vibrio to attach to their chitinous exoskeletons. This symbiotic relationship enhances the bacterium's ability to survive in an aquatic environment, as the exoskeleton provides the bacterium with carbon and nitrogen.

Copepods are known for extensive and varied type of parasitism. In this process they show all degrees of modifications right from slight reduction to complete disappearance. Several marine animals such as anemones, annelids, crustaceans mollusks, tunicates, fishes and even whales and sharks too are being parasitized by the copepods. They can be ectoparasites or endoparasites. Members Lernaeopodidae and Lernaeidae family (Or: Copepoda) are well known ectoparasites. Copepods of Family Caligidae are ectoparasites found on the gills, buccal cavity, and opercular cavity [31].

Copepods are multicellular animals, more abundant than any other groups including insects and nematodes [32]. Though they are mostly inhabit in natural and man-made aquatic systems, they can also inhabit nutrient-rich black oozes of abyssal ocean depths to the nutrient-poor waters of the highest mountain tarns. Some of them are found on canopies of some rain forests, hot springs, leaf-litter, in caves, between sand grains (Figure 1).

They also exhibit symbiotic associations with other animal and plant species. Their density can be as high as 92,000 individuals/L [33].

Copepods form a subclass belonging to the subphylum Crustacea (crustaceans). Copepods
are divided into ten orders. Some 13,000 species of copepods are known, and 2,800 of them
live in freshwaters [34].

Group	Size Range	Example
Megaplankton	(>20 mm)	Metazoans; e.g. Jellyfish; Ctenophores; Salps (e.g. Cyclosalps, Members of genus Thalia) Pelagic Tunicates (e.g. Sea Tulip, Sea Squirts or Sea Pork); Cephalopodes (e.g. Octopus, squid, Cuttle fish)
Macroplankton	(2–20 mm)	Metazoans; Chaetognaths (eg: Sagitta); Euphausids (e.g.: Antarctic krill), Medusae (e.g. Coelenterates); ctenophores; salps, doliolids (e.g. Doliolum) Tunicata Cephalopoda
Mesoplankton	(0.2 -2 mm)	Metazoans; e.g. copepods; Medusae; Cladocera; Ostracoda; Chaetognaths; Pteropods; Tunicata; Heteropoda
Microplankton	(20–200)	Large eukaryotic protists; most phytoplankton; Protozoa (Foraminifera); ciliates; Rotifera; juvenile metazoans - Crustacea (copepod nauplii)
Nanoplankton	(2–20 µm)	Small eukaryotic protists; Small Diatoms; Small Flagellates; Pyrrophyta; Chrysophyta; Chlorophyta; Xanthophyta
	(0.2–2 µm)	Small eukaryotic protists; bacteria; Chrysophyta

Table 1. Classification of plankton based on the size of organisms [30].

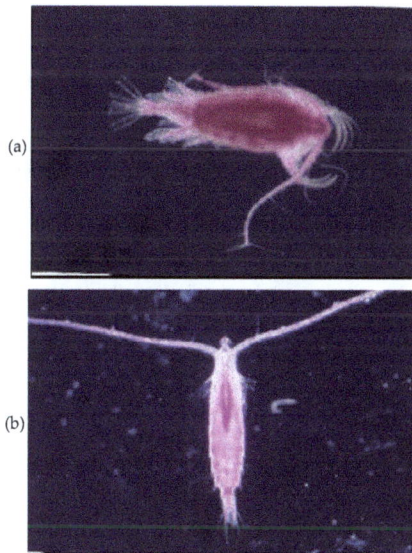

Figure 1. (a) and (b). Representative specimens of copepods: *Euchaeta marina* (a), and *Rhinocalanus cronutus* (b).

Copepods are known to carry pathogenic strains of *Vibrio* and have the potential to play important roles in cholera transmission [35]. This acute bacterial infection of the intestine caused by a few strains of bacterium *Vibrio cholerae* is transmitted through consumption of contaminated water. The bacteria needs chitinous surface of copepods to replicate. In Asia and Africa due to seasonal blooms of phytoplankton, which happen to be the food of the main food source of copepods, increases the amount of cholera-causing bacteria in waterways. When people consume bacteria infected copepod colonized water, they get cholera. The bacteria cause severe watery diarrhea, known as "rice water" diarrhea, and vomiting. Fluid loss can lead to severe dehydration and death within 24 hours of the onset of symptoms if dehydration is not treated. Poor sanitation, mixing up of sewage containing feces from cholera infected patients further contaminates water sources, allowing cholera to continue to propagate.

Apart from this aspect they are vectors of relevant human diseases. Fasciolasis also known as Distomatosis and Liver rot is an important disease caused by trematode helminthes viz., *Fasciola hepatica* (the common liver fluke or sheep live fluke) and *Fasciola gigantica*. This disease belongs to the plant-borne trematode zoonoses. In Europe, the Americas and Oceania only *F. hepatica* is common while in Asia and Africa both species have found in common. Estimated loss by this disease is pegged around US$3.2 billion per annum. As around 2.4 million people are infected ad over 180 million people are at risk, WHO has considered this disease as an emerging human disease. *Fasciola hepatica* is a parasitic flatworm (Cl: Trematoda, Ph.: Platyhelminths), that infects the liver of various mammals, including humans. *F. hepatica* is distributed worldwide, and has been known as an important parasite of sheep and cattle for hundreds of years, causing great economic losses in sheep and cattle. Thus has been the subject of many scientific investigations and may be the best known of any trematode species. They have a wide range of definitive host, which includes many herbivorous mammals, including humans. They have freshwater snails such as *Galba truncatula*, (in which the parasite can reproduce asexually) as an intermediate host for completion of their life cycle. For completion of liver fluke they pass through cercaria and miracidium larval stages, which are also considered as planktonic stages. Though a freshwater snail is required as a intermediate host, for the *F. hepatica* to complete its life cycle, Species in the family Lymnaeidae include: *Austropeplea tomentosa, Austropeplea ollula, Austropeplea viridis, Radix peregra, Radix lagotis, Radix auriculari, Radix natalensis, Radix rubiginosa, Omphiscola glabra, Lymnaea stagnalis, Stagnicola fuscus, Stagnicola palustris, Stagnicola turricul, Pseudosuccinea columella, Lymnaea viatrix, Lymnaea neotropica, Fossaria bulimoides, Lymnaea cubensis, Galba truncatula, Lymnaea cousini, Lymnaea humilis, Lymnaea diaphana, Stagnicola caperata* and *Lymnaea occulta* that serve as naturally or experimentally intermediate hosts of *Fasciola hepatica*.

Adult specimens live in bile passages of the liver of many kinds of mammals in general and ruminants in particular. Humans are also occasionally infected. In fact, fascioliasis is one of the major causes of hypereosinophilia in France. The flukes feed on the lining of biliary ducts. Their eggs are passed out of the liver with bile and into the intestine to be voided with feces. If they fall into water where the eggs complete their development and turn into miracidia, which hatch in 9 to 10 days during warm weather. During cold season it takes longer period. On hatching, miracidia have 24 hours in which find a suitable snail host. Mother sporocysts produce first generation rediae, which in turn produce daughter rediae that develop in snail's digestive gland. From the snail, minute cercariae emerge, which swim through pools of water to pasture and encyst as metacercariae on near-by vegetation. When ruminants feed on this vegetation or when human eat uncooked/semi cooked food prepared out of these plants from the pasture, the metacercar iae find their way into ruminants or in human beings. In the liver, due to low pH, these encysted metacercaria start excystement. Later, these parasites break free of the metacercariae and burrows through the duodenum and intestinal lining into the peritoneal cavity. Though the newly excysted juvenile does not feed at this stage. After some days, once they find the liver parenchyma, they start feeding. This immature stage in the liver tissue is the pathogenic stage, causing anaemia and clinical signs sometimes observed in infected animals. The parasite feeds on liver tissue for a period of about six weeks, and later moves into bile duct, where it matures into an adult and begins to produce eggs. Under mild infection, these organisms can produce up to 25,000 eggs per day per fluke and can produce and deposit up to 500,000 eggs onto a pasture by a single sheep.

Trypanosomiasis also called as Chagas disease is caused in several vertebrates like horses, buffalo, dogs, cats and also human beings by parasitic protozoan trypanosomes of the genus *Trypanosoma*. It is reported that around 500,000 men, women, and children in 36 countries of sub-Saharan Africa suffer from human African trypanosomiasis and around 21,000 die due to this disease. The main casual agents are *Trypanosoma brucei gambiense* and *Trypanosoma brucei rhodesiense*.

Basically there are two types of trypanosome species viz. salivarian species and the stercorarian species trypanosoma exists. Stercorarian trypanosomes infect the insects like triatomid kissing bug, develop in its posterior gut and infective organisms are released into the faeces and deposited on the skin of the host. The organism then penetrates and can disseminate throughout the body. Insects become infected when taking a blood meal. While the second type, namely Salivarian trypanosomes develop in the anterior gut of insects, most importantly the Tsetse fly and infective organisms are inoculated into the host by the insect bite before it feeds.

As trypanosomes progress through their life cycle they undergo a series of morphological changes as is typical of trypanosomatids. The life cycle often consists of the trypomastigote form in the vertebrate host and the trypomastigote or promastigote form in the gut of the invertebrate host. Intracellular lifecycle stages are normally found in the amastigote form. The trypomastigote morphology is unique to species in the genus *Trypanosoma*.

The role of copepods as intermediate hosts of the fish parasite *Diphyllobothrium latum* is well known [36]. The life cycle of this tapeworm include copepod, and fish as first and second hosts, respectively. Human consumers of raw or lightly processed fish are final hosts. The debilitating disease, dracunculosis is vectored by freshwater copepods such as *Mesocyclops kieferi*, *M. aspericornis*, *Thermocyclops incisus*, *T. inopinus* and *T. oblongatus* of the Guinea worm, *Dracunculus mediensis* [35]. Though stomach digestive juices destroy the copepods, the larvae of the Guinea worm survive and penetrate the stomach or small intestinal wall, migrating to the subcutaneous tissue of the abdomen and thorax.

Other adverse impacts on human health of copepods include their potential as important allergens [37].

2.2. Relevance of edible fish

This section deals, mainly, with the relevance on contaminants on fish, due to the relationship between the environment and human populations through diet.

Contaminants are among the anthropogenic stresses with negative impact on water quality, thus contributing for general decline on several fish species which economical value is well recognised [38]. Moreover, hazardous chemicals alter the chemical composition of water, thus may render them susceptible to infectious diseases, being a source for several zoonotic diseases agents.

Fish is considered as one of the best indicators of heavy metal contamination in coastal milieu [39]. A number of fish species has been used as relevant bio-indicators in monitoring programs around the world. For example, skipjack tuna (*Katsuwonus pelamis*) has been used for global monitoring of wide range pollutants (eg. PCBs and organochlorine pesticides, polybrominated diphenyl ethers, polychlorinated dibenzo-p-dioxins, furans, and coplanar polychlorinated biphenyls [40-43]. Red mullets (*Mullus barbatus*) were used as sentinel organisms from anthropogenic impacted areas at Mediterranean Sea [44]. The Atlantic cod, *Gadus morhua* has been used in the Barents Sea sub-Arctic location for PAHs and metals monitoring [28]. *Anguilla anguilla*, *Platichthys flesus* and *Dicentrarchus labrax* are other bioindicadors of contaminants in different geographical areas [45-48].

Bottom feeders such as mullets, and flounders concentrate contaminants to a higher degree than other species.

To evaluate the biological responses of contaminants on fish a wide range of techniques have been used namely histopathology, and biochemistry of enzymes. Biomarkers such as DNA integrity and detoxification enzyme status in fish tissues have also frequently been used. Other biomarkers of aquatic pollution including fish phagocytes-induced ROS, peroxidative damage, and oxidative stress were reported on the European eel *Anguilla anguilla* [49, 50]. A battery of biomarkers together with gonad histology was used to characterize the responses of red mullets (*Mullus barbatus*) to anthropogenic pollutants [44].

The effects of some stressors were evaluated on *Platichthys flesus*, using several biomarkers [46]. Different patterns of response, namely enzymatic, genotoxic, and cytotoxic were observed on fish from impacted areas, underlying the role of reliable biomarkers for future biomonitoring studies. Other studies reported on biological responses of this flatfish to chemical stress including gene expression, genotoxicity, cholinesterase, and growth rate [51].

Novel biomarkers at molecular level, such as alterations in the expression of *xpf* gene and some of the genes found by SSH, such as HGFA were described in *Dicentrarchus labrax* and *Liza aurata* exposed to environmental contaminants [52].

Adverse changes on liver of *Poecilia vivipara* assessed semi-quantitatively using the (Histopathological Alterations Index – HAI) were described and the possibility of relationship to pesticides, heavy metals, sewage and others factors were postulated [53]. Other potential markers on environmental pollution were illustrated by analyse of matrix metalloproteinases on fish bile from *Mugil liza* and *Tilapia rendalli* [54].

High concentration values of heavy metals exceeding the permissive levels and the allowable maximum concentrations of these pollutants on organs of edible fish were reported in different species worldwide, suggesting that fishes could cause serious problems to human health, due to bioaccumulation over time; for example high levels of the most hazardous metals on muscular tissue of *Oreochromis niloticus* were reported (1.315 Cd 2.053 Pb 1.159 Hg mg/kg) representing an hazard at human health point of view [55]. Among nine commercially important species, the concentration of Mn, Fe, and Pb in a few species exceeded the WHO guideline values for safe human consumption [39]. For example muscle samples of *Lepturacanthus savala* displayed maximum levels of Pb (2.29 μg g-1). Similarly, chemical analyzes on four species (*Sarda sarda, Mulus barbatus ponticus, Trachurus trachurus* and *Merlangius merlangus* using flame and graphite furnace atomic absorption spectrometry revealed acceptable values of trace element levels. However, lead and cadmium (e.g. 0.28 ± 0.03 μg/g Pb and 0.35 ± 0.04 μg/g Cd/ *Sarda sarda*) in fish samples were higher than the recommended legal limits [56].

High mercury levels in organs of *Liza aurata* inhabiting a contaminated estuary were reported, and human risk associated to the ingestion of fish was not excluded [57].

Other reports mention lower concentration of some pollutants on fish tissues, namely muscle, being suitable for human diet. However, the influence of chemical interactions must be considered. For example heavy metal concentrations in different tissues of *Labeo rohita* and *Ctenopharyngodon idella* of Upper Lake of Bhopal were within the recommended limit values for fish consumption [58]. Although the results of this study confirm the safety for human health, these authors alert for the need of further preventive measures, since it is quite evident that there was accumulation of heavy metals in fish tissues.

Studies on heavy metals and metalloid (mercury, cadmium, lead, and arsenic) levels in the muscles of three relevant economically pelagic species (*Sardine pilchardus, Scomber japonicus* and *Trachurus trachurus*) from the Northeast and Eastern Central Atlantic Ocean revealed different patterns of contamination according to feeding behaviour [59]. Values of As>Pb>Hg>Cd for sardine, and As>Hg>Pb>Cd for chub mackerel and horse mackerel were reported. This elegant survey also estimated the potential public health risks via consumption of the mentioned species. From those studies it was concluded the safety for human consumption in terms of the amounts of cadmium and lead although moderate intake was recommended due to possible health risks derived from arsenic and mercury.

Another survey, aiming to evaluate potential risk–benefit of fish consumption was conduct-ed using 24 common fish species collected from Chinese markets on 2007 [60]. Nutritional value and contaminants levels (DDT, PCB_7, arsenic and cadmium) were evaluated. Al-though mercury concentration in common carp exceeded the upper limit of the Chinese na-tional standard these studies indicated that fish, particularly marine oily fish can be regularly consumed to achieve optimal nutritional benefits, without causing significant con-taminant related health risks. Nevertheless, potential health warning was referred for peo-ple consuming large amounts of fish, namely wild fish.

Some physiological alterations such as, breathing, gastrointestinal, and skin disorders were reported as associated to individuals consuming As-contaminated fish daily and the poten-tial risk of arsenicosis among poor people was underlined [61].

Some of the examples above mentioned illustrate the significance of pollutants release into the environment on edible fish species which may represent a warning for public health. Therefore, these findings may lead to public health interventions and policy initiatives for safeguarding human health.

2.3. Experimental studies with laboratory mice

The following section presents some examples of our experimental studies conducted with laboratory mice, aiming to illustrate the effects of some hazardous compounds at different levels of biological response (cellular, tissue, and/or physiological). Efforts aiming a cross-disciplinary interaction were done and several techniques were used, such as histology, transmission electron microscopy, and flow cytometry. These approaches complemented with chemical analysis of the toxicants or its metabolits on tissues exemplify the relationship between contamination, and injury.

Apart from our experience using this model the scientific evidence of adverse health effects from ubiquitous anthropogenic pollutants (eg. metals, metaloids, and pesticides) on both an-imal species and humans has been largely documented, thus, contributing to identify poten-tial harmful chemicals for human health.

Some environmental toxicants have been shown to exhibit deleterious effects on testis, namely spermatogenesis, and fertility.

There is growing evidence that lead ($PbCl_2$) and cadmium compounds ($CdCl_2$) adversely af-fects spermatogenesis and fertility parameters of mice indicated by severe degenerative changes on seminiferous tubules, and poor quality of semen [62, 63]. Histopathological stud-ies were also conducted in order to explore the extension of damage. In addition, flow cy-tometry (FCM) studies were performed using buffered formalin fixed and paraffin embedded paraffin samples of testicular tissue from mice exposed to cadmium and lead chloride per se, in order to establish the ploidy level of germ cells. Significant alterations in germ cell percentages in mice exposed to cadmium were detected by FCM, supporting the histopathological data [62]. However, no alterations in the percentages of testicular germ cells detected by FCM were evident in animals exposed to lead chloride, excepting of an in-crease in the percentage of cells in S phase.

Further reports, by using several biomarkers at subcellular level of sperm physiology such as DNA fragmentation, and chromatin integrity, assessed by the terminal deoxylnucleotidyl transferase-mediated deoxyuridine triphosphate (dUTP) nick-end labelling (TUNEL), and sperm chromatin structure assays (SCSA), respectively, coupled to other techniques for evaluation of sperm function authors demonstrated that lead chloride affects physiological parameters such as motility, morphology, and acrosome status, although no significant genotoxic effects were noted [63]. In fact, sperm DNA is in general resistant due to its highly compacted nature. Those reports also evidenced the role of flow cytometry as a powerful tool for quantitative analyses of different cell types and an insight on cell cycle status, added to the measurement of DNA content of cell subpopulations in the testis.

More recently the genotoxic effects induced by cadmium were reported using a panel of suitable microsatellites as markers of genetic instability [64].

The effects on testis after co-exposure to lead and cadmium were also described on mice through a histological approach [65]: seminiferous epithelium degeneration, exfoliation of germ cells into the lumen, distorted morphology of tubules was accompanied by atrophy. Work in progress in our laboratory demonstrated adverse effects of this mixture on other target organs such as kidney, spleen, and liver, comparing with respective controls (Figures 2 and 3). Degenerative aspects were noted on renal cortical area; splenic sections denoted cell loosening and numerous macrophages; hepatic parenchyma displays several haemorrhagic foci. Overall, the histopathological study revealed several adverse changes pointing obviously for dysfunctions.

Another illustration of a toxicant targeting the male reproductive function of mice was the research conducted with sodium arsenite [66]. Awareness was directed to spermatogenesis, a multipart process involving delicate cells such as germ cells, often targets of a wide range of contaminants. Impairment of spermatogenesis was found on testis sections, complemented with biochemical parameters. Those issues have been established as suitable in the evaluation of physiological disorders in mice.

Further studies aiming to explore and characterize possible recovery of sperm morphology and functional parameters after withdrawal of the toxicant revealed several changes at ultrastructural level, namely irregular pattern of chromatin, and altered acrosome [67]. In addition, a molecular approach demonstrated high DNA fragmentation index revealing abnormal chromatin structure. In this work, as in present studies on this topic, transmission electron microscopy studies were pertinent to identify fine changes on cell organelles (Figure 4).

Work in progress also demonstrated the effects of sodium arsenite on splenic structure of dosed animals (Figure 5). The degree of lesions was irregular: some areas of the spleen evidenced reduced cellular concentration (Figure 5a) and disruption (Figure 5b), respectively, within white pulp comparing with controls (data not shown). In addition, an increase of megakaryocytes was observed, probably due to the required phagocytic activity.

Histopathology coupled with ultrastructural studies were sensitive tools for the detection of adverse effects of sodium arsenite on target organs (eg. testis) allowing information on the nature of the lesions, and its eventual recovery.

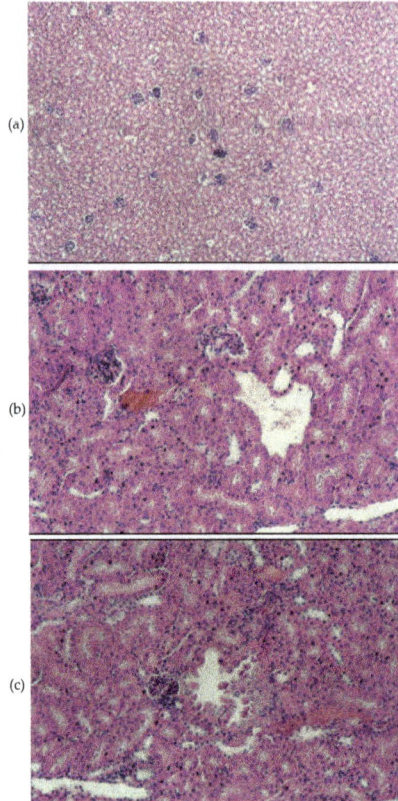

Figure 2. Representative histological section from kidneys of controls where regular pattern of organization is observed (a), and lead and cadmium co-exposure on mice ((b), and (c)). Figures (b), and figure (c) display haemorrhagic focus, and strong dilation of intertubular spaces. Cell detachment is evident. Haematoxylin & eosin staining (HE). Original magnification: Figure (b) – 40x; Figure (c), and 5 – 100x.

The relevance of toxicity of some chromium compounds, namely hexavalent chromium generated by production industries such as leather tanning, and chrome plating, were investigated on mice [68-70]. In these studies Cr(VI), a proved strong carcinogenic, was investigated in vivo in order to evaluate Cr(VI), and Cr(V) reduction effects on the target organs such as testis, liver, and kidneys. For example it was demonstrated that Cr(V), in the form of $[CrV-BT]^{2-}$ is a male reprotoxicant, causing several histological and ultrastructural changes in mice spermatogenesis [68]. One of the most representative lesions was the loss of acrosome sperm integrity, as demonstrated by electron microscopy studies. Adverse effects were also observed on cauda epididymis, namely epithelial vacuolation. Altogether, these lesions confirm the potent toxicity of this compound.

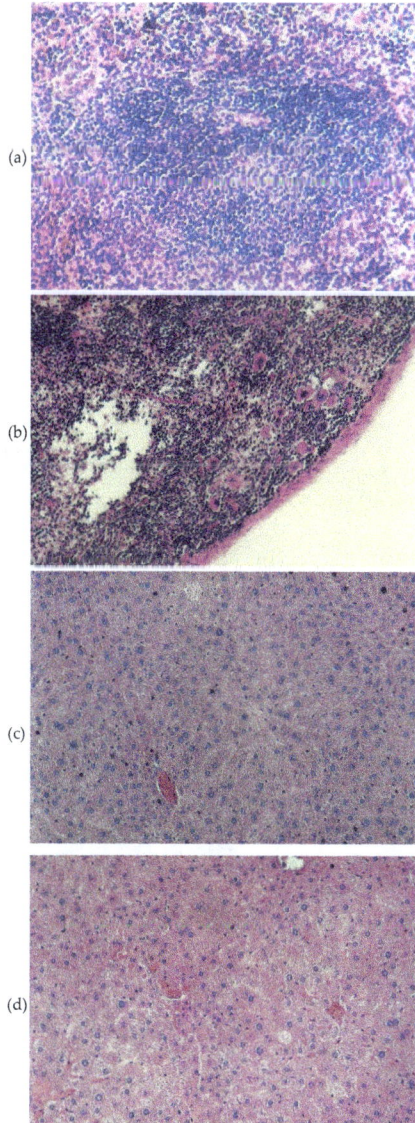

Figure 3. Representative histological sections from spleen, and liver from controls (Figures a,c), and cadmium-lead exposed mice (Figures b,d). A great number of megakaryocytes are evident in spleen (Figure b); WP – White pulp. Several hemorrhagic areas are seen in hepatic parenchyma (Figure d). Original magnification: Figures a-d – 100x; haematoxylin & eosin staining.

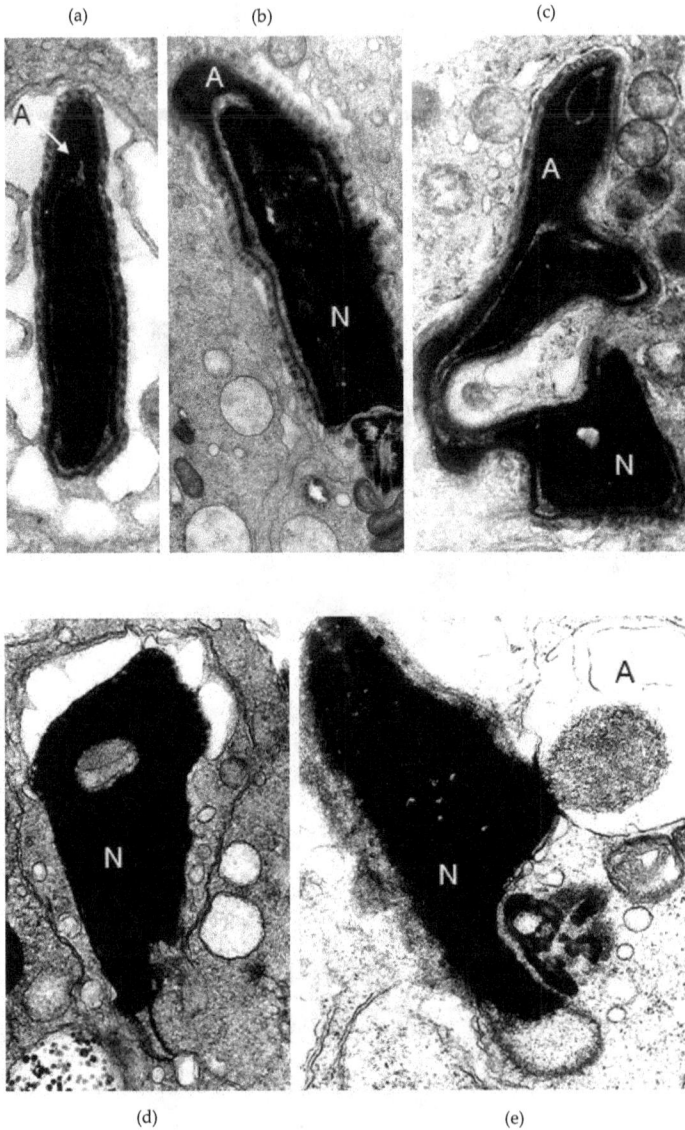

Figure 4. Transmission electron micrographs from spermatozoa and late spermatids in control (a) and sodium arsenite exposed animals during seven days where some morphological irregularities are seen (b-e). N – nucleus; A – acrosome; double staining with uranyl acetate and lead citrate. Original magnification : Figures a -c – x6,700; Figure d – x10,000 ; Figure e – x14,000.

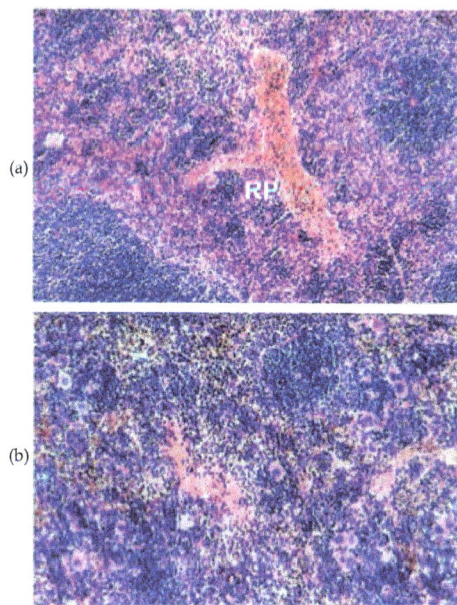

Figure 5. Representative sections of spleen from sodium arsenite dosed group, displaying injury of red pulp (RP) (a), and altered morphology pattern of white pulp (b). Original magnification Figure 5 –x100; haematoxylin & eosin staining.

In a subsequent study the reproductive toxicity on testis and sperm cell's function was evaluated on mice exposed to potassium chromate through a wide range of approaches for a more comprehensive analysis of its effects [70]. Chromium contents on mice testes were determined by inductively coupled plasma mass spectrometry (ICP-MS), and higher levels of chromium were found on K_2CrO_4 exposed group. Histology data of testis were supported by the analysis of testicular cellular subpopulations by flow cytometry. Multiple abnormalities were noted on sperm cells after one cycle of spermatogenic process, such as decreased motility, and percentage of cells with intact acrosome, revealing a premature acrosome reaction. Although no DNA damage on sperm cells assayed by SCSA was observed, altogether those results underlined the reprotoxic effects of hexavalent chromium compounds. Although no histopathological changes on testis or epididymis were noted, a reduction in seminiferous tubules diameter occurred on exposed animals, as determined by software based on deformable models (Snakes) as previously reported [71]. These authors have demonstrated the suitability of this method for evaluation of seminiferous tubules diameter in mice exposed to chromium compounds, one of the relevant parameters for testis damage. Also, the functional properties of Sertoli cells from mice exposed to Cr(V) were investigated using ultrastructural tracer techniques [72]. Horseradish peroxidase added in vitro to the medium was used to follow the route of macromolecules. Seminiferous tubules were then placed into this medium, and the marker penetrated freely on the blood-testis barrier compared to controls, evidencing the toxicity induced by the reduction of Cr(VI) compounds.

Other organs such as kidneys were also affected by hexavalent chromium [69].

Similar approaches were conducted to clarify the nephrotoxicity of chromium copper arsenate (CCA), and its constituents *per se* using mice as models [73-75]. Although this mixture (CCA type C - 34.0% As_2O_5, 47.5% CrO_3 and 18.5% CuO, w/w) was broadly used in the past, as a wood preservative, elevate levels of residues as arsenic still remain in the environment posing a great hazard for public health. For example, CCA, arsenic pentoxide, and chromium trioxide were studied per se on kidneys, based on histopathology, and histochemistry. Correlating histology, and histochemistry with the chromium and arsenic analyses (ICP-MS and GFAAS) on kidney, the synergetic effect of the components (pentavalent arsenic and hexavalent chromium) within the mixture conducted to acute tubular necrosis. The histochemistry assay confirmed the presence of carbohydrate, and proteins filling the tubular lumen; the degeneration of epithelial cells (both in cortex and medulla) was also noted. In addition, higher values of arsenic in CCA-exposed group when noted to those submitted to As_2O_5 one of the components of CCA.

Some of the abovementioned studies based case-by-case underline the contribution of animal research for the understanding of the adverse effects of harmful chemicals on human health.

3. Conclusion and future perspectives

Globally, the field of environmental epidemiology has gained substantial attention in current days due to the adverse effects on human health induced by the myriad of pollutants persisting in air, oceans and freshwater, and agriculture soils. In addition, natural resources which safeguard and support human life are also affected by contaminants. A growing body of research focuses on how the environment can damage human life, through the understanding of toxicity signs in other animal species among different taxa. In this concern, a wide range of biological responses were described (eg. reduction of the population, changes in reproductive pattern, and loss of some species). Surveillance programs have been conducted around the world using key species for contaminants monitoring. These studies showed that accumulation and biomagnification of current hazardous chemicals occurs in many species.

Zooplankton can very well act as bio indicators for probable and possible spread of diseases. Breaking the link between such kind of zooplankton and the hosts will result in non-completion of the life cycle of several such disease causing agents which are threatening the human kind. This will also help in having a healthy world.

Other relevant aspect to report is the overall benefits on human health populations due to regular fish consumption. Trials conducted worldwide based on the nutrients value suggests that fish intake based on policy recommendation lowers the risk of some diseases. Several international regulatory agencies such as the Codex Alimentarius Commission, and European Commission, Council and Parliament and Food and Agriculture Organization/ World Health Organization conventioned maximum limits for numerous contaminants on edible fish.

On the other hand, the accumulation of harmful residues in fish fillets, even below the maximum limit, may alert for future surveillance. A comprehensive risk–benefit evaluation of fish intake is essential and consumption advisories for specific populations such as pregnant women, and children are required.

The last part of this chapter outlines the contribution of laboratory studies using mice for the knowledge of biological mechanisms and toxicity of several hazardous chemicals. The use of laboratory rodents in biomedical research still remains useful to identify potential responses of harmful chemicals under controlled conditions. However, ethics in animal care and procedures must be considered.

The examples mentioned in this chapter highlight that changes occurring in lower levels of biological organization such as copepods, fish, and mammals, added to the environment surrounding affecting humans, may predict, or may alert to potential harmful effects on human health highlighting the role of environmental epidemiology as an emergent discipline. In fact, monitoring health problems within fauna, and health hazards may contribute for searching new solutions, thus improving the quality of live. An integrated monitoring of species from different taxa with trophic relevance permit a more comprehensive outlook of environmental health problems, and is an important step forward to protect wildlife and human health. However, these approaches comparing effects among different species that might occurs in humans as well, needs a special attention in extrapolating result in animals to humans.

In conclusion, this chapter clearly shows that, the contribution of the need for further local, and global multi-and inter-disciplinary research involving critical representative trophic chain species within impacted areas, since they offer important data. The valuable information of human biomonitoring combined with watchfulness on different species and humans sharing the same environment is needed. A continued focus to promote coordination of biobanks, and data harmonisation is encouraged aiming to formulate public health strategies in the future. In addition, new technologies including analytical methods for detection of contaminants, and multiplicity of biomarkers at different biological levels of organization represent decisive advances in this field.

Acknowledgements

This work was funded by the Research Centre on Ceramic and Composite Materials (CICE-CO) from Aveiro University (Portugal). Pest-C/CTM/LA0011/2011- FCT is acknowledged. Thanks to Mr. Aldiro Pereira for preparing photographs. Thanks to Mr. Aldiro Pereira for preparing photographs.

Author details

Maria de Lourdes Pereira[1], Irvathur Krishnananda Pai[2] and Fernando Garcia e Costa[3]

*Address all correspondence to: mlourdespereira@ua.pt

1 Departament of Biology & CICECO, Aveiro University, Aveiro, Portugal

2 Department of Zoology, Goa University, Goa, India

3 Departament of Morphology & Function, CIISA, Faculty of Veterinary Medicine, Technical University of Lisbon, Portugal

References

[1] Smol J.P. A planet in flux. Nature 2012; 483, S12-S15.

[2] Merrill R.M. Introduction to Environmental Epidemiology. In: Environmental Epidemiology: Principles and Methods, Jones & Bartlett Learning; 2008. p3-25.

[3] Kah M, Levy L & Brown C. Potential for effects of land contamination on human health. 1. The case of cadmium. Journal of Toxicology & Environmental Health B Critical Reviews 2012; 15(5), 348-363.

[4] Eisler R. Mercury hazards to living organisms. CRC Press, Boca Raton; 2006.

[5] Mudgal V., Madaan N., Mudgal A., Singh R.B. & Mishra S. Effect of Toxic Metals on Human Health. The Open Nutraceuticals Journal 2010; 3, 94-99.

[6] Jomova K. & Valko M. Advances in metal-induced oxidative stress and human disease. Toxicology 2011; 283, 65–87.

[7] Harmanescu M., Alda L.M., Bordean D.M., Gogoasa I., & Gergen I. Heavy metals health risk assessment for population via consumption of vegetables grown in old mining area; a case study: Banat Country, Romania. Chemistry Central Journal 2011; 5: 64-74.

[8] Huss J. Health hazards of heavy metals and other metals. Council of Europe. Doc. 12613, 12 May 2011. http://assembly.coe.int/Documents/WorkingDocs/Doc11/EDOC12613.pdf (accessed 6 September 2012).

[9] Cooksey C. Health concerns of heavy metals and metalloids. Science Progress 2012; 95(1), 1–16.

[10] Argos M., Ahsan H., Graziano J.H. Arsenic and human health: epidemiologic progress and public health implications. Reviews on Environmental Health 2012. http://www.ncbi.nlm.nih.gov/pubmed/22962196 (accessed 7 September 2012).

[11] Morais S., Costa F.G. & Pereira M.L. Heavy Metals & Human Health. In: Jacques O. (ed.) Environmental Health - Emerging Issues and Practice, 1st Ed.; InTech; 2012a. p227-246.

[12] Morais S., Costa F.G. & Pereira M.L. Thoughts on Evaluation of Heavy Metals Toxicity. In: James C. (ed.) Advances in Chemistry Research 14, Taylor; Nova Science Publishers; Inc. 2012b. https://www.novapublishers.com/catalog/product_info.php? products_id=30588&osCsid= (accessed 2 September 2012).

[13] Environmental Protection Agency. Pesticides and Food: Health Problems Pesticides May Pose. http://www.epa.gov/pesticides/food/risks.htm (accessed 7 September 2012).

[14] Tchounwou P.B. Editorial. International Journal of Environmental Research & Public Health 2010; 7, 2131-2135.

[15] Schulz C., Calafat A.M., Haines D., Becker K.B. & Kolossa-Gehring M. Editorial. International Conference on Human Biomonitoring, Berlin 2010. International Journal of Hygiene & Environmental Health 215; 91– 92.

[16] Meeting report. Human biomonitoring: Political benefits—Scientific challenges. September 26–28, 2010. International Journal of Hygiene & Environmental Health 2012; 215: 247– 252.

[17] van der Schalie W.H., Gardner Jr. H.S., Bantle J.A., De Rosa C.T., Finch R.A., Reif J.S., Reuter R.H., Backer L.C., Burger J., Folmar L.C. & Stokes W.S. Animals as Sentinels of Human Health Hazards of Environmental Chemicals. Environmental Health Perspectives 1999; 107: 309-315.

[18] Reif J.S. Animal sentinels for environmental and public health. Public Health Reports 2011; Supplement 1, 126, 50-57.

[19] Loos M., Schipper A.M., Schlink U., Strebel K. & Ragas Ad.M.J. Receptor-oriented approaches in wildlife and human exposure modelling: a comparative study. Environmental Modelling & Software 2010; 25: 369–382.

[20] Fossi M.C., Casini S., Caliani I., Panti C., Marsili L., Viarengo A., Giangreco R., di Sciara G.N., Serena F., Ouerghi A. & Depledge M.H. The role of large marine vertebrates in the assessment of the quality of pelagic marine ecosystems. Marine Environmental Research 2012; 77, 156-158.

[21] Tanabe S. & Ramu K. Monitoring temporal and spatial trends of legacy and emerging contaminants in marine environment: Results from the environmental specimen bank (es-BANK) of Ehime University, Japan. Marine Pollution Bulletin 2012; 64, 1459–1474.

[22] Costa R.A., Petronilho J. M. S., Soares A. M. V. M. & Vingada J. V. The use of passerine feathers to evaluate heavy metal pollution in Central Portugal. Bulletim of Environmental Contamination & Toxicology 2011; 86, 352–356.

[23] Galante-Oliveira S., Oliveira I., Santos J.A., Pereira M.L., Pacheco M. & Barroso C. Factors affecting RPSI in imposex monitoring studies using Nucella lapillus (L.) as bioindicator. Journal of Environment Monitoring 2010; 12, 1055-1063.

[24] Todd B.D., Bergeron C. M. & Hopkins W.H. Use of toe clips as a nonlethal index of mercury accumulation and maternal transfer in amphibians. Ecotoxicology 2012; 21, 882–887.

[25] Marques S.M., Antunes S.C., Pissarra H., Pereira M.L., Gonçalves F. & Pereira R. Histopathological changes and erythrocytic nuclear abnormalities in Iberian green frogs (Rana perezi Seoane) from a uranium mine pond. Aquatic Toxicology 2009, 91, 187-195.

[26] Bron J.E., Frisch D., Goetze E., Johnson S.C., Lee C.M. & Wyngaard G. A. Observing copepods through a genomic lens. Frontiers in Zoology, 2011; 8:22, 1-15.

[27] Zorita I., Apraiz I., Ortiz-Zarragoitia M., Orbea A., Cancio I., Soto M., Marigómez I. & Cajaraville M.P. Assessment of biological effects of environmental pollution along the NW Mediterranean Sea using mussels as sentinel organisms. Environmental Pollution 2007; 148, 236-250.

[28] Nahrganga J., Brooks S.J., Evenseta A., Camusa L., Jonssona M., Smitha T.J., Lukinaa J., Frantzena M., Giarratano E. & Renauda P.E. Seasonal variation in biomarkers in blue mussel (Mytilus edulis), Icelandic scallop (Chlamys islandica) and Atlantic cod (Gadus morhua) — Implications for environmental monitoring in the Barents Sea. Aquatic Toxicology 2012. http://www.sciencedirect.com/science/article/pii/S0166445X12000227# (accessed 2 September 2012).

[29] Galloway, T.S. Biomarkers in environmental and human health risk assessment. Marine Pollution Bulletin (2006); 53, 606–613.

[30] Battish S.K. Freshwater zooplankton of India. New Delhi, India, Oxford and IBH publishing Co; 1992.

[31] Nair N.B. & Thumpy D.M., A textbook of Marine Ecology, New Delhi, India. The MacMillan Company: 1990.

[32] Humes A. How many copepods? In: F.D. Ferrari & B.P. Bradley (eds.). Ecology and morphology of copepods: proceedings of Fith International Conference on Copepoda, 292/293, London: Springer: 1-7, 1994.

[33] Buskey E.J., Peterson, J.O. & Ambler J.W. The swarming behavior of the copepod Dioithona oculata: In situ and laboratory studies. Limnology and Oceanography 1996; 41: 513-521.

[34] Boxhall, G.A. & Defaye D. Global diversity of copepods (Crustacea: Copepoda) in freshwater. Hydrobiologia 2008; 595 (1): 195–207.

[35] Bron J., Boore J., Boxshall G., Bricknell I., Frisch D., Goetze E., Hansen B., Johnson S., Lee C.E., Lee J., Lenz P., Skern R., Willet C. & Wyngaard G. Copepod Genome Initia-

tive. White Paper for the Development of Large-Scale Genomics Resources for Copepods. World Association of Copepodologists, 2009; July 2nd.1-53.

[36] Piasecki, W.,Goodwin A.E., Eiras J.C. & Nowak B.F. Importance of Copepoda in
Freshwater Aquaculture. Zoological Studies 2004; 43(2): 193-205.

[37] Muthiah, R., Kagen S., Burton, R. S. Copepods: Worldwide Sources of Allergens -
Partial Sequences of Three Unique Proteins. Journal of Allergy & Clinical Immunolo-
gy 2005; 115(2): PS91.

[38] ICES, 2010. Report of the ICES Advisory Committee, ICES Advice 2010; Book 9, pp.
115–123.

[39] Biswas S., Prabhu R.K., Hussain K.J., Selvanayagam M., & Satpathy K.K. Heavy metals concentration in edible fishes from coastal region of Kalpakkam, southeastern
part of India. Environmental Monitoring Assessment 2012; 184, 5097–5104.

[40] Ueno D., Takahashi S., Tanaka H., Subramanian A., Fillman G., Nakat H., Lam
P.K.S., Zheng J., Muchtar M., Prudente M., Chung K.H. & Tanabe S. Global pollution
monitoring of PCBs and organochlorine pesticides using skipjack tuna as a bioindicator. Archives of Environmental Contamination and Toxicology 2003; 45: 378–389.

[41] Ueno D., Kajiwara N., Tanaka H., Subramanian A., Fillmann G., Lam P.K.S., Zheng
G.J., Muchtar M., Razak H., Prudente M., Chung K.H. & Tanabe S. Global pollution
monitoring of polybrominated diphenyl ethers using skipjack tuna as a bioindicator.
Environmental Science & Technology 2004; 38: 2312–2316.

[42] Ueno D., Watanabe M., Subramanian A., Tanaka H., Fillmann G., Lam P.K., Zheng
G.J., Muchtar M., Razak H., Prudente M., Chung, K.H. & Tanabe S. Global pollution
monitoring of polychlorinated dibenzo-p-dioxins (PCDDs), furans (PCDFs) and coplanar polychlorinated biphenyls (coplanar PCBs) using skipjack tuna as bioindicator. Environmental Pollution 2005; 136: 303–313.

[43] Ueno D., Alaee M., Marvin C., Muir D.C., Macinnis G., Reiner E., Crozier P., Furdui
V.I., Subramanian A., Fillmann G., Lam P.K., Zheng G.J., Muchtar M., Razak H., Prudente M., Chung K.H. & Tanabe S. Distribution and transportability of hexabromo-
cyclododecane (HBCD) in the Asia-Pacific region using skipjack tuna as a
bioindicator. Environmental Pollution 2006; 144: 238–247.

[44] Zorita I., Ortiz-Zarragoitia M., Apraiz I., Cancio I., Orbea A., Soto M., Marigómez I.
& Cajaraville M.P. Assessment of biological effects of environmental pollution along
the NW Mediterranean Sea using red mullets as sentinel organisms. Environmental
Pollution 2008; 153 157-168.

[45] Pacheco M., Santos M.A., van Der Gaag M.A., The ecotoxicological relevance of Anguilla anguilla L. as a proposed model for brackish-water genetic toxicological studies. Science of Total Environment 1993; (Suppl.) Part 1: 817–822.

[46] Napierska D., Janina Barsiene J., Mulkiewicz E., Podolska P. & Rybakovas A. Biomarker responses in flounder Platichthys flesus from the Polish coastal area of the Baltic Sea and applications in biomonitoring. Ecotoxicology 2009; 18, 846–859.

[47] Dabrowska H., Ostaszewska T., Kamaszewski M., Antoniak A., Napora-Rutkowski L., Kopko O., Lang T., Fricke N.F., Lehtonen K.K. Histopathological, histomorphometrical, and immunohistochemical biomarkers in flounder (Platichthys flesus) from the southern Baltic Sea. Ecotoxicology and Environmental Safety 2012; 78, 14–21.

[48] Abreu S.N., Pereira E., Vale C. & Duarte A.C. Accumulation of Mercury in Sea Bass from a Contaminated Lagoon (Ria de Aveiro, Portugal). Marine Pollution Bulletin 2000; 40(4), 293-297.

[49] Ahmad I., Pacheco M. & Santos M.A. Anguilla anguilla L. oxidative stress biomarkers: An in situ study of freshwater wetland ecosystem (Pateira de Fermentelos, Portugal). Chemosphere 2006; 65: 952–962.

[50] Santos M.A., Pacheco M. & Ahmad I. Responses of European eel (Anguilla anguilla L.) circulating phagocytes to an in situ closed pulp mill effluent exposure and its association with organ-specific peroxidative damage. Chemosphere 2006; 63, 794–801.

[51] Evrard E., Devaux A., Bony S., Burgeot T., Riso R., Budzinski H., Du M.L., Quiniou L. & Laroche J. Responses of the European "flounder Platichthys flesus to the chemical stress in estuaries: load of contaminants, gene expression, cellular impact and growth rate. Biomarkers, 2010; 15(2): 111–127.

[52] Nogueira P., Pacheco M., Pereira M.L., Mendo S. & Rotchell J.M. Novel potential molecular biomarkers of aquatic contamination in Dicentrarchus labrax and Liza aurata. In: Hamamura N., Suzuki S., Mendo S., Barroso C.M., Iwata H. and Tanabe S. (eds.) Interdisciplinary Studies on Environmental Chemistry — Biological Responses to Contaminants. Terrapub; 2010. p127–138.

[53] Paulo D.V., Fontes F.M. & Flores-Lopes F. Histopathological alterations observed in the liver of Poecilia vivipara (Cyprinodontiformes: Poeciliidae) as a tool for the environmental quality assessment of the Cachoeira River, BA. Brazilian Journal of Biology 2012; 72, 131-140.

[54] Hauser-Davisa R.A., Lima A.A., Ziolli R.L. & Campos R.C. First-time report of metalloproteinases in fish bile and their potential as bioindicators regarding environmental contamination. Aquatic Toxicology 2012; 110-111: 99-106.

[55] Authman M.M.N., Wafa T. Abbas, W.T. & Gaafar A.Y. Metals concentrations in Nile tilapia Oreochromisniloticus (Linnaeus, 1758) from illegal fish farm in Al-Minufiya Province, Egypt, and their effects on some tissues structures. Ecotoxicology & Environmental Safety 2012; 84: 163–172.

[56] Mendil D., Demirci Z., Tuzen M. & Soylak M. Seasonal investigation of trace element contents in commercially valuable fish species from the Black sea, Turkey. Food and Chemical Toxicology 2010; 48: 865–870.

[57] Mieiro C.L., Pacheco M., Pereira M.E. & Duarte A.C. Mercury distribution in key tissues of fish (Liza aurata) inhabiting a contaminated estuary-mplications for human
and ecosystem health risk assessment. Journal of Environmental Monitoring 2009; 11:
1004–1012.

[58] Malik N., Biswas A.K., Qureshi T.A., Borana K. & Virha R. Bioaccumulation of heavy
metals in fish tissues of a freshwater lake of Bhopal. Environmental Monitoring Assessment 2010; 160, 267–276.

[59] Vieira C., Morais S., Ramos S., Delerue-Matos C. & Oliveira M.B.P.P. Mercury, cadmium, lead and arsenic levels in three pelagic fish species from the Atlantic Ocean:
intra- and inter-specific variability and human health risks for consumption. Food &
Chemical Toxicology 2011; 49, 923-932.

[60] Du Z.Y., Zhang J., Wang C., Li L., Man Q., Lundebye A.K. & Frøyland L. Risk–benefit
evaluation of fish from chinese markets: nutrients and contaminants in 24 fish species from five big cities and related assessment for human health. Science of the Total
Environment 2012; 416, 187–199.

[61] Shah A.Q., Kazi T.G., Baig J.A. & Afridi H.I. Correlation between arsenic concentration in fish and human scalp hair of people living in arsenic-contaminated and non-
contaminated areas of pakistan. Biology of Trace Elements Research 2011; 144(1-3):
197-204.

[62] Oliveira H., Loureiro J., Filipe L., Santos C., Ramalho-Santos J., Sousa M. & Pereira
M.L. Flow cytometry evaluation of lead and cadmium effects on mouse spermatogenesis. Reproductive Toxicology 2006a; 22, 529–535.

[63] Oliveira H., Spanò M., Santos C. & Pereira M.L. Lead affects mice sperm motility and
acrosome reaction. Cell Biology & Toxicology 2009; 25, 341–353.

[64] Oliveira H., Lopes T., Almeida T., Pereira M.L. & Santos C. Microsatellite instability
in mice exposed to cadmium. Human & Experimental Toxicology 2012. doi:
10.1177/0960327112445937.

[65] Pereira M.L., Rodrigues N.V. & Garcia e Costa F. Histomorphological evaluation of
mice testis after co-exposure to lead and cadmium. Asian Pacific Journal of Repro-
duction 2012; 1: 35-38.

[66] Ferreira M., Matos R.C., Oliveira H., Nunes B., & Pereira M.L. Impairment of mice
spermatogenesis by sodium arsenite. Human and Experimental Toxicology 2012; 31,
290-302.

[67] Pereira M.L. & Garcia e Costa F. Cytotoxic effects of sodium arsenite on mice sperm
cells: conference proceedings. 10th International Congress on Cell Biology, July 25-28,
2012, Rio Convention & Exhibition Centre, Brazil; 2012.

[68] Pereira M.L., das Neves R.P., Oliveira H., Santos T.M. & de Jesus J.P. Effect of Cr(V)
on reproductive organ morphology and sperm parameters: an experimental study in
mice. Environmental Health 2005; 27, 4-9.

[69] Oliveira H., Santos T.M., Ramalho-Santos J. & Pereira M.L. Histopathological effects of hexavalent chromium in mice kidney. Bulletin of Environmental Contamination and Toxicology 2006b; 76, 977–983.

[70] Oliveira H., Spano M., Guevara M.A., Santos T.M., Santos C. & Pereira M.L. Evaluation of in vivo reproductive toxicity of potassium chromate in male mice. Experimental & Toxicologic Pathology 2010; 62: 391-404.

[71] Guevara M.A., Silva A., Oliveira H., Pereira M.L. & Morgado F. Segmentation and morphometry of histological sections using deformable models: a new tool for evaluating testicular histopathology. In: Sanfeliu A, Shulcloper JR, editors. Progress in pattern recognition, speech and image analysis: Ciarp 2003. Lecture Notes in Computer Science 2003; 2905, 282–290.

[72] Pereira M.L., Santos T.M., Garcia e Costa F. & Pedrosa de Jesus J. Functional Changes of mice Sertoli cells induced by Cr(V). Cell Biology & Toxicology 2004; 20: 285-291.

[73] Matos R.C., Vieira C., Morais S., Pereira M.L. & Pedrosa de Jesus J.P. Nephrotoxicity of CCA-treated wood: a comparative study with As_2O_5 and CrO_3 on mice. Environmental Toxicology & Pharmacology 2009a; 27, 259–263.

[74] Matos R.C., Vieira C., Morais S., Pereira M.L. & Pedrosa de Jesus J.P. Nephrotoxicity effects of the wood preservative chromium copper arsenate on mice: histopathological and quantitative approaches. Journal of Trace Elements in Medicine & Biology 2009b; 23, 224-230.

[75] Matos R.C., Vieira C., Morais S., Pereira M.L. & Pedrosa de Jesus J.P. Toxicity of chromated copper arsenate: A study in mice. Environmental Research 2010; 110, 424-427.

Chapter 4

Pathogen Management in Surface Waters: Practical Considerations for Reducing Public Health Risk

Matthew R. Hipsey and Justin D. Brookes

Additional information is available at the end of the chapter

1. Introduction

Pathogen contamination of water systems is a major public health challenge in both developing and developed countries across the globe [1-9]. The pathogens of concern to human health vary between aquatic systems depending on the nature of the pathogen source and the intended use of the water. Due to their persistence in the environment and resistance to conventional treatment technologies, the (oo)cysts of the protozoan organisms *Cryptosporidium* spp. and *Giardia* spp. are a typical concern in water bodies used for drinking water [10-11]. In poorly treated drinking water storages and recreational waters (both fresh and marine), other problem organisms include bacteria such as *Salmonella* spp., *Shigella* spp., *Vibrio* spp. *Clostridium* spp. and *Staphylococcus aureus,* and numerous human enteric viruses such as those from the genera *Enterovirus*, *Hepatovirus*, *Rotavirus* and *Norovirus* [12-13]. Accordingly, the nature of disease caused by these organisms is also widely variable (Table 1).

Most concern is given to allochthonous enteric microorganisms, those that enter surface waters via external loading. However, depending on the environmental context, some autochthonous pathogens, those that develop internally, may also be important (*e.g. Vibrio cholerae*). The allochthonous sources typically occur when heavy rains wash infected material from surrounding agricultural and/or urban catchments into the runoff waters that ultimately supply the waterbody, or when effluent is discharged directly into watercourses (Figure 1). Inputs to lakes and rivers from recreational users can also lead to a significant increase in pathogen concentrations [14]. These major pathogen sources present a risk to humans through three main routes of exposure: direct consumption of microorganisms within drinking water, recreational contact, and consumption of microorganisms that have bio-accumulated within the tissues of consumable shellfish (Figure 2).

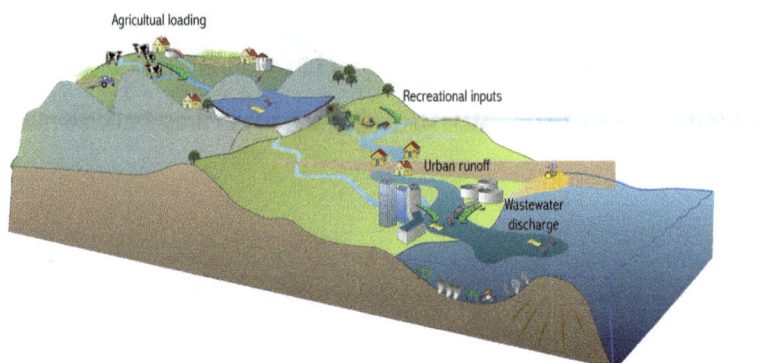

Figure 1. Schematic overview of allochthonous microbial sources and receiving aquatic environments from the catchment to the ocean.

Disease	Agent	Symptoms
Amebiasis	Protozoan (*Entamoeba histolytic*)	Abdominal pain, fatigue, weight loss, diarrhoea
Campylobacteriosis	Bacterium (*Campylobacter jejuni*)	Fever, Abdominal pain, fatigue, diarrhoea
Cholera	Bacterium (*Vibrio cholerae*)	Fever, Abdominal pain, vomiting, diarrhoea
Cryptosporidiosis	Protozoan (*Cryptosporidium parvum*)	Abdominal pain, vomiting, diarrhoea
Diarrhoeagenic *Escherichia coli*	Bacterium (*Escherichia coli* O157:H7)	Acute bloody diarrhoea, abdominal cramps
Giardiasis	Protozoan (*Giardia lamblia*)	Abdominal pain, vomiting, diarrhoea
Hepatitis	Virus (Hepatitis A)	Fever, chills, abdominal pain, jaundice
Salmonellosis	Bacterium (*Salmonella* sp.)	Fever, abdominal cramps, bloody diarrhoea
Shigellosis	Bacterium (*Shigella* sp.	Fever, diarrhoea, bloody stools
Viral Gastroenteritis	Virus (rotavirus etc.)	Vomiting, diarrhoea, headache, fever

Table 1. Summary of common water-borne diseases.

Pathogen distribution and transport in surface waters is a function of the pathogen load in the source water (*e.g.* agricultural runoff or direct wastewater discharge), the settling or entrainment characteristics of the particles that they may attach to, and resuspension from sediment-associated organisms by turbulence at the benthic boundary layer. The distribution of organisms will also be impacted by predation [15] and degradation due to sunlight exposure, or mortality due to undesirable physico-chemical conditions [16]. For some organisms, in situ growth may also need to be considered.

Contamination of rivers, lakes and reservoirs that are primarily used for drinking water is a particular challenge for environmental scientists and water managers charged with supplying water that minimises the risk of infection to downstream consumers. The nature of the contamination and the mechanisms that control contaminant dynamics may vary considerably due to either site-specific or contaminant-specific properties and hence there is a need to better understand how to assess and mitigate the risks.

As indicated above, microbial contaminants such as the (oo)cysts of the pathogens *Crytpo-sporidium* or *Giardia*, are mainly derived from allochthonous (external) sources, whereas others may be generated autochthonously (internally) within the water storage. It is therefore not surprising that a fundamental principle of drinking water supply is to use high quality, protected source waters as a means of reducing the potential load of drinking water contaminants and thus reducing treatment costs and subsequent health risks to consumers. In reference [17], it was reported that the mean concentration of *Cryptosporidium* oocysts in protected reservoirs (0.52/100L) and pristine lakes (0.3 – 9.3/100L) was considerably lower compared to polluted rivers (43 – 60/100L) and polluted lakes (58/100L), which demonstrates the merit of this strategy. However, with increasing pressures on catchments, aquatic systems are not always sufficiently protected and pathogen risks must therefore be appropriately managed. In developing countries this is further confounded since both drinking and recreational waters may be subject to substantial direct and unregulated effluent discharges that are difficult to control at the source.

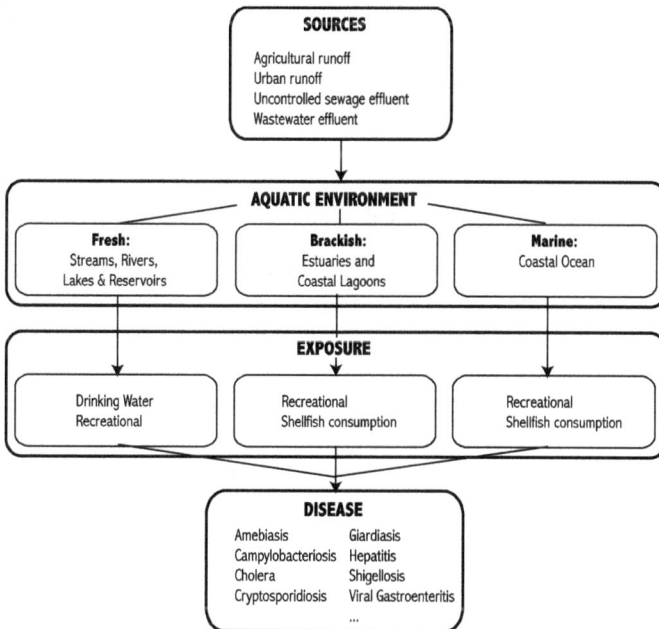

Figure 2. Conceptual breakdown of routes of exposure of microbial pollutants.

When planning management measures or policies it is important to consider that the presence or absence of pathogens within the aquatic environment does not always translate directly to a high risk to human health. For example, *Cryptosporidium* and *Giardia* (oo)cysts have been identified at hazardous levels in Lake Kinneret, which has historically supplied around half of Israel's water, however no major outbreaks were reported in Israel during an equivalent period [5]. Conversely, outbreaks of cryptosporidiosis have been documented where the water met guidelines based on standard bacterial indicator concentrations [3-4]. It must therefore be recognized that contaminant data and risk assessment procedures need to consider the wider management framework that encompasses the entire system, from source to exposure. To obtain a more realistic assessment of the overall contaminant risk it is necessary to understand the critical variables controlling contaminant fate and distribution once they enter the aquatic environment.

Allen *et al.* [18] went further, and described pathogen monitoring alone as being of little value and highlighted several cases where monitoring had misled regulatory authorities as to the actual risk, including both false positives and false negatives. They highlight several technical and administrative barriers why this is the case, and instead suggest that the human and financial resources would be better invested in enhancing treatment processes and gaining a better understanding of the system (such as the major pathogen sources and sinks, and inactivation processes). Within a drinking water system this is fairly clear since there are many points at which the quality of the source water can be controlled before the public is ultimately exposed, but for other environmental waters there is only limited ability for intervention. However, aquatic systems have an inherent natural assimilative capacity and, there are a number of beneficial water quality changes that can occur when water is stored in reservoirs, which may ultimately attenuate pathogen concentrations [16,19]. Reduced water movement increases the rate of sedimentation of particulate material. This reduces turbidity and may also result in the sequestering of the microbes associated with the particles. Many of the pathogens of concern are attenuated by environmental conditions with mortality linked to temperature, grazing by protozoa, and incident ultra violet radiation being the most critical factors. Of particular importance is having a good knowledge of the hydrodynamic processes that control water transport in the aquatic environment as this will ultimately determine the length of time the water is retained and the environmental conditions that it will be subjected to. In reservoirs, issues such as the thermal stratification and the short-circuiting of inflows have been identified as being significantly important [20].

The question then becomes whether or not it is possible to optimise the performance of aquatic systems as barriers to pathogen transmission by manipulating river or reservoir conditions. The climatic and hydrological conditions that lead to the development of a specific contamination threat are highly diverse and it is necessary to have a clear understanding of the origin and dynamics of the potential contaminants in relation to environmental conditions in order to understand the most appropriate control methodologies to implement of the range that are available. Further, it is often the case where multiple contaminants occur within a single storage or system, and the optimum solution for minimising risk is a compromise between minimising exposure to individual contaminants and may involve implementation of several management options. As a result it is necessary to manage the associated risks through development of a suitable risk management framework. To address the complexities and variability inherent in pathogen transmission requires a detailed quantitative understanding of contaminant fate and distribution through surface water systems, yet this is rarely achieved in practice and there is a need for improved assessment and mitigation of pathogen threats.

The aim of this chapter is to describe how to best gather specific information to support structured risk assessment programs for dealing with pathogen distribution in surface water systems. With this knowledge we summarise several control measures and discuss how they may be implemented within a structured framework to minimise the risk of contamination to humans. It is important to understand the key dynamics of contaminants, as described next, to provide the necessary context for the risk management framework and control measures.

2. Controls on fate and transport of microbial contaminants

Hydrodynamic controls on pathogen distribution: Hydrodynamics are a key driver in shaping distribution of pathogens in aquatic systems [21] and determine the horizontal transport, rates of dispersion and dilution, and their vertical distribution. In lakes and reservoirs horizontal transport is predominantly driven by basin-scale circulation patterns including wind-driven currents, inflows and basin-scale internal waves [22]. Although wind-driven currents only influence the surface layer, inflows can occur at any depth in a stratified water column [23], and internal waves can generate significant internal currents that may act in different directions at different depths. In stratified lakes and reservoirs, internal waves have been shown to be responsible for the vertical advection of pathogens past offtake structures resulting in periodic variations in water quality [24].

Dispersion describes both the turbulent dispersion (for example in the surface mixed layer) and shear dispersion due to the presence of a horizontal or vertical velocity shear, (*e.g.* rivers or in tidally forced systems). In river-floodplain systems sharp velocity gradients between the floodplain and main river cause substantial horizontal dispersion and mixing.

Since the source of most pathogens to reservoirs is via catchment inflows or engineered outfalls, the behaviour of inflowing water as they enter the water column is of particular importance. Inflow dynamics are controlled by their density and momentum relative to that of the ambient water. For example, warm inflows will flow over the surface as a buoyant surface flow, and cold dense inflows will sink beneath the ambient water where they will flow along the bottom towards the deepest point. In either case, as it propagates the gravity current will entrain ambient water, increasing its volume, changing its density and diluting the concentration of pathogens and other properties. A further complication is introduced where the density difference is derived from particulate matter (turbidity current), in which case the settling of these particles will influence the density and propagation of the inflow [25]. The speed at which the inflowing water travels, its entrainment of ambient water and resulting dilution of its properties, and its insertion depth are all of critical importance in determining the hydrodynamic distribution of pathogens. Prediction therefore requires a detailed numerical solution, often in three dimensions, which can resolve processes controlling momentum, mixing, and thermodynamics.

Kinetics: As particles are advected and mixed throughout a waterbody they are also subject to 'non-conservative' behaviour, *i.e.* growth or decay. Organisms become inactivated as they are exposed to the range of biotic and abiotic pressures that face them within the aquatic environment. In particular, organisms are known to be sensitive to temperature, salinity, pH, oxygen, turbidity, sunlight, and they are also subject to predation by larger autochthonous microorganisms [15]. Some bacteria may also be able to support growth through assimilation of nutrients from the water [26-30].

Sedimentation & association with particles: The settling rate of free-floating organisms is relatively small [31]. Association with inorganic and organic aquatic particles however can considerably increase the losses due to sedimentation, with particle settling being affected by their size and density according to Stoke's law [32-33]. Pathogens may be associated with particles via adsorption at the surface, or they may be physically enmeshed within the organic matrix of faecal material. Differences in dynamic aggregation rates between different organism classes (*i.e.* protozoan, bacterial, viral) are thought to be an important determinant when deciding the applicability of surrogates [21].

Resuspension: Since pathogens may remain viable for significant periods in aquatic sediments [34-36], the resuspension and subsequent re-distribution of pathogens and indicator organisms can potentially be an important process. Sediment resuspension occurs when the shear stress due to currents and turbulent velocity fluctuations reaches a critical level. In rivers and estuaries, large currents are capable of generating significant critical bed-shear that exceeds the critical level regularly. In lakes and stratified environments such high velocities are reached less frequently, but can be caused by large underflow events and by basin-scale internal waves motions, for example after a period of significant wind forcing. Turbulent motions within the benthic boundary layer driven by currents and internal wave breaking [37] result in the resuspension of particulate material [38]. In environments with an active surface wave field such as the coastal ocean and estuarine environments, then oscillatory currents due to wind-wave action will also be important in periodically redistributing pathogen-laden sediments near coastal cities [39-40].

3. Hazard analysis and risk assessment framework

In drinking supply reservoirs the major contaminant risks not only originate from the introduction of pathogens, but also from the release of dissolved iron and manganese from sediment, growth of cyanobacteria and subsequent release of associated toxins, and from natural organic matter (NOM) reaction with the chlorine used for treatment. Risk management of pathogens therefore cannot be considered in isolation. The timescale over which these hazards generate varies from days to weeks, or even months. Problems associated with iron, manganese and cyanobacteria typically develop with the evolution of thermal stratification. It may take a number of days or weeks for cyanobacteria to grow to concentrations that may cause a taste and odour or toxin problem. Problematic concentrations of iron and manganese develop under anoxic conditions from long periods of stratification typically ranging from weeks to months. On the other hand, the greatest risk of transport of pathogens from catchment to the treatment plant is after significant inflow events, which may present a water quality issue within the timescale of hours to days depending upon the reservoir size and flow magnitude. Similarly the highest loading of NOM and turbidity occurs during inflow events.

In addition to the variable time scales that must be considered when deciding control measures and developing a risk management framework, the potential for large spatial heterogeneity must also be considered. In long, drowned-valley reservoirs, the concentration of a contaminant introduced from upstream may pass through a long reach of standing water and be progressively attenuated prior to reaching the offtake location(s), depending on the hydrodynamics and stratification at the time of the event. If the shape of the supply is more circular then circulation patterns may be more complex and considerable variability and patchiness may develop and influence the observed trends. For cyanobacteria and metal contaminants, the dynamics are strongly governed by vertical gradients in temperature and other physicochemical properties that will vary based on meteorological conditions.

In many cases there maybe coinciding water quality issues that pose different risks and require the implementation of control measures that minimize exposure to one threat but which may actually increase exposure to another. For example, in a single reservoir, cyanobacterial toxins may exist in the surface, pathogens within an inflow intrusion at mid-depth, and anoxia and soluble metals in the deepest regions. In such instances care must be taken to ensure the management strategies that are implemented are well founded and the individual risks are well quantified. In these more complicated situations cost-benefit analyses may help guide the most appropriate action and help assess the relative benefits for public health, also set within context of reducing treatment costs at the downstream treatment facility.

Informed management not only requires knowledge on the spatial distribution, but also the temporal variability of threats. As the threat changes, so may the most suitable control measure, and it is therefore logical that any management framework that is implemented is adaptable and able to respond to changes in risk. To be effective in this regard, monitoring must also be flexible and reflect the nature of the risk at any given time [41].

Catchment-reservoir systems are complex and it is important to note that given the high variability in these systems one can never reduce all risk(s) to zero, however by strategic identification of potential problems, one can mitigate risk with knowledge of some basic hydrodynamics, the evolution of hazards, and careful monitoring. In drinking water supplies that are deemed critical and face multiple pressures, more sophisticated options such as real-time management systems are emerging to assist with the assessment of risks and the ongoing monitoring of the implemented control measures.

Successful risk management of water supply reservoirs and recreational waters requires a systematic approach to contaminant monitoring and prediction in order to reduce the risk of exposure to the public. This is best achieved through a quantitative understanding of the critical processes involved in contaminant distribution and transport, such as dilution rates and time scales for inactivation or contaminant decay. Such information would enable water managers to quantify the risk to water quality associated with a contaminant threat in source water, revise monitoring protocols to detect the organisms or chemicals of concern, and to manage water treatment or recreational closures proactively based upon detected or, ideally, modelled (anticipated) risk. Due to their flexibility, such 'adaptive' management strategies are more effective than their rigid counterparts [42], yet they are rarely adopted due to numerous uncertainties in our understanding and due to poor numerical model predictions.

The critical fist step in developing an adaptive management strategy for water supply is identifying the hazards of concern, articulating the hydrodynamic and biogeochemical conditions that lead to the development of the hazard and understand how these are influenced by the prevailing meteorology and hydrology (Figure 3). Within a drinking water supply reservoir the important processes can be summarised as loads entering the reservoir; transport, growth or attenuation with the reservoir and the distribution of the hazard relative to the offtake (Figure 3). Each of the parameters contributing to risk can be monitored and the processes measured and modelled.

4. Management framework

Routine monitoring and targeted measurement of the major processes systematically builds up a bank of knowledge to support reservoir management and detect and mitigate risks in a timely fashion. The aim is to measure the processes and hazards identified in Figure 3 which contributes to knowledge of the system (Figure 4).

System knowledge can be used to inform on catchment hydrology and contaminant loads, reservoir behaviour and can help focus the monitoring effort on the key variables. Monitoring for those variables will vary depending upon the timescales for which different hazards present, the cost associated with monitoring and the ease at which the parameter can be monitored. Typically these fall with three classes; routine monitoring for analytes that are sampled and then measured within a laboratory, online monitoring where sensors are deployed in the reservoir and log key parameters at relatively short time intervals (typically 10 min) and ad hoc monitoring in response to an event, such as a rain event inflow.

This monitoring serves two purposes; it allows for detection of the hazard so the appropriate risk assessment can be undertaken, and it also allows the managers to draw correlations between when the hazard is present and the reservoir and catchment conditions at the time. Upon detection of the hazard the situation needs to be assessed with respect to what risk it poses to water quality. This stage of the management framework can draw upon expert knowledge, specific process understanding derived from online monitoring and simulation of the event with hydrodynamic models. Armed with this knowledge and a prediction about the severity of the event, decisions on the operational response can be made. Points of control include attenuation of inflows in engineered wetlands and biofilters, alteration of the inflow dynamics, in reservoir treatment or manipulation of the offtake depth to select the best quality water to send to the treatment plant.

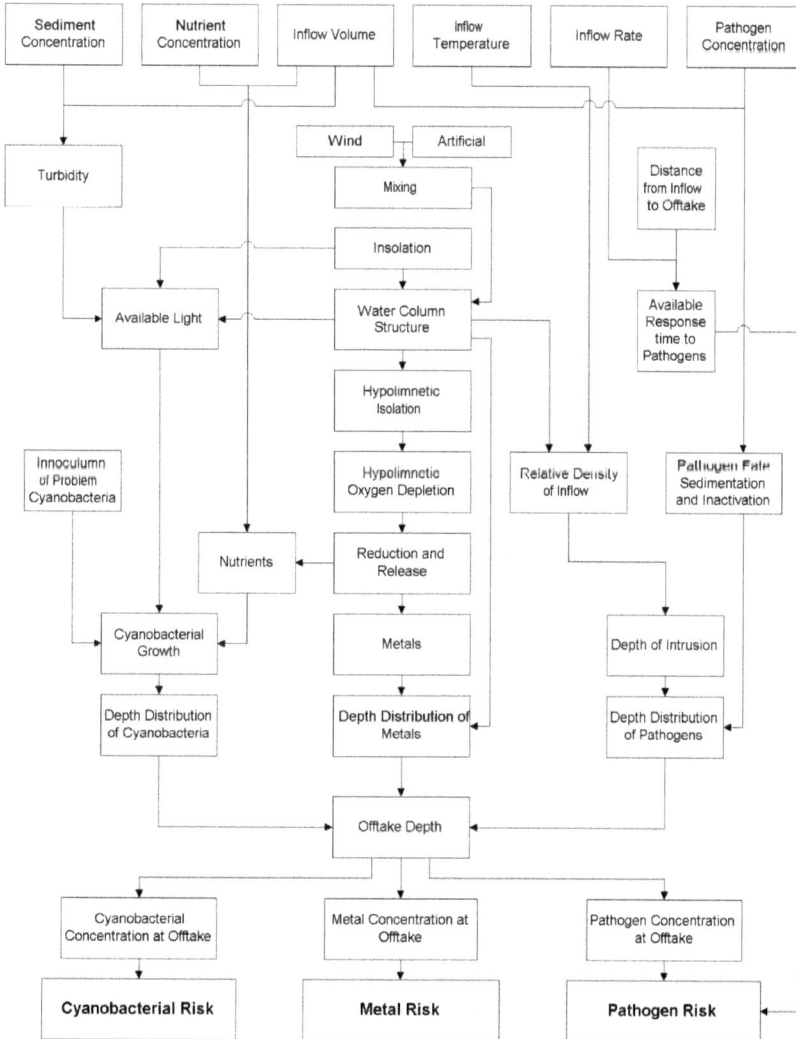

Figure 3. Conceptual model of the major hazards challenging drinking water supplies and their links to meteorology, hydrodynamics and biogeochemistry.

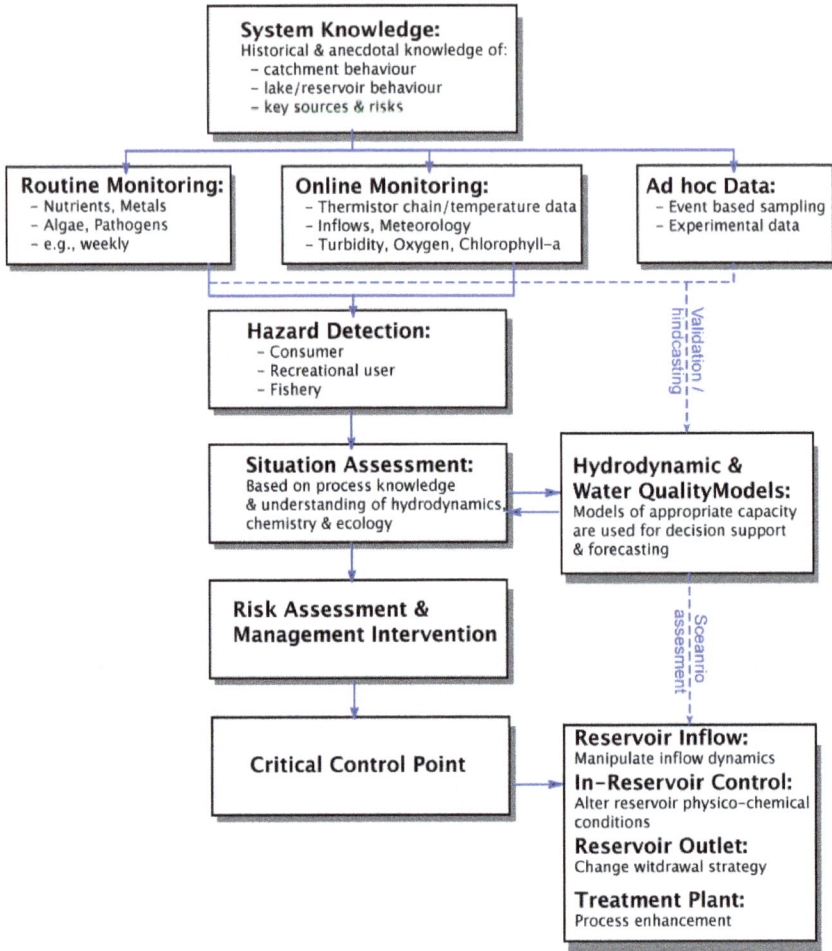

Figure 4. Management framework for assessing and responding to health threats to drinking water sources (modified from [20]).

5. Gathering information for risk assessment

The above risk assessment framework is built around suitable streams of information that are used to inform decision making and guide mitigative measures. There are numerous types of information that contribute to the understanding of an aquatic system, ranging from static information that characterises the domain, to routinely collected water quality samples and real-time sensors, through to strategically collected data related to a particular threat. In addition to general environmental or direct microbial data measurements, microbial surrogates (or bio-indicators) also have an important place in risk assessments. The application of hydrodynamic and water quality models have also significantly increased in recent years to supplement direct measurements. The hydrodynamic models are now well developed and tested and there are now numerous published models of pathogen dynamics in aquatic systems. These various information sources are discussed in this section.

5.1. System characterisation and baseline monitoring

Catchment: In most cases, the quality of water and public health risks that may exist within a lake, river or reservoir used for drinking water will reflect land-use practices and their distribution within the surrounding catchment. Any risk determination or control measure assessment must therefore give careful consideration to the nature of the activities within the catchment and identify key sources of contaminants or contaminant precursors and whether they are point-source or diffuse in nature. This analysis need not be complex and may simply involve plotting topography, land-use type, vegetation and soil type within a Geographical Information System (GIS), and assessing them within the context of the stream and drainage network and proximity to the water supply. The distribution of land-use activities that provide large quantities of contaminants will vary widely depending on the site-specific catchment properties and it is therefore not possible to generalise risk profiles with certain land-use activities. Using the case of *Cryptosporidium* within areas used for dairying as an example, animal husbandry practices vary from farm to farm, and how these activities are managed relative to the stream will largely determine the downstream pathogen numbers. Nonetheless it is useful information to have to help identify potential contaminant 'hot-spots'. Areas of urbanisation are generally major sources of diffuse inputs and easily identifiable.

Other attributes that should not be overlooked included catchment vegetation distribution, since this influences contaminant attenuation, runoff quality and concentrations of natural organic matter and suspended material. More specific indicators such as riparian integrity can also be considered as it is well documented that this correlates with turbidity [43] and pathogen attenuation [44-45]. When considering catchment properties that may contribute to downstream contaminant loading, it is important to not only look for potential sources of contaminants, but also to search for opportunities to implement management measures. Preventing contaminant loading by reducing the source may in fact be the most cost-effective and sustainable solution rather than purely relying on engineering interventions or avoidance procedures in downstream locations [42].

Rivers & Reservoirs: For most situations it is critical to understand the nature of inflows entering a river reach, lake or reservoir. They are of direct relevance from a health point of view as they are the mechanism for seeding downstream water bodies with pathogens washed from the catchment. The relationship between flow and pathogens is well established and different phases of the hydrograph may be identified from a risk perspective [46]. For example, the first-flush concept highlights that risk is concentrated around times of large rainfall events and is therefore linked with the stochastic nature of climatic drivers for the location of interest. As pathogen concentrations vary with flow stage, so to do factors such as suspended particles, dissolved organic carbon and other variables such as predatory microorganisms. Highly turbid water is effective at attaching bacteria and viruses [33], but may be ineffective at removing protozoan (oo)cysts. Dissolved organic carbon is also critical in attenuating UV light, which is an important mechanism for inducing mortality in a range of microbial organisms.

In addition to the river flow rate measurement (or stage-height should a suitable height-flow rating relationship exist), it is essential to regularly measure the temperature and salinity (or electrical conductivity) of the inflow for characterisation of its density for later comparison with the stratification profile present at downstream stations. Depending on the nature of the site, the characteristic concentration of suspended particles in the inflow water may also be insightful since highly turbid waters not only influence sedimentation, but also can impact the density and ultimate fate of the inflow water [25]. This may be easily measured using an optical turbidity probe, or ideally an *in situ* particle analysis instrument (e.g., [47]). Developing a relationship between the particle size distribution and the optical turbidity signal is also able to provide further information about the dynamics of suspended sediment [25].

In stratified water bodies such as estuaries and deep lakes or reservoirs, the fate of inflowing water is largely determined by the stratification profile and the domain morphology. The vertical structure of density, and how it varies seasonally, will ultimately determine whether the inflow water will flow along the surface, along the bottom thalweg of the site, or at some level in between (Figure 5). It will also control the travel time, and level of entrainment that the inflow water experiences within the ambient water profile. The environmental conditions the pathogens experience will also vary accordingly and this may impact on the ability of the site to attenuate pathogens successfully or otherwise [23]. To best understand the vertical structure it is essential to have vertically resolved information of temperature (and salinity where relevant), and ideally a thermistor chain with a surface meteorological station to understand the dynamics of wind mixing and surface heat fluxes.

The information detailed above permits the development a clear picture of how the system is interfacing with the surrounding catchment and the key controls on transport processes. This can be improved by collection of water quality samples that provide specific information on microbiological concentrations in the water. They should generally be collected upstream and at various locations along the waterbody. Given that they are more resource intensive (both cost and time) than typical environmental measurements, it is essential they are targeted to specific points of concern and the monitoring program should be designed within the context of the transport dynamics.

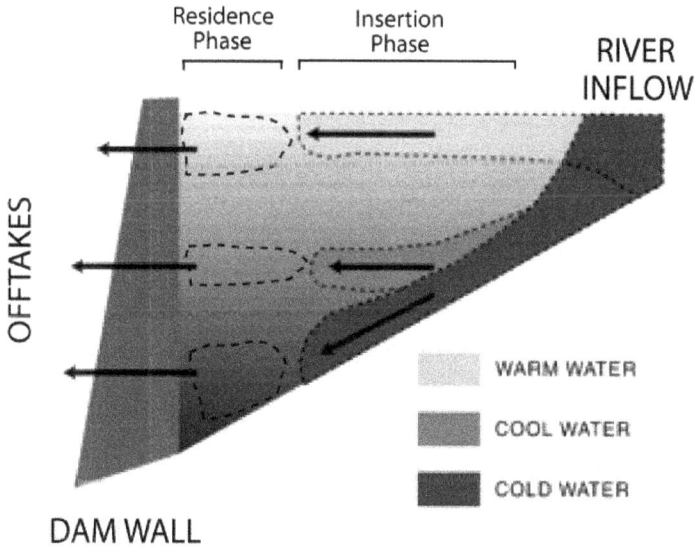

Figure 5. Schematic of inflow scenarios that may be observed entering a lake or reservoir, illustrating the surface overflow, interflow and underflow.

5.2. Real-time sensors

Often *ad hoc* monitoring, such as that described above, will miss 'events' that occur at a frequency below the monitoring interval unless they are specifically programmed to coincide with the event. Generally, the timescales of horizontal transport in rivers and lakes during flood events are significantly less than the routinely implemented monitoring frequencies. Remotely deployable sensors are therefore attractive to supplement other sources of information. Logistical challenges may also make deployable sensors better value as they save travel and manpower expenses, although maintenance and regular calibration is essential for these to be reliable and useful.

Instrumentation used to collect *in situ* data are available from numerous sources. Real-time sensors for meteorology, temperature, conductivity, turbidity and chlorophyll-a are commercially available from numerous vendors to provide high temporal resolution data, which in many cases, may be transmitted automatically to managers via telemetry. Such instrumentation is already being used widely across the globe to support decision-making activities. Advances in sensor technology continue and sensors are now available for examining *in situ* concentrations for nutrients, metals and other contaminants although they are yet to be widely adopted. As these become more widely available, practitioners will be able to take advantage of high-resolution time-series of many physical and chemical constituents. Even without the implementation of more advanced sensors, real-time information of core environmental properties (temperature, salinity, oxygen and turbidity) can provide considerable insight into the dynamics that will ultimately control pathogen fate and transport.

5.3. Strategic data collection

Strategic sampling may be undertaken to improve process understanding about the dynamics of the system. For example, routine sampling may not be able to provide sufficient information on hydrodynamic or biogeochemical processes at a scale required to truly assess the risk of a threat developing. Commonly, site-specific experimental data is collected to supplement other information on items such as the particle size distribution of suspended sediment, fine to medium scale horizontal and vertical mixing processes, and important ecological processes.

It is often the case that routine monitoring programs do not accurately portray the actual risk and strategic data can help to build knowledge about a system and improve the management practices. As an example, the reservoir shown in Figure 5 would typically be monitored by the managing water utility by collecting microbial samples at the inflow and at the surface near the centre of the basin. Although noticeable inflow concentrations would be recorded, surface grab samples from the main body of lake would be near the minimum level of detection, and it would therefore be assumed the reservoir had sufficiently attenuated the inflowing load. Experimentation of pathogen transport by [21] has showed that in fact in the case the reservoir may have attenuated little of the incoming load, and that significant concentrations existed below the surface layer [48]. Furthermore, most microbial monitoring programs are based on regular, often weekly, sampling. Although this is a good idea, and is acceptable for the case where there is a constant pollution source, for lakes and reservoirs fed by rivers, the highest risk is from large runoff events. It is therefore also recommended that event based monitoring be implemented. Even for large reservoirs that have considerable residence times, it can take just a few days for contaminated inflow water to reach the extraction point (e.g., [20,23,49]).

Often models (discussed below) can be used to assist in the design of an effective and targeted monitoring programme that reflects the dynamics of the system and can more accurately portray the risk. Sophisticated monitoring programmes also include capacity to logically adapt the monitoring regime as a particular threat is observed to develop. This approach acknowledges that we are more interested in the spatial and temporal variability in the contaminant of concern as the probability of exposure increases, and accordingly the monitoring effort intensifies to ensure the actual risk is being portrayed accurately.

5.4. Surrogate measurements for indicating threats to health

Often it is not possible or practical to directly detect the presence of a certain contaminant within a water body and so surrogates or other indirect indicators of the dynamics may be defined. In particular, the complexity, cost and time constraints associated with the direct enumeration of pathogens to identify their distribution in large water bodies, frequently limits the ability of water managers to detect the intrusion of poorer quality water inflows into the aquatic environment. As a result, there is considerable discussion in regulatory organizations and water utilities as to the value of using surrogates, such as microbial indicator organisms or even physical properties such as turbidity, as a way of detecting the presence of microbial contamination and hence the threat of actual pathogenic organisms. Microbial indicators have the advantage of being low-risk, present in high concentrations relative to other organisms of concern and simple and cheap to enumerate.

The most widely used indicator organisms of microbial pollution are the enteric coliform bacteria, which are gram-negative bacilli that belong to the family *Enterobacteriaceae* (*e.g. Klebsiella* spp., *Enterobacter* spp. *Citrobacter* spp., *Escherichia coli*). Specific coliform measurements include total coliforms, faecal coliforms, and in particular the specific organism *E. coli* [50]. The latter two are the most common since they are abundant in the faeces of humans and other warm blooded animals, and are hence thought to be a reliable indicator of faecal pollution. Total coliforms are used less frequently since they include organisms from soil and cold-blooded animals. Except for certain strains of pathogenic *E. coli* (*e.g.* O157), coliform bacteria are not a threat to human health, but their high abundance means that they are easy to detect, thereby alerting regulatory authorities to pollution events that may contain other organisms of concern. Other routinely used indicator bacteria include the gram-positive cocci, including Enterococci and faecal streptococci. However, it is now apparent that these bacterial indicators are not suitable for assessing the risk posed by protozoan pathogens and some enteric viruses [21,51-52].

Various bacteriophages are used as index organisms for enteric viruses [53-56]. The single-stranded F-specific RNA (F$^+$ RNA) bacteriophages (*e.g.* strains *MS-2*, *F2* and *Q beta*) and the double-stranded somatic coliphages (*e.g.* strains *T$_2$*, *T$_7$* and *ϕX174*) are routinely measured in fresh and coastal waters. However, faecal bacteriophages are not always suitable index organisms since they are present in a range of animal as well as human faeces, whereas human enteric viruses only originate from human faeces. There have also been reports of human enteric viruses being detected in waters in the absence of bacteriophages [57]. The rationale for their use as model organisms is based on their similar size and morphology, along with the low cost, ease and speed of detection compared to human enteric virus assays. The ideal host bacteria would be of human faecal origin only, consistently present in sewage in sufficient numbers for detection, and only lysed by phages that do not replicate in another host or the environment. While bacteriophages to *Bacteroides fragilis* strain HSB40 appear to be human specific and do not replicate in the environment [58], their phage numbers are too low for general use. Due to their high abundance, studies have focused on the coliphage systems, including the double and single-stranded DNA and RNA-containing phages listed above, and for a range of bacterial hosts. The F$^+$ RNA coliphages attach to the sides of the bacterial pili that only occur on exponentially growing specific (F$^+$) strains of *E. coli* or an engineered *Salmonella typhimurium* (strain WG49), and are therefore the current models of choice [53,57].

The use of spores of the gram-positive bacilli *Clostridium perfringens* has been suggested as a good indicator of human faecal contamination and may correlate with human parasitic protozoa and enteric viruses [21,58-59]. However, two confounding factors must be considered; first, *C. perfringens* spores are very persistent [35] and second, they may be excreted by various animals [60]. Hence, they may show little relationship with parasitic protozoa in animal-impacted raw waters, and could be misleading about the likely presence of infective human viruses.

Particle counting and turbidity levels have also been identified as potential surrogates of microbial pollution and weak epidemiological evidence exists that suggests waterborne illness from drinking water may be associated with the raw water turbidity [61]. The use of turbidity alone to predict pathogen presence is difficult because turbidity is dependent on a range of processes that are independent of pathogen presence. For example, it is well established that many young calves are infected with *Cryptosporidium* [62], however, calving is timed to coincide with the period when feed is abundant and cows are on a rising plane of nutrition. Consequently, calving and high oocyst numbers occur when catchments are well vegetated, yet this is typically when turbidity is low. Additionally, surrogates such as turbidity are influenced by catchment specific factors such as soil-type distribution and non-grazing land-use such as horticulture that do not correlate with pathogen input. In shallow systems, turbidity may be caused through resuspension of sediment during high wind events or strong currents, and therefore may exist unrelated to any catchment or wastewater discharges. Nonetheless, turbidity is a readily measurable parameter that warrants investigation as a potential early warning mechanism of increased risk.

While no single water quality indicator can reliably assess the bacterial, protozoan and viral contamination of aquatic environments in all circumstances, it is feasible that a suite of surrogates may be identified that will estimate levels of microbial contamination within defined circumstances, such as within a storage reservoir with well characterized inputs [21]. To understand how they relate to each other, it is necessary to develop a process-based understanding of surrogate organisms in order to develop a model of their behaviour and assess their dynamics relative to their pathogenic counterparts [16].

5.5. Role of numerical models

Although the processes influencing enteric organism fate and distribution are fairly well established, much uncertainty remains as to the relative importance of each process on a system-wide scale, and the spatial and temporal variability that is present. Furthermore, a detailed understanding of how pathogen dynamics vary between systems, which may differ in their loading, salinity, temperature and trophic status, remains elusive. As a result, *ad hoc* monitoring routines are often employed that rarely give an indication of the true risk. Numerical models are attractive since they offer to integrate the myriad of interacting and non-linear processes and place them within a system-wide context.

The use of numerical models to augment existing monitoring and risk-management activities is becoming increasingly widespread since they are able to highlight dominant processes controlling organism dynamics, and can be used to fill knowledge gaps and test catchment management scenarios or examine engineering interventions. There have been several models used to simulate different components of microbial pollution reported in the literature that range in sophistication and that are relevant for different surface water environments, including freshwater lakes and reservoirs [16,63-64], streams and rivers [65], and estuaries and coastal lagoons [66-68].

Models are used by a range of organizations for a variety of applications:

- *as a scientific tool to explore the dominant processes within a given system* – for managers interested in understanding the spatial and temporal variability in the dynamics that control enteric organism behaviour, and conducting pathogen budgets and exploring sensitivities;

- *to guide the design targeted monitoring programs* – the model can be run to provide information about expected transport and kinetic controls to ensure that the sampling locations and frequency is focused on the areas that present the largest risk;

- *to quantify differences between species* – the model can be used to 'correct' the observed microbial indicator organism data so that the true risk by actual pathogenic organisms can be quantified;

- *to quantify the impact of proposed management scenarios* – scenarios such as catchment remediation, climate change and engineering interventions can be compared to the base case system as part of a cost-benefit analysis prior to any remedial action;

- *to support real-time decision-making* – the model can be used to provide now- and fore-casts of conditions within an aquatic system to enable managers to alter pumping regimes or issue recreational closures.

Models for assisting with the understanding of contaminant dynamics within a system range from simple web-based tools to full three-dimensional (3D) hydrodynamic-water quality models. To demonstrate their ability to describe pathogen transport dynamics, here we focus on a case-study of a medium sized Australian reservoir, Myponga Reservoir in South Australia, where pathogen transport dynamics have been measured and modelled using various approaches. The model developed to simulate pathogen kinetics is shown in Figure 6.

INFLOW: This is a simple web-based tool written in JavaScript (http://www.cwr.uwa.edu.au/) developed by [23], that estimates the entrainment experienced by a riverine intrusion as it enters and progresses through a standing body of water (*e.g.* lake or reservoir) and the final insertion depth and inflow thickness. The model simply requires the inflow parameters including temperature, salinity and channel parameters (*e.g.* bed slope, roughness), and reservoir information such as the vertical temperature and salinity profiles. This information is used to estimate whether the inflow will act as an overflow, interflow or underflow (Figure 5), the approximate entrainment rate (and hence the dilution), and the timescale for transport and insertion. In addition, since the model is able to estimate the time-scale of transport, a simplified loss-model (simplified version of Figure 6) is included that estimates the loss due to settling and inactivation. Therefore, with relatively simple input information, the user is able to assess reservoir risk reduction of pathogen concentrations by dilution, settling and inactivation. This tool is only applicable where the lake is weakly forced at the surface, and doesn't tell you what happens to the contaminated inflow water once it has inserted. However, the simplicity of knowing if the water will travel at the surface, mid-regions or at depth and an approximate dilution factor is a surprisingly powerful management tool.

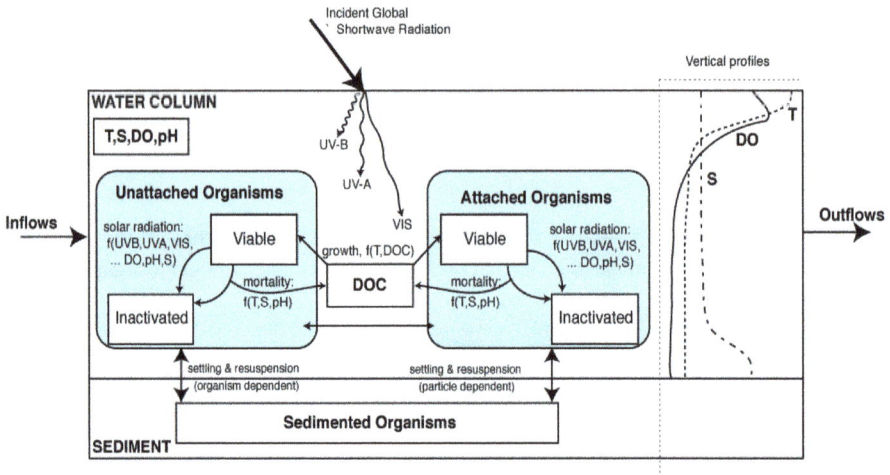

Figure 6. Schematic indicating organism dynamics showing the major pools and kinetic processes that occur in response to sunlight (UV-B, UV-A and VIS), temperature (T), salinity (S), dissolved oxygen (DO), pH and available carbon (DOC) (modified from [16]).

CAEDYM: The Computational Aquatic Ecosystem Dynamics Model (CAEDYM) is a comprehensive water quality model available from the Centre for Water Research at The University of Western Australia [69], able to couple with a 1D lake stratification model (DYRESM) and a 3D hydrodynamic model (ELCOM). ELCOM is specifically designed for modelling circulation patterns in stratified lakes and reservoirs and can be easily run on a desktop computer. The pathogen sub-model includes inactivation due to different solar radiation bandwidths (including UV), natural mortality, sedimentation and aggregation onto suspended particles, and resuspension as described in [16]). ELCOM-CAEDYM is well suited to applications where topographic effects may be important or where lake circulation is a dominant process over inflow forcing. For example, if the source is a recreational area or a lakeside canal estate, then three-dimensional effects may be important in determining the mixing of the contaminated water around the lake. Similarly, if the source is a discrete effluent discharge, then the prevailing hydrodynamics will need to be well understood in order to accurately characterize the risk of the contaminated water reaching an off-take or recreational area. As an example, the application to Myponga Reservoir (Figure 7) describes a contaminated inflow entering from a side tributary before it begins to interact with a large peninsula and migrate into the main basin. Output from the model highlights the strong vertical gradients that result. Hipsey et al [16] use this platform to further investigate the controls on *E. coli* dynamics over a range of time-scales for different sized reservoirs and showed that a different combination of transport and kinetic processes could ultimately shape the response of the microbial concentrations observed at the offtake.

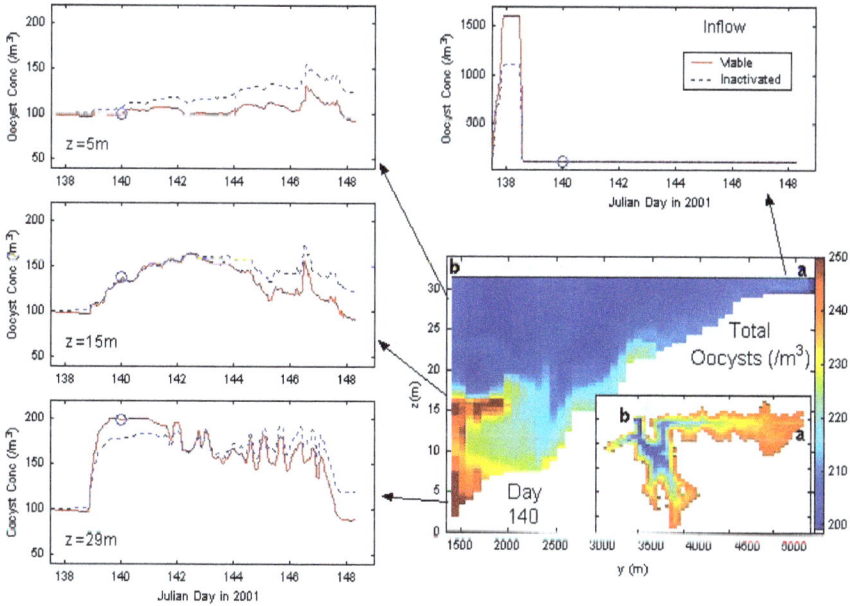

Figure 7. ELCOM-CAEDYM *Cryptosporidium* concentrations (oocysts/10L) presented as a slice through Myponga Reservoir (bottom-right, colour scale reflects oocyst concentration), South Australia (see inset), following a large runoff event, and highlighting *Cryptosporidium* oocyst concentrations as a function of time for three depths near the offtake (left).

DYRESM, is a 1D hydrodynamic model that has been shown to accurately capture the temperature and salinity dynamics of large and small lakes and reservoirs [70]. It accommodates horizontal motions caused by inflows and outflows, in addition to a Lagrangian vertical mixing model and a surface thermodynamics module. CAEDYM couples with DYRESM and includes the same detailed microbial sub-model as outlined in Figure 6. The horizontal averaging used in DYRESM-CAEDYM significantly improves computational efficiency and means that seasonal or even multi-decadal simulations can be performed with reasonable run-times. This model is therefore well suited to applications that look at the long-term impact of different watershed management or climate change scenarios for example, and its ease of use makes it particularly useful to reservoir and lake managers.

GLM-FABM: The General Lake Model (GLM) is coupled with the open-source ecological model FABM as described in [71]. The model GLM is similar to DYRESM but based on [72], and a simplified version of the pathogen kinetic model [16] is implemented within FABM. Output from the model as applied to Myponga Reservoir for the year of 2003 (Figure 8) demonstrates how the incoming oocyst load manifests in the water column concentrations and highlights the temporal and vertical variability that may be expected. The figure indicates the variability seen in the off-take *Cryptosporidium* concentrations at three different depths, and demonstrates the potential benefits of selective withdrawal and adaptive reservoir management to minimize the potential risks.

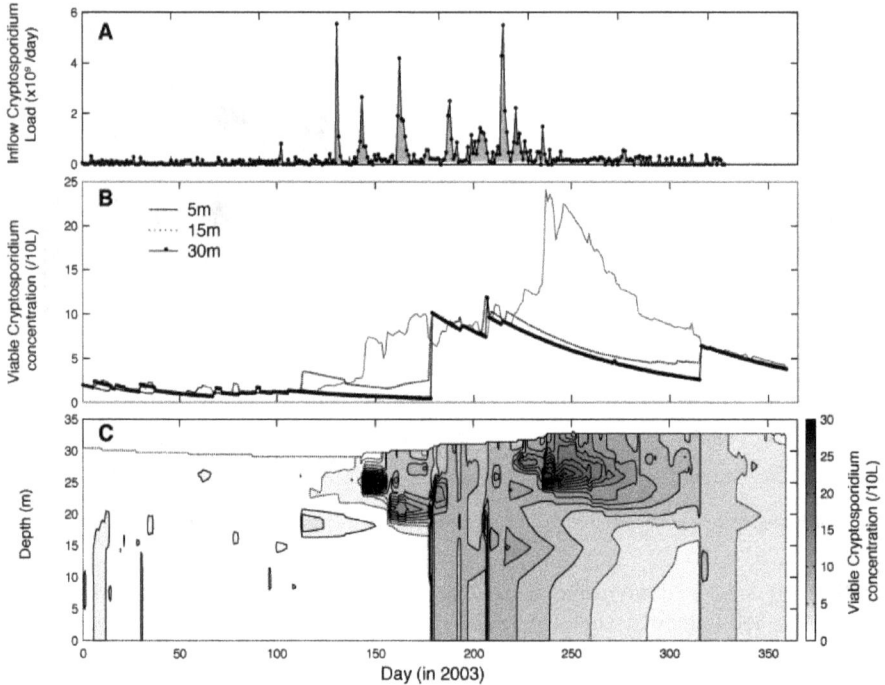

Figure 8. Time-series of A) viable inflow oocyst load as estimated from data; B) simulated concentrations of viable oocysts at the dam wall for three different depths, and C) the viable oocyst concentrations (oocysts/10L) throughout the water column as simulated by GLM-FABM.

6. Control measures and considerations to minimise exposure

There are a range of control measures that can be implemented to mitigate the risk of contaminants passing through to delivery systems. Here we provide a broad overview of the different approaches and their relevance to different contamination issues. The different control methods can be characterised based on the nature of the intervention:

- reducing the delivery of contamination to the exposure point (water storage);

- improved attenuation of the contaminant within the storage;

- and optimal extraction of water to reduce exposure.

The methods around these are discussed next, including a discussion on operational monitoring and the potential for real-time management of water bodies for risk minimization.

6.1. Catchment management

Most contamination within drinking water storages is linked to the surrounding catchment land-use. The contamination can either originate from the catchment and enter the tributaries to the storage, or a precursor of the contamination may originate within the catchment that is later transformed to the end product that constitutes a health risk. There is therefore much scope to reduce contamination within drinking waters through strategic assessment and management of catchment land-use and the condition of tributary streams.

For *Cryptosporidium* and other pathogens the biggest threat is when heavy rains wash viable cells from agricultural catchments within the surrounding river basin into the floodwaters that feed the reservoirs [73-74], or in some cases when effluent from wastewater treatment plants is discharged directly into upstream watercourses (75-76). For many reservoirs, prevention of the contaminant source from entering the hydrological network is the ultimate method for reducing downstream health risks. In particular this involves improving agricultural practices and the best example is related to improvement of the methods used in animal husbandry. Farm-scale alleviation techniques such as improved drainage and runoff recharge may prevent or delay contaminated runoff from entering the stream network. At the sub-catchment scale, policies for suitable riparian management are also recommended since it has been shown that suitable riparian buffers can act to filter contaminated farm water from entering streams [46].

In urban environments, principles of Water Sensitive Urban Design (WSUD) are increasingly being adopted with numerous innovations in the design of stormwater management features including biofilters and constructed wetlands at critical catchment points [77].

6.2. Inflow manipulation

A significant critical control point for managing contaminant transfer into the main reservoir body is through strategic engineering based interventions where catchment tributaries meet a standing water body. Several flow management options exist here that can reduce the delivery of contaminants, including:

- *flow diversions* – as seen in pathogen concentrations over the course of an inflow event, higher values occur at the leading edge of the peak in the hydrograph, and so there is potential for 'first-flush' flows to be diverted away from the water body under consideration. After the initial peak in cell numbers are reduced, then the flow diversion can be removed. The disadvantage of this approach is the potential loss of valuable water, however it could be considered as an environmental flow.

• *sedimentation basins, or 'pre-reservoirs'* –can be used to slow incoming water down and encourage sedimentation of particulates. The water that overflows the basin is usually of a higher quality and passes into the main water body with a lower concentration. There are potential complications with this approach, particularly considering that oocysts have a long life in the sediment and a very high may mobilise previously sedimented organisms in a single event.

• *constructed wetlands* – like pre-reservoirs are useful at slowing the inflowing water and enhancing attenuation (e.g., [78]), also mentioned above.

To assess the efficiency of any of these controls and the loading reduction, it is a simple case of measuring water at the outlet relative to the influent water.

6.3. In-lake controls

Aside from manipulating the inflow concentrations (above) or offtake strategy (below), there is some potential to manipulate concentrations by using in-lake interventions. However, there are no standard methods for controlling the concentration of pathogens within standing waters and these are more commonly applied for management of nuisance cyanobacteria, for example, but also offer potential to support management of high pathogen loads. The most common method for managing stratified waters is destratification, generally achieved through the introduction of compressed air on the lake bottom. The air-water mixture with lowered specific weight causes a rising water curtain, destroying stratification. Similarly, impellers have also be suggested as a method to disperse contaminated water that is concentrated within highly important areas to regions where they are less of a concern. They operate by enhancing the water exchange rate (potentially the littoral water exchange rate, depending upon the flushing technique and the location of the devices), which, if important enough, can prevent the formation of high concentration patches. Some flushing devices also increase also vertical mixing and this may impact on incident light received by organisms.

Where hypolimnetic contaminants become unmanageable, for example following a large, dense flood intrusion, then historically there has been examples of hypolimnetic release or purging to remove these from the system. It can be done in natural lakes by pipes called Olszewski-tubes [79], and by selecting an appropriate height of the discharge on the dam for reservoirs. However, this potentially involves losing valuable water resources and may also lead to enhanced downstream contamination.

Morillo *et al* [80] numerically demonstrated the use of a suspended geo-textile curtain to manipulate the flow path of contaminated inflow water, thereby increasing time taken for natural attenuation processes to occur. These curtains change the internal flow-paths by compartmentalisation, and either slow down or redirect highly contaminated inflow pulses. They may also contribute to address other contamination concerns, since they can have an impact on the nutrient distribution and the residence time of the lake [80-81]. In addition to controlling the path of inflowing water, they constitute a barrier to internal waves, and thus can prevent enhanced mixing due to seiching and subsequent sediment resuspension.

However, such measures are logistically difficult and may incur considerable cost, and for pathogens in particular, management of the offtake location usually remains a more practical and effective means to reduce risk.

6.4. Adapting the location of drinking-water offtakes and bathing sites

The vertical variability in reservoir water quality can be exploited to select an offtake depth with the lowest contaminant concentrations. Selective withdrawal is a widely used method for controlling transmission of contaminants downstream of surface storages. This is mostly applicable for reservoirs with sufficient depth and the capability in the dam offtake structure for multiple offtake depths.

The simple INFLOW model described above enables prediction of the depth at which the riverine inflow will occur and the anticipated dilution as it travels through the reservoir. Consideration should be given to the time of transport. Appropriate monitoring is necessary to ensure stratification and intrusion type is known to the operator. The speed at which an inflow travels through a lake, the degree of entrainment of ambient lake water, the dilution, and the insertion depth are all important in determining the distribution of pathogens in lakes and reservoirs. Consequently it is important to know the depth of the riverine intrusion so water can be harvested outside of this intrusion.

Similarly, where bathing sites are situated around the system of interest, the best solution is temporary closure upon detection of high concentrations with the monitoring data, or from the model predictions.

6.5. Real-time management systems

Given the complexity of managing environmental waters it is not surprising that there has been a considerable proliferation of decision support systems (DSS) in the water resources sector over the past several decades. In general DSSs integrate databases, models, and data visualization tools through a user-friendly interface. The complexity of the models and the databases ranges greatly depending on the intended use. A distinction exists between 'real-time' DSSs that provide advanced warning of deleterious impacts and 'non-real-time' DSSs that serve as planning and operational development tools. Real-time flood prediction DSSs have emerged as commonplace technology, which provide advance warning to save life and property. However, the development of real-time systems for water quality concerns has been less common, but is increasing as data acquisition systems and the associated cyber-infrastructure associated with such developments improves.

The purpose of the DSS is to accurately predict the fate and transport of floods and contaminant dynamics. Because these types of incidents have high spatial and temporal variability in inland standing waters, complex three-dimensional simulations are often also implemented. In this case the DSS performs all of the tasks to maintain simulations of the current conditions in an automated manner so that when incidents occur, the system provides useful predictions to aid in mitigation measures (Figure 9).

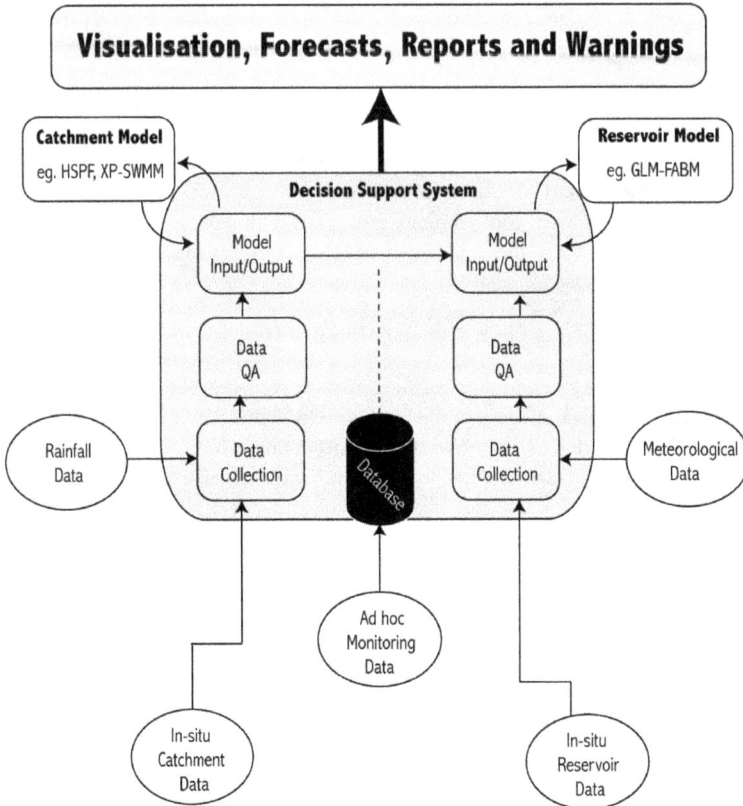

Figure 9. Framework for a Decision Support System (DSS) that has inputs from a range of monitoring programs which inform and input to hydrodynamic and management models to visually represent predictions of risk, and report exceedance of contaminant thresholds and send warnings to managers.

7. Conclusions

It is apparent that contaminant risk to drinking water supply needs to consider a broad management framework that encompasses the entire system, from source to exposure. Reducing the corporate and human health risk associated with these contaminants requires a realistic assessment of the overall contaminant risk which can only be achieved with an understanding of the critical variables controlling contaminant fate and distribution once they enter the aquatic environment. Whilst it is near impossible to reduce the pathogen risk to zero, it is possible to manage the load of pathogens entering the water body, understanding and predicting where they go within a drinking water supply reservoir and managing the withdrawal of water to ensure the best quality of water is treated and distributed for potable supply. Sanitation and water treatment have dramatically reduced the burden of water borne disease on the human population. However, the water industry cannot afford to be complacent or not implement risk management strategies for contaminants in drinking water supply catchments and reservoirs. Failure to do so has significant cost, can lead to outbreaks and at worst cost human lives [82]. Tragically water borne disease still takes an enormous toll in developing countries but with implementation of some of the simple technologies and approaches presented here, an integrated risk management framework, and in combination with treatment and disinfection, this toll can be reduced.

Author details

Matthew R. Hipsey[1] and Justin D. Brookes[2]

1 School of Earth and Environment, The University of Western Australia, Nedlands, Australia

2 School of Earth and Environmental Science, The University of Adelaide, Adelaide, Australia

References

[1] Herwaldt, B. L, Craun, G. F, Stokes, S. L, & Juranek, D. D. (1992). Outbreaks of waterborne disease in the United States: 1989-90, *J. Amer. Water Works Assoc.* , 64(4), 129-135.

[2] Moore, A. C, Herwaldt, B. L, Craun, G. F, Calderon, R. L, Highsmith, A. K, & Juranek, D. D. (1994). Waterborne disease in the United States, 1991-1992, *J. Amer. Water Works Assoc.* , 86(2), 87-99.

[3] MacKenzieW. R., Hoxie, N. J., Procter, M. E., Gradus, M. S., Blair, K. A., and Peterson, D. E., (1994). A massive outbreak of Milwaukee *Cryptosporidium* infection transmitted through the public water supply, *N. Engl. J. Med.* , 331(3), 161-167.

[4] Lisle, J. T, & Rose, J. B. (1995). *Crytposporidium* contamination of water in the USA and UK- a mini review, *Aqua* , 44(3), 103-117.

[5] Zuckerman, U, Gold, D, Shelef, G, & Armon, R. (1997). The presence of *Giardia* and *Cryptosporidium* in surface waters and effluents in Israel, *Water Sci. Technol.* 25(11-12): 381-384.

[6]   Gibson, C. J, Haas, C. N, & Rose, J. B. (1998). Risk assessment of waterborne proto-
      zoa: current status and future trends, *Parasitol.* , 117, 205-212.

[7]   Hsu, B. M, Huang, C, Hsu, Y. F, & Hsu, C. L. L. (2000). Examination of *Giardia* and
      Cryptosporidium in water samples and faecal specimens in Taiwan, *Water Sci. Tech-
      nol.* , 41(7), 87-92.

[8]   Howe, A. D, Forster, S, Morton, S, Marshall, R, Osborn, K. S, & Wright, P. (2002).
      Cryptosporidium oocysts in a water supply associated with cryptosporidiosis out-
      break, *Emerg. Infect. Dis.* , 8(6), 619-624.

[9]   Belkin, S, & Colwell, R. R. eds., (2005). *Oceans and health: pathogens in the marine envi-
      ronment*, Springer, New York, 464p.

[10] Robertson, L. J, Campbell, A. T, & Smith, H. V. (1992). Survival of *Cryptosporidium
      parvum* oocysts under various environmental pressures, *Appl. Environ. Microbiol.* ,
      58(11), 3494-3500.

[11] Castro-hermida, J. A, Garci, a-P. r. e. s. e. d. o, Almeida, I, & Gonzalez-warleta, A. M.,
      Correia Da Costa, J. M., Mezo, M., (2008). Contribution of treated wastewater to the
      contamination of recreational river areas with *Cryptosporidium* spp. and *Giardia duode-
      nalis. Water Res.* , 42, 3528-3538.

[12] Soller, J. A, Schoen, M. E, Bartrand, T, Ravenscroft, J. E, & Ashbolt, N. J. (2010). Esti-
      mated human health risks from exposure to recreational waters impacted by human
      and non-human sources of faecal contamination. *Water Res.* , 44(16), 4674-4691.

[13] Fong, T, & Lipp, E. K. (2006). Enteric viruses of humans and animals in aquatic envi-
      ronments: health risks, detection, and potential water quality assessment tools, *Mi-
      crobiol. Mol. Biol. Rev.* , 69(2), 357-371.

[14] Sunderland, D, Graczyk, T. K, Tamang, L, & Breysse, P. N. (2007). Impact of bathers
      on levels of *Cryptosporidium parvum* oocysts and *Giardia lamblia* cysts in recreational
      beach waters. *Water Res.* , 41(15), 3483-3489.

[15] Bichai, F, Payment, P, & Barbeau, B. (2008). Protection of waterborne pathogens by
      higher organisms in drinking water: a review. *Can. J. Microbiol.* 2008, 54(7): 509-524.

[16] Hipsey, M. R, Antenucci, J. P, & Brookes, J. D. process-based model of microbial pol-
      lution in aquatic systems, Water Resour. Res. 44: W07408.

[17] Edzwald, J. K, & Kelley, M. B. (1998). Control of *Cryptosporidium-* from reservoirs to
      clarifiers to filters, *Water Sci. Technol.* , 37(2), 1-8.

[18] Allen, M. J, Clancy, J. L, & Rice, E. W. (2000). The plain, hard truth about pathogen
      monitoring, *J. Amer. Water Works Assoc.* 92(9), 64-76.

[19] Kay, D, & Mcdonald, A. (1980). Reduction of coliform bacteria in two upland reser-
      voirs: the significance of distance decay relationships, *Water Res.* , 14, 305-318.

[20] Brookes, J. D, Antenucci, J. P, Hipsey, M. R, Burch, M. D, Ashbolt, N, & Ferguson, C. M. (2004). Fate and transport of pathogens in lakes and reservoirs, *Environ. Intl.* , 30, 741-759.

[21] Brookes, J. D, Hipsey, M. R, Burch, M. D, Regel, R. H, Linden, L, Ferguson, C. M, & Antenucci, J. P. (2005). Relative value of surrogate indicators for detecting pathogens in lakes and reservoirs, *Environ. Sci. Technol.* , 39(22), 8614-8621.

[22] Wuest, A, & Lorke, A. (2003). Small-scale hydrodynamics in lakes. *Ann. Rev. Fluid Mech.* , 35, 373-412.

[23] Antenucci, J, Brookes, J. D, & Hipsey, M. (2005). A simple model for quantifying *Cryptosporidium* transport, dilution, and potential risk in reservoirs. *Journal of the American Water Works Association* , 97(1), 86-93.

[24] Deen, A, Craig, R, & Antenucci, J. P. (2000). The Sydney Water contamination incident of monitoring and modelling. *In "Hydro 2000: 3rd International Hydrology and Water Resources Symposium".* Institution of Engineers Australia, Perth, Australia., 1998.

[25] Chung, S. W, Hipsey, M. R, & Imberger, J. (2009). Modelling the propagation of turbid density inflows into a stratifuied lake: Daecheong Reservoir, Korea. Environ. Model. Softw. , 24, 1467-1482.

[26] Evison, L. M. (1988). Comparative studies on the survival of indicator organisms and pathogens in fresh and sea water, *Water Sci. Technol.* 20(11-12): 309-315.

[27] Lopez-torres, A. J, Prieto, L, & Hazen, T. C. (1988). Comparison of the in situ survival and activity of *Klebsiella pneumoniae* and *Escherichia coli* in tropical marine environments, *Microb. Ecol.* , 15, 41-57.

[28] Camper, A. K, Mcfeters, G. A, Characklis, W. G, & Jones, W. L. (1991). Growth kinetics of coliform bacteria under conditions relevant to drinking water distribution systems, *Appl. Environ. Microbiol.* , 57(8), 2233-2239.

[29] Ashbolt, N, Dorsch, M. R, Cox, P. T, & Banens, B. Blooming *E coli*, what do they mean?' *In Coliforms and E. coli: problem or solution?* (D. Kay and C. Fricker, eds.), The Royal Society of Chemistry, Cambridge, UK., 78-85.

[30] Solo-gabriele, H. M, Wolfert, M. A, Desmarais, T. R, & Palmer, C. J. (2000). Sources of *Escherichia coli* in a coastal subtropical environment, *Appl. Environ. Microbiol.* , 66(1), 230-237.

[31] Brookes, J. D, Davies, C, Antenucci, J, & Hipsey, M. (2006). Association of *Cryptosporidium* with bovine faecal particles and implications for risk reduction by settling within water supply reservoirs. *Water and Health* , 4, 87-98.

[32] Reynolds, C. S. (1984). *The ecology of freshwater phytoplankton*, Cambridge Univ. Press, Cambridge, 390p.

[33] Hipsey, M. R, Brookes, J. D, Regel, R. H, Antenucci, J. P, & Burch, M. D. (2006). In situ evidence for the association of total coliforms and *Escherichia coli* with suspended inorganic particles in an Australian reservoir, *Water Air Soil Pollut.* 170(1-4): 191-209.

[34] Gerba, C. P, & Mcleod, J. S. (1976). Effect of sediments on the survival of *Escherichia coli* in marine waters, *Appl. Environ. Microbiol.*, 32(1), 114-120.

[35] Davies, C. M, Long, J. A. H, Donald, M, & Ashbolt, N. J. (1995). Survival of fecal microorganisms in marine and freshwater sediments, *Appl. Environ. Microbiol.*, 61(5), 1888-1896.

[36] Howell, J. M, Coyne, M. S, & Cornelius, P. L. (1996). Effect of sediment particle size and temperature on fecal bacteria mortality rates and the fecal coliform/fecal streptococci ratio, *J. Environ. Qual.*, 25, 1216-1220.

[37] Lemckert, C. J, & Imberger, J. (1998). Turbulent benthic boundary layer mixing events in fresh water lakes', *In Physical Processes in Lakes and Oceans* (J. Imberger, ed.), American Geophysical Union, Washington., 54, 503-516.

[38] Michallet, H, & Ivey, G. N. (1999). Experiments on mixing due to internal solitary waves breaking on uniform slopes, *J. Geophys. Res.* 104(C6): 13467-13478.

[39] Beach, R. A, & Sternberg, R. W. (1992). Suspended sediment transport in the surf zone: response to incident wave and longshore current interaction, *Mar. Geol.*, 108, 275-294.

[40] Grant, S. B, Litton, R. M, & Ahn, J. H. (2011). Measuring and modeling the flux of fecal bacteria across the sediment-water interface in a turbulent stream. *Water Resour. Res.* 47: W05517.

[41] Hobson, P, Fabris, R, Develter, E, Linden, L. G, Burch, M. D, & Brookes, J. D. (2010). Reservoir inflow monitoring for improved management of treated water quality-A South Australian experience. *Water Resour. Manag.*, 24(14), 4161-4174.

[42] Bryan, B. A, Kandulu, J, Deere, D. A, White, M, Frizenschaf, J, & Crossman, N. D. (2009). Adaptive management for mitigating Cryptosporidium risk in source water: a case study in an agricultural catchment in South Australia. *J Environ. Manage.*, 90(10), 3122-3134.

[43] Pusey, B. J, & Arthington, A. J. (2003). Importance of the riparian zone to the conservation and management of freshwater fish: a review. *Mar. Freshwater Res.*, 54(1), 1-16.

[44] Ferguson, C. M, Davies, C. M, Kaucner, C, Krogh, M, Rodehutskors, J, Deere, D. A, & Ashbolt, N. (2007). Field scale quantification of microbial transport from bovine faeces under simulated rainfall events. *J. Water Health*, 5, 83-95.

[45] Winkworth, C. L, Matthaei, C. D, & Townsend, C. R. (2008). Recently planted vegeta-tion strips reduce giardia runoff reaching waterways. *J. Environ. Qual.* , 37(6), 2256-2263.

[46] Bach, P. M, Mccarthy, D. T, & Deletic, A. (2010). Redefining the stormwater first flush phenomenon. *Water Res.* , 44(8), 2487-2498.

[47] Agrawal, Y. C, & Pottsmith, H. C. (2000). Instruments for particle size and settling velocity observations in sediment transport. *Mar. Geol.* , 168, 89-114.

[48] Hipsey, M. R, Brookes, J. D, Antenucci, J. P, Burch, M. D, & Regel, R. model of Cryp-tosporidium dynamics in lakes and reservoirs: a new model for risk management. *Intl. J. River Basin Manage.* , 2(3), 181-197.

[49] Romero, J. R, Antenucci, J. P, & Imberger, J. (2004). One- and three- dimensional bio-geochemical simulations of two differing reservoirs, *Ecol. Model.* , 174(1), 143-160.

[50] Baudisova, D. (1997). Evaluation of *Escherichia coli* as the main indicator of faecal pol-lution, *Water Sci. Technol.* 35(11-12): 323-336.

[51] Helmi, K, Skraber, S, Burnet, J, Leblanc, L, Hoffmann, L, & Cauchie, H. (2011). Two-year monitoring of *Cryptosporidium parvum* and *Giardia lamblia* occurrence in a recrea-tional and drinking water reservoir using standard microscopic and molecular biology techniques. *Environ. Monit. Assess.* , 179, 163-175.

[52] Ashbolt, N. J, Grabow, W. O. K, & Snozzi, M. (2001). Indicators of microbial water quality', *In WHO | Water Quality: Guidelines, Standards and Health. Risk assessment and management for water-related infectious disease* (L. Fewtrell and J. Bartram, eds.). IWA Publishing, London.

[53] Havelaar, A. H, Van Olphen, M, & Drost, Y. C. (1993). F-specific RNA bacteriophages are adequate model organisms for enteric viruses in fresh water, *Appl. Environ. Mi-crobiol.* , 59(9), 2956-2962.

[54] Armon, R, & Kott, Y. (1995). Distribution comparison between coliphages and phages of anaerobic bacteria (*Bacteroides fragilis*) in water sources, and their reliability as faecal pollution indicators in drinking water, *Water Sci. Technol.* 31(5-6): 215-222.

[55] Tartera, C, Lucena, F, & Jofre, J. (1989). Human origin of *Bacteroides fragilis* bacterio-phage present in the environment, *Appl. Environ. Microbiol.* , 55, 2696-2701.

[56] Cornax, R, & Morinigo, M. A. (1991). Significance of several bacteriophage groups as indicator of sewage pollution in marine waters, *Water Res.* , 25(6), 673-678.

[57] Grabow, W. O. K, Taylor, M. B, & De Villiers, J. C. (2001). New methods for the de-tection of viruses: call for review of drinking water quality guidelines, *Water Sci. Technol.* , 46(12), 1-8.

[58] Payment, P, & Franco, E. (1993). *Clostridium perfringens* and somatic coliphages as in-
      dicators of the efficiency of drinking water treatment for viruses and protozon cysts,
      Appl. Environ. Microbiol. , 59(8), 2418-2424.

[59] Ferguson, C. M, Coote, B. G, Ashbolt, N. J, & Stevenson, I. M. (1996). Relationships
      between indicators, pathogens and water quality in an estuarine system, *Water Res.* ,
      30(9), 2045-2054.

[60] Leeming, R, Nichols, P. D, & Ashbolt, N. J. (1998). Distinguishing sources of faecal
      pollution in Australian inland and coastal waters using sterol biomarkers and micro-
      bial faecal indicators'. Water Services Association of Australia, Melbourne.

[61] Juranek, D. D, & Mackenzie, W. R. (1998). Drinking water turbidity and gastrointesti-
      nal illness, *Epidemiol.* , 9(3), 228-231.

[62] Ongerth, J. E, & Stibbs, H. (1989). Prevalence of *Cryptosporidium* infection in dairy
      calves in western Washington, *Am. J. Vet. Res. 50*, 1069-1070.

[63] Auer, M. T, & Niehaus, S. L. (1993). Modeling fecal coliform bacteria- I. Field and lab-
      oratory determination of loss kinetics, *Water Res.* , 27(4), 693-701.

[64] Jin, G, Englande, A. J, & Liu, A. (2003). A preliminary study on coastal water quality
      monitoring and modeling, *J. Environ. Sci. Health A*, 38(3), 493-509.

[65] Wilkinson, J, Jenkins, A, Wyer, M, & Kay, D. (1995). Modelling faecal coliform dy-
      namics in streams and rivers, *Water Res.* , 29(3), 847-855.

[66] Salomon, J. C, & Pommepuy, M. (1990). Mathematical model of bacterial contamina-
      tion of the Morlaix Estuary (France), *Water Res.* , 24(8), 983-994.

[67] Steets, B. M, & Holden, P. A. (2003). A mechanistic model of runoff-associated fecal
      coliform fate and transport through a coastal lagoon, *Water Res.* , 37, 589-608.

[68] Mccorquodale, J. A, Georgiou, I, Carnelos, S, & Englande, A. J. (2004). Modeling coli-
      forms in storm water plumes, *J. Environ. Eng. Sci.* , 3, 419-431.

[69] Hipsey, M. R, & Hamilton, D. P. (2008). Computational Aquatic Ecosystem Dynamic
      Model: CAEDYM Science Manual v3.3. Centre for Water Research Report, Perth,
      Australia, 140pp.

[70] Gal, G, Imberger, J, Zohary, T, Antenucci, J. P, Anis, A, & Rosenberg, T. (2003). Simu-
      lating the thermal dynamics of Lake Kinneret. Ecol. Model. , 162, 69-86.

[71] Hipsey M. R, Bruce L. C, Boon C, Bruggeman J, Bolding K, & Hamilton D. P. (2012).
      GLM-FABM - Model Overview and User Documentation. The University of Western
      Australia Technical Manual, Perth, Australia. 44pp.

[72] Hamilton, D. P, & Schladow, S. G. (1997). Water quality in lakes and reservoirs. Part I
      Model description. *Ecol. Model.* , 96, 91-110.

[73] Atherholt, T. B. LeChevalier, M. W., Norton, W. D., and Rosen, J. S., (1998). Effect of rainfall on Giardia and Crypto, *J. Amer. Water Works Assoc.*, 90(9), 66-80.

[74] Walker, M. J, Montemagno, C. D, & Jenkins, M. B. (1998). Source water assessment and non-point source of acutely toxic contaminants: A review of research related to survival and transport of *Cryptosporidium parvum, Water Resour. Res.*, 34(12), 3383-3392.

[75] Rajala, R. L, & Heinonen-tanski, H. (1998). Survival and transfer of faecal indicator organisms of wastewater effluents in receiving lake waters, *Water Sci. Technol.*, 38(12), 191-194.

[76] Medema, G. J, & Schijven, J. F. (2001). Modelling the sewage discharge and dispersion of *Cryptosporidium* and *Giardia* in surface water, *Water Res.*, 35(18), 4307-4316.

[77] Li, Y. L, Deletic, A, Alcazar, L, Bratieres, K, Fletcher, T. D, & Mccarthy, D. T. (2012). Removal of *Clostridium perfringens, Escherichia coli* and *F-RNA coliphages* by stormwater biofilters. *Ecol. Engng.*, 49, 137-145.

[78] Wu, C. Y, Liu, J. K, Cheng, S. H, Surampalli, D. E, Chen, C. W, & Kao, C. M. (2010). Constructed wetland for water quality improvement: a case study from Taiwan. *Water Sci Technol.*, 62(10), 2408-18.

[79] Olszewski, P, & Sikorowa, A. (1973). Drawing off of hypolimnion waters as a method for improving the quality of lake waters. In: International Symposium on Eutrophication and Water Pollution Control, October 16-20, 1973, Castle Reinhardsbrudnn: , 136-141.

[80] Morillo, S, Imberger, J, & Antenucci, J. P. (2006). Modifying the residence time and dilution capacity of a reservoir by altering internal flow-paths. *Intl. J. River Basin Manage.*, 4(4), 255-271.

[81] Asaeda, T, Pham, H. S, Priyanthac, D. G. N, Manatunge, J, & Hocking, G. C. (2001). Control of algal blooms in reservoirs with a curtain: a numerical analysis. *Ecol. Engng.*, 16(3), 395-404.

[82] Hrudey, S, & Hrudey, E. J. (2004). Safe drinking water: lessons from recent outbreaks in affluent nations. IWA publishing 1-84339-042-6, 486.

Chapter 5

Cyanobacterial Toxins in Food-Webs: Implications for Human and Environmental Health

John Berry

Additional information is available at the end of the chapter

1. Introduction

Cyanobacteria (or "blue-green algae") are among the oldest known groups of organism on Earth, with fossil records spanning approximately 3.5 billion years, and inhabit nearly every ecological niche on the planet. In addition to their conspicuous occurrence as aquatic "blooms" (e.g. visible scums on ponds and lakes; Fig. 1), as well as various colonial or macrophytic forms, in marine and freshwater habitats, these photosynthetic prokaryotes are widely found in terrestrial soils, and as part of numerous symbiotic relationships with a range of organisms including animals, plants and fungi. To illustrate the extent of their global abundance and importance, approximately 50% of all primary productivity, and related oxygen production, occurs in the ocean, and the majority of this is derived from two genera of cyanobacteria, *Synechococcus* and the picophytoplankton, *Prochlorococcus* (Ting et al., 2002). Likewise, nitrogen-fixing cyanobacteria, and particularly the genus, *Trichodesmium*, are the largest source of nitrogen in ocean systems (Carpenter and Romans, 1991). Moreover, several lines of evidence (see, for example, Paerl and Huisman, 2009) point to an increase in the abundance, distribution and persistence of cyanobacterial blooms in marine and freshwater system, specifically driven by regional and global changes in climate (e.g. elevated water temperature, stratification of the water column, changes in interseasonal weather patterns). The latter, in particular, underscores the potential of cyanobacteria – and specifically toxin-producing cyanobacterial blooms (discussed below) – as a rapidly emerging concern for public health.

Alongside their global biological importance, the cyanobacteria are widely recognized as producers of a chemically diverse array of biologically active secondary metabolites (see, for example, reviews by Gerwick et al., 2001; Tan, 2007; Tan, 2010). Considerable work over the past four decades (see Tan, 2007) has, in particular, focused on exploring this chemical diversity as a source of bioactive compounds with possible relevance to biomedicine, and specifically development of potential chemotherapeutics. Furthermore, a rather convincing body of evidence (Proksh et al., 2002; Simmons et al., 2008) also suggests that many of the pharmacologically active marine natural products, originally isolated from various marine animal sources – and including several currently either in clinical trials, or being commercially developed as drugs - may, in fact, originate from cyanobacterial (or other microbial) sources as a result of trophic transfer (e.g. herbivory, filter-feeding), and symbiotic or commensal relationships.

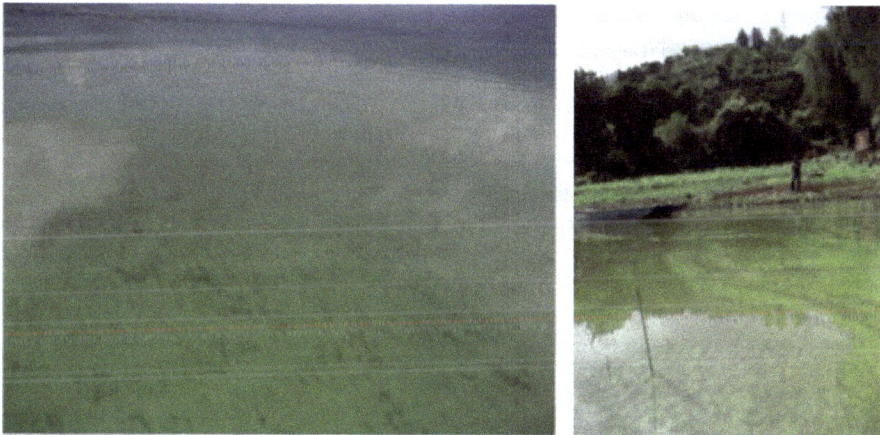

Figure 1. Bloom of toxin-producing cyanobacteria on Lake Patzcuaro (Michoacan, Mexico), and subsistence fishing occurring within the bloom. Photo courtesy of Alan Wilson (Auburn University).

In addition to their potential in biomedicine, however, a number of these bioactive metabolites have been identified as naturally occurring toxins, and have been associated – as so-called "cyanotoxins" - with various human and environmental health concerns. Perhaps most notably, in freshwater systems, cyanobacterial populations can proliferate to the extent that they form large "blooms," typically manifesting as "films" or "scums" on lakes, ponds and other freshwater systems (see Fig. 1). When comprised of toxin-producing representatives, their occurrence is generally categorized as "harmful algal blooms" (HABs), or frequently as "cyanoHABs" (to distinguish from similar blooms of several, unrelated, but likewise toxigenic, marine microalgae). In particular, toxins from cyanoHABs - or even simply high abundance of cyanobacterial cells – can contaminate water, and exposure to toxins via drinking water, recreational exposure and related routes has been linked to various cases of human and animal intoxication, as well as possible sub-acute and/or chronic health effects (e.g. increased rates of certain cancers, effects on fetal development). As these direct routes of exposure are beyond the scope of this chapter, and have been thoroughly covered by many previous authors, the reader is direct to several good reviews on the topic (e.g. Rao et al., 2002; Stewart et al., 2006; Funari and Testai, 2008).

Although the vast majority of studies related to the health impacts of cyanobacteria have focused on direct exposure to cyanotoxins via drinking water and related routes, there is a growing body of evidence to suggest that toxic cyanobacterial metabolites can bioaccumulate in aquatic food-webs, and may consequently pose additional health concerns as food-borne contaminants. The relatively limited number of studies on food-borne cyanobacterial contaminants may be attributed, in part, to the perceived lack of a mechanism for their bioaccumulation. Unlike more lipophilic contaminants, many of the recognized, water-soluble cyanotoxins would, as such, not be expected to biomagnify by otherwise well-documented mechanisms (i.e. storage, and subsequent transfer, in fatty tissues of animals) to higher trophic levels most frequently consumed by humans. However, despite the lack of a clear means transfer of these hydrophilic toxins in food webs, numerous studies have, indeed, demonstrated presence and apparent bioaccumulation in a range of trophic levels. Also likely limiting the attention paid to cyanobacterial toxins in food-webs is the fact that best documented cases of intoxication have been generally limited to direct exposure to these toxins, and specifically acute human or animal poisonings with clear links to consumption of contaminated water, or various related route, whereas there are - at present - few, if any, clear cases of recognized human intoxication by food-borne cyanotoxin. That said, growing recognition that cyanobacterial toxins may contribute to a sub-acute and/or chronic health effects – ranging from increased rates of cancers, neurodegeneration and development toxicity - which are considerably more difficult to identify, would suggest that, despite the lack of currently documented toxicoses, health threats posed by diet-derived toxins remains a very real concern.

The following chapter will present the current state of knowledge regarding the bioaccumulation of cyanobacterial toxins in the food web, and the possible role of these food-borne toxins as it relates to human and environmental health. To begin, the chapter will present a brief summary of the recognized cyanobacterial toxins, and their known toxicology and health effects. Subsequently, the current evidence related to the bioaccumulation, trophic transfer and bioavailability of these cyanobacterial toxins in food webs will be reviewed, along with related methodologies (including methodological limitations and innovations) for investigating these aspects. In addition to the widely recognized water-soluble cyanotoxins, cyanobacteria produce a host of bioactive metabolites, including a number of lipophilic representatives. Accordingly, the discussion will include a consideration of the less characterized bioactive metabolites that, despite relatively unknown health effects, may represent – due to their potential for biomagnification –relevant food-web contaminants. Finally, the chapter will summarize the current state of knowledge regarding the impacts of cyanobacterial toxins as it relates to human and environmental (i.e. ecosystem, animal) health.

2. Recognized cyanobacterial toxins: Chemistry and toxicology

2.1. Hepatotoxins

Detoxification of a wide range of toxic metabolites occurs - via multiphasic enzymes, and associated processes (e.g cellular transporter and "pumps") - in the liver or equivalent organ systems in animals. Accordingly, many toxic metabolites are actively transported (for subsequent detoxification) to, and thus accumulate primarily in, hepatocytes. Not surprising, therefore, two of the most commonly recognized cyanobacterial toxins are, in fact, associated with hepatotoxicity. However, aside from active transport of these toxins to – and consequent toxicity in - hepatocytes, it is becoming increasingly clear that the same metabolites may accumulate in a range of tissues (even if not associated with acute toxicity in these cells), and may – along with their generally uncharacterized toxicology in these tissues - be thusly transferred to higher trophic levels.

2.1.1. Microcystins (MCs) and nodularin (NOD)

Perhaps the most widespread, and consequently well studied, of the cyanobacterial toxins, microcystins (MCs) and nodularin (NOD) are, respectively, hepatotoxic hepta- and penta-peptide toxins. Both share structural similarity (Fig. 2), specifically characterized by a peptide macrocyle incorporating common and unusual amino acids. However, the former (i.e. MCs) represents a chemically diverse group of toxins, comprised of more than ninety variants (Welker and Van Dohran, 2006). Although structural variation throughout the macrocycle of the MCs has been reported, the primary differences occur in "X" and "Y" positions (Fig. 2), as per the accepted nomenclature for the group. As an example, the most common, and generally considered the most toxic, of these variants is MC-LR in which the X and Y positions, respectively, are occupied by leucine (L) and arginine (R) residues. Although chemical variations exist, both NOD and most MC variants are characterized by a relatively well-conserved unusual β-amino acid, 3-amino-9-methoxy-2,6,8-trimethyl-10-phenylde-ca-4,6-dienoic acid (Adda), which is involved (see below) in the toxicology of these metabolites (Gulledge et al., 2003). Finally, whereas NOD is generally limited to a single late summer blooming species, *Nodularia spumigens*, the MCs are produced by a taxonomically wide array of cyanobacterial species including, most notably, the widespread species, *Microcystis aeruginosa*, but also a growing list of other diverse taxa (e.g. *Aphanizomenon, Oscillatoria, Planktothrix, Anabaena, Nostoc*).

Toxiologically, both NOD and the MCs are inhibitors of Ser/Thr type 1 and 2A protein phosphatases (PPases). Data generally suggest that Adda of NOD and MCs are involved in the binding of the metabolite to the active site of PPases (Nishiwaki-Matsumishi et al., 1991; Gulledge et al., 2003). To demonstrate this, several analogues of the MCs, specifically comprised of only a single amino acid (i.e. Gly, or L- or D-Ala) coupled via peptidyl linkage to the carboxylic acid of the N-acetylated Adda, were synthesized (Gulledge et al. 2003) and evaluated for toxicity. Although orders of magnitude lower than intact MC-LR, these analogs retained substantial PPase inhibitory activity, suggesting that Adda significantly contributes to the toxicophore of the MCs and NOD. On the other hand, the unusual amino acid, N-methyldehydroalanine (Mdha), found in many MC variants has been shown to covalently bind via a Michael addition to Cys_{273} of type 1/2A Ser/Thr PPases (MacKintosh et al., 1995). Accordingly, it has been suggested that this distal (to Adda) amino acids is, therefore, also involved in irreversible binding of the toxin to the PPase targets, as well as considerable

underestimation of bioaccumulation (as a non-extractable "bound" form) in organisms
exposed to the toxin (see 4.2 *Methodologies for evaluating cyanobacterial toxins in food-webs*, below).

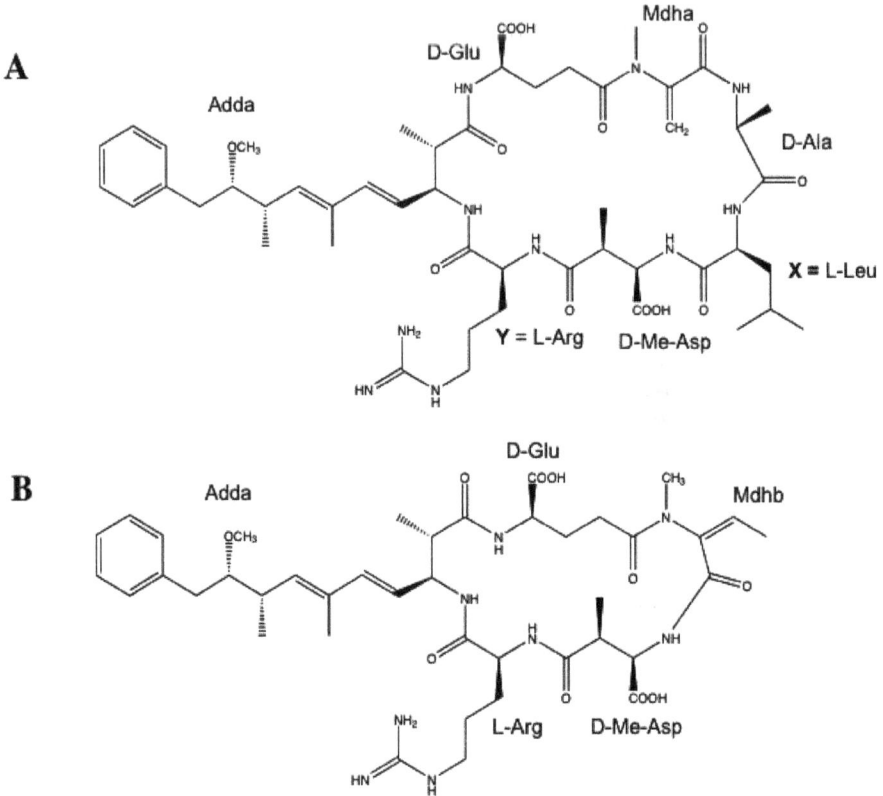

Figure 2. Chemical structures of hepatotoxic microcystins (A) and nodularin (B). In the former, structural variability is
primarily based on variation in the "X" and "Y" amino acid positions indicated; for reference, the common variant, MC-
LR, in which X and Y positions are leucine (L) and arginine (R) is shown.

Given the importance of PPases in a wide range of cellular functions, inhibition of these
enzymes, following exposure to NOD/MCs, can result in a range of acute toxicoses. Accumulating primarily in hepatocytes (i.e. liver) and associated organ systems, inhibition of PPase by
MCs and NOD most typically manifests as acute failure and hemorrhaging in these systems.
However, recent studies, specifically pointing to the presence of similar active transporters in
mammalian (e.g. rat) brains, have proposed a possible connection between MC uptake and
apparent inhibitory effects on short- and long-term memory (Maidana et al., 2006). Moreover,
emerging evidence supports an additional role of MCs in various chronic health effects, and
particularly, as recognized tumor promoters, increased rates of certain cancers. Most notably

studies in China (Yu, 1995; Ueno et al., 1996; Yu et al., 2001) have linked chronic exposure to MC through ingestion of contaminated surface (i.e. ditch) waters to endemically high rates of primary liver cancers. These studies suggest, in particular, that health concerns associated with exposure to even quite low (e.g. sub-picogram per day) doses of cyanobacterial toxins, such as MC/NOD, may promote negative health effects that might not clearly manifest as acute intoxication. This may be particularly germane to discussion of the bioaccumulation of these toxins since there have been to-date no known cases of overt intoxication from food-borne MCs or NOD, whereas the possible long-term effects associated with chronic exposure to these toxins (and others, e.g. BMAA) in the diet continues to present a possible concern.

2.1.2. Cylindrospermopsin (CYN)

Cylindrospermopsin (CYN) is a zwitterionic tricyclic alkaloid, specifically containing a unique hydroxyuracil (Fig. 3). It was first identified following a relatively large intoxication event (the so-called "Palm Island Mystery") in Queensland, Australia. In this original case, children from more than one hundred families on Palm Island, and nearby mainland community of Towns-ville, were stricken with severe gastroenteritis. Subsequent studies (Bourke et al., 1983; Hawkins et al., 1985) linked the illness to the Solomon Dam – the primary water reservoir for the community – and identified several bloom-forming species of cyanobacteria. Among these, a toxic (in mouse bioassay) strain of the species, *Cylindrospermopsis raciborskii*, was identified (Hawkins et al., 1985). More than ten years after the incident, CYN was identified as the toxic principle of the *C. raciborkii* blooms in the reservoir (Ohtani et al., 1992), and following subsequent stereoselective synthesis (Heintzelman et al., 2001), assigned the structure shown in Figure 3. Originally thought to be a strictly tropical species, *C. raciborskii*, has been subsequently shown to occur worldwide in both tropical and temperate freshwater systems, possibly the result of recent expansion in its geographic distribution (Gugger et al., 2005). Moreover, since its initial identification from *C. raciborskii*, CYN has been subsequently found to be produced by several other members of the Nostocales, including the closely related *Aphanizomenon* and *Anabaena* (Banker et al., 1997; Spoof et al., 2006; Preußel et al., 2006), as well as at least one member of the Stigonometales (i.e. *Umezakia*; Harada et al., 1994), suggesting relatively widespread production of the toxin.

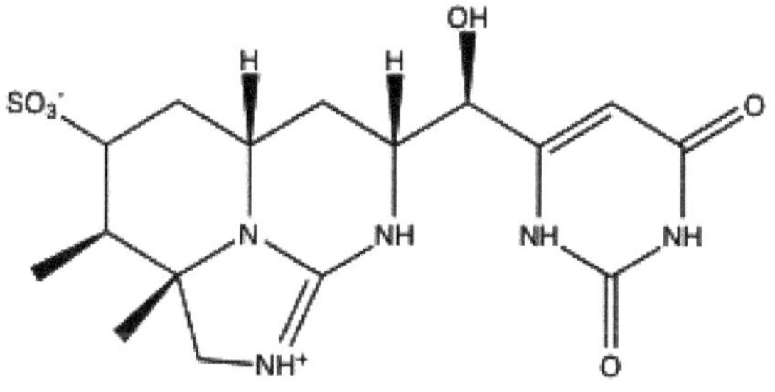

Figure 3. Chemical structure of the hepatotoxin, cylindrospermopsin (CYN).

Toxicological studies primarily suggest that CYN is an inhibitor of protein synthesis (Terao et al., 1994; Froscio et al., 2001). Specifically, Terao et al. (1994) demonstrated ribosomal detach-ment (from endoplasmic reticula) in hepatocytes treated with CYN, and *in vitro* studies using the rabbit reticulocyte translation system showed that CYN inhibits protein synthesis at nanomolar concentrations (e.g. $IC_{50} = 120$ nM; Froscio et al., 2001). However, a range of possible mechanisms of toxicity, and associated biomarkers of the toxin, have been additionally identified and/or proposed. In accordance with inhibition of protein synthesis, Runnegar et al. (1994, 1995) showed a reduction of the tripeptide, glutathione (GSH), in rat hepatocytes exposed to CYN, particularly via apparent inhibition of GSH synthesis, leading to a presump-tive reduction in the detoxifying capacity of cells. Studies (e.g. Shaw et al., 2000; Humpage et al., 2005) have similarly pointed to possible interaction of CYN with cytochrome P450, and suggested a role of this detoxifying enzyme system. Based on structural similarity to nucleo-tides, specifically as guanidine alkaloid, and more specifically the hydroxyuracil moiety contained in the tricyclic structure (Fig. 3), it has been suggested that CYN may additionally exert toxicity by means of interaction with DNA and/or RNA. Indeed, CYN has been found to form covalent linkages with DNA, leading to consequent chromosomal strand breakage (Shaw et al., 2000; Shen et al., 2002), as well as other apparent genotoxic effects (Bazin et al., 2010). This is notable as the uracil moiety of CYN has been shown as required for toxicity (Banker et al., 2001). Finally, *in vivo* studies, particularly in the mouse model, point to a range of histo-pathological effects, particularly in cells of the liver, but additionally in several organ systems (e.g. kidney, adrenal glands, lungs, intestines), following exposure via intraperitoneal or oral exposure (Hawkins et al., 1985; Shaw et al, 2000; Humpage and Falconer, 2003). Moreover, recent studies (in mice) show that long-term oral exposure to low-doses of CYN leads to measurable effects (e.g. reduced hematocrit levels; Sukenik et al., 2006), and, likewise, exposure to CYN during gestation induces fetal toxicity (Rogers et al., 2007), indicating that (similar to MCs) sub-acute effects may occur with relatively low doses, but may be missed by simple assessment of intoxication.

2.2. Neurotoxins

Several of the prominent cyanobacterial toxins are known to presumably cross the blood-brain barrier, and have been consequently associated with neurotoxicity. Neurotoxic cyanotoxins have been particularly identified based on observation of acute toxicity following exposure to these toxins (see below). However, in at least one case (i.e. BMAA; see below), toxicity has been associated with possible chronic neurodegeneration.

2.2.1. Anatoxin-a (ATX-a) and anatoxin-a(s)

Although chemically unrelated, two of the most active neurotoxins produced by cyanobacteria are related both in name and mode of action. First identified from species of *Anabaena*, anatoxin-a (ATX-a) is a tropane alkaloid (Fig. 4) with structural, but not pharmacological, similarity to cocaine. In contrast, the relatively less common anatoxin-a(s), so-named due to hyper-*salivation* associated with its neurotoxicity, is a phosphate ester of N-hydroxyguanine (Fig. 4), likewise, isolated primarily from *Anabaena* spp. Although structurally very different, the two metabolites (along with a few chemically related variants, e.g. homoanatoxin-a) share related toxicological mechanisms of action. Known as the "very fast death factor," ATX-a and its analogues are potent inhibitors of nicotinic acetylcholine receptors (nAChRs), specifically mimicking the endogenous neurotransmitter, acetylcholine, whereas anatoxin-a(s) inhibits related acetylcholinesterases (Aráoz et al., 2010). Interestingly, ATX-a is not degraded by acetylcholinesterases, and thus irreversibly inhibits nAChRs (Aráoz et al., 2010). With regards to food-webs, it should be noted that – compared to other cyanobacterial toxins – the "ana-toxins" are relatively unstable chemically, as well as being generally limited in their distribution and occurrence, and thus rather few studies have reported their bioaccumulation (e.g. Mejean et al., 2010; Osswald et al., 2011). That said at least one case of apparent bioaccumulation of ANTX-a and its analogue (i.e. homoANTX-a) is, in fact, among the very few cases of acute intoxications being possibly linked to food-borne cyanotoxins (see 3. *Evidence for bioaccumulation of cyanobacterial toxins in aquatic food-webs*, below).

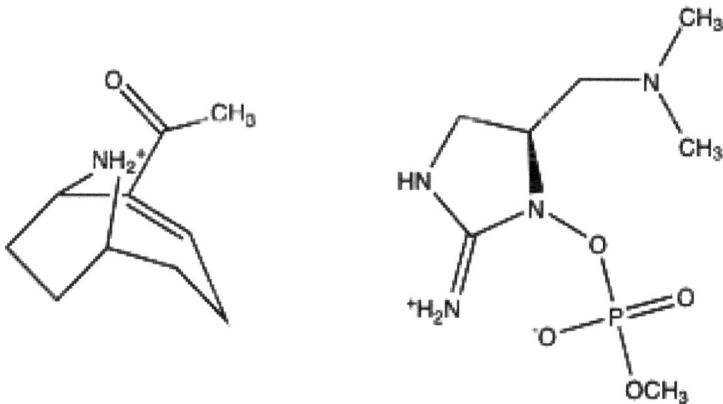

Figure 4. Chemical structure of the neurotoxins, anatoxin-a (ATX-a, left) and anatoxin-a(s) (right).

2.2.2. Saxitoxin (STX) and "Paralytic Shellfish Toxins" (PSTs)

Potent inhibitors of voltage-gated sodium channels, saxitoxin (STX) and several chemically related metabolites have been frequently associated with contamination of shellfish, and consequent toxicity (i.e. "paralytic shellfish poisoning" [PSP]), as the so-called "paralytic shellfish toxins" (PSTs). Specifically, in marine systems, the origins of STX/PSTs have been identified as *Alexandrium* and several related species of dinoflagellates. However, in the late 1960s, apparent STX was identified (Jackim and Gentile, 1968) in the cyanobacterial species, *Aphanizomenon flos-aquae*. Over the subsequent four decades, STX and related PSTs have been identified from a wide range of cyanobacterial genera (e.g. Mahmood and Carmichael, 1986; Humpage et al., 1994; Negri et al., 1995; Carmichael et al., 1997; Lagos et al., 1999; Beltran and

Neilan, 2000; Pomati et al., 2000; Smith et al., 2011) including members of the Nostocales (e.g. *Anabaena, Scytonema, Cylindrospermopsin*) and Oscillatoriales (e.g. *Lyngbya, Planktothrix*).

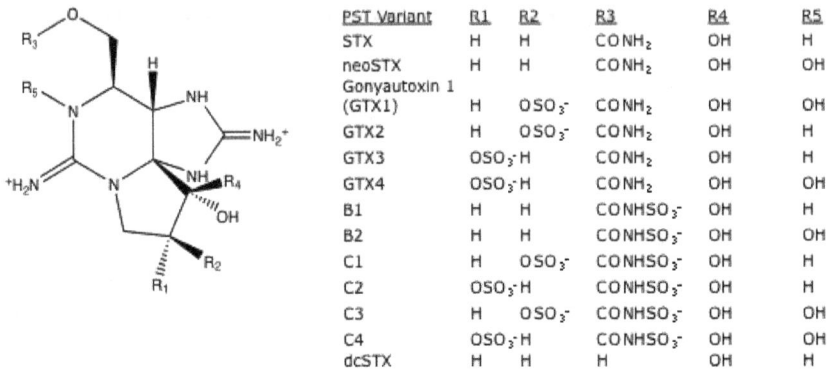

PST Variant	R1	R2	R3	R4	R5
STX	H	H	$CONH_2$	OH	H
neoSTX	H	H	$CONH_2$	OH	OH
Gonyautoxin 1 (GTX1)	H	OSO_3^-	$CONH_2$	OH	OH
GTX2	H	OSO_3^-	$CONH_2$	OH	H
GTX3	OSO_3^-H		$CONH_2$	OH	H
GTX4	OSO_3^-H		$CONH_2$	OH	OH
B1	H	H	$CONHSO_3^-$	OH	H
B2	H	H	$CONHSO_3^-$	OH	OH
C1	H	OSO_3^-	$CONHSO_3^-$	OH	H
C2	OSO_3^-H		$CONHSO_3^-$	OH	H
C3	H	OSO_3^-	$CONHSO_3^-$	OH	OH
C4	OSO_3^-H		$CONHSO_3^-$	OH	OH
dcSTX	H	H	H	OH	H

Figure 5. Chemical structure of saxitoxin (STX) and selected variants of the related "paralytic shellfish toxins" (PSTs).

STX/PSTs are potent inhibitors of voltage-gated sodium channels in neuronal cells, specifically acting on (via binding to, and consequent blockage of) sodium passage through channel pores (Aráoz et al., 2010). Inhibition of sodium channels, by blocking sodium influx involved in the propogation of action potentials in neurons, leads to the aforementioned PSP syndrome which manifests in a range of neurotoxic symptoms including numbness, tingling, weakness and difficulty breathing as a result of the neuromuscular paralysis (Etheridge, 2010). Interestingly, STX/PST binds to the nearly identical location as the equally potent neurotoxin, tetrodotoxin (TTX), associated with poisoning by consumption of several species of pufferfish (Stevens et al., 2011), and STX has, in fact, been identified alongside TTX in pufferfish (Nakamura et al., 1984; discussed below). Notably, despite the identification of STX/PSTs from numerous cyanobacteria species found in freshwater sytems, as well as apparent bioaccumulation of presumptively cyanobacteria-derived toxin in fish and shellfish consumed by humans, reported poisoning by the PSTs has been generally limited to ingestion of shellfish contaminated by apparent marine dinoflagellate sources.

2.2.3. β-Methylamino-L-alanine (BMAA)

As perhaps the best studied case of apparent long-term toxicity resulting from a cyanobacterial toxin bioaccumulated within food webs, the non-essential, non-protein amino acid, β-methylamino-L-alanine (BMAA; Fig. 6) has been linked to high rates of the otherwise rare amyotrophic lateral sclerosis (ALS), and possibly other related neurodegenerative diseases (e.g. Parkinson's Disease, Alzheimer's Disease). Indeed, the first reports of BMAA as a neurotoxic cyanobacterial metabolite specifically stemmed from studies of extraordinarily high rates of ALS amont the indigenous Chamorro populations on the island of Guam. BMAA was originally identified as a plant-derived natural product, and specifically found in non-flowering plants of the genus, *Cycas* (Vega & Bell, 1967). However, the origin of the metabolite was ultimately traced to an endosymbiotic species of the cyanobacterial genus, *Nostoc*, found within roots these cycads. The occurrence of BMAA in this cycad species (Spencer et al., 1987), and its apparent biomagnification by fruit bats (or "Flying Foxes") which consume the fruits of the cycad, which are, in turn, consumed as a delicacy by the Chamorro of Guam (Cox et al., 2003; discussed below), has been suggested to provide a route of exposure to the neurotoxin, and was consequently linked to ALS among the Chamorro. Indeed, subsequent studies have accordingly identified both apparent biomagnification of the metabolite in this rather short "food chain" (i.e. an approximately 10^4-fold increase from cyanobacteria to cycad to fruit bat), as well as measurable levels of BMAA in the brains of Chamorro patients that died from ALS and related syndromes (Cox et al., 2003).

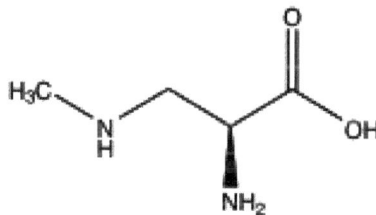

Figure 6. Chemical structure of β-Methylamino-L-Alanine (BMAA).

Toxicologically, BMAA is a recognized agonist of glutamate receptors. Staton and Bristow (1997) found that BMAA excited glutamate receptors, leading to apoptotic and necrotic cell death, in cerebellar granule cells. Subsequent studies (e.g. Rao et al., 2006; Lobner et al., 2007; Cucchiaroni et al., 2010) have confirmed a similar effect in a range of relevant neurons (e.g. spinal motor neurons, cortical neurons, dopaminergic substantia nigra pars compacta cells). More recently, however, it has been proposed that BMAA – as an amino acid – may become erroneously incorporated via translation into proteins. One of the hallmarks of several related neurodegenerative diseases (including ALS, Alzheimer's Disease, Parkinson Disease/Dementia) is the formation of misfolded protein aggregates, and it has consequently been proposed that the possible mis-incorporation of BMAA may represent an alternative mechanism of action for this putative toxin.

Although first identified in the Chamorro/ALS case, potential health concerns associated with BMAA have continued to grow with recent reports of a widespread occurrence of the metabolite among cyanobacteria, and its bioaccumulation in a wide range of systems, as well as additional epidemiological findings that link the compound to a complex of related neurodegenerative diseases. In a study by Cox et al. (2005) chemical analysis of a wide range of cyanobacteria, including marine, freshwater and terrestrial representatives, indicated that as many as 95% of the genera produce BMAA, and pointed to a potentially widespread occurrence of the metabolite. Since this study, the analytical techniques used with respect to BMAA have rapidly evolved (see 5. *Methodologies for analyis of cyanobacterial toxins in food-webs*, below). Accordingly, several investigators (e.g. Li et al., 2012) have, in fact, argued - specifically based on re-evaluation of the analytical methods previously used - that these prior estimates regarding occurrence among cyanobacteria are perhaps exaggerated. However, despite this standing controversy, a growing number of studies have concurrently pointed to the apparent bioaccumulation of the metabolite in food webs and relevant human foods (discussed below) which, along with increasing experimental evidence to support toxicological effects related to neuronal and memory function (e.g. Karlsson et al., 2009 and 2009b; Liu et al., 2009; Purdie et al., 2009 and 2009b; Karlsson et al., 2011), and links to additional clusters of these disease, have continued to fuel emerging hypotheses regarding BMAA and neurodegeneration. With regards to the latter, *post mortem* studies have identified BMAA in the brain tissues of patients who had died from ALS and Alzheimer's Diesease (AD), but not from either strictly hereditary neurodegenerative disease (e.g. Huntington's Disease) or unrelated causes (Pablo et al., 2009). Several studies have, likewise, suggested links between BMAA and so-called "sporadic" occurrence of these diseases ranging from Canadian AD patients (Murch et al., 2004) to clusters of ALS associated with exposure to water blooms in New England (Caller et al., 2009) to sporadic occurrence among Gulf War veterans purportedly exposed to BMAA through cyanobacteria in desert dust (Cox et al., 2009). As these questions regarding occurrence of BMAA among cyanobacteria, as well as its toxicological relevance, continue to be answered, it is becoming clear that understanding the potential role of food-web bioaccumulation, as a route of exposure to this metabolite, will be particularly critical.

3. Evidence for bioaccumulation of cyanobacterial toxins in aquatic food-webs

Toxins from a number of marine HAB species – particularly including diverse eukaryotic taxa within the dinoflagellates and diatoms (Bacilliariophyta) – bioaccumulate and/or biomagnify in marine food-webs, and have been clearly linked to contamination of fish and seafood, and consequent intoxication of humans and wildlife (Van Dolah, 2000). Notably, marine algal toxins are (1) frequently associated with commercially important seafood species, including filter-feeding/grazing shellfish (e.g. clams, mussels) and several plantivorous fish species, and/or (2) alternatively characterized by relatively high lipophilicity enabling uptake and storage in fat tissues as a means of biomagnifications to higher trophic levels, including marine fish species eaten by humans (Van Dolah, 2000). Relevant examples of the former include dinophysotoxins and various other metabolites associated with "diarrhetic shellfish poisoning"   (DSP), domoic acid associated with "amnesic shellfish poisoning" (ASP) and contamination of shellfish by so-called PSP toxins (i.e. STX and other PSTs, see above) derived from dinoflagellates (e.g. *Alexandrium* spp.). Examples of the latter, on the other hand, include biomagnification of ciguatoxin, and several chemically related lipophilic metabolites (e.g. maitotoxin), by various top-level predator species of fish in relation to the well documented "ciguatera poisoning."

Compared to marine HAB toxins, bioaccumulation of cyanobacterial toxins in food webs, and its consequent relevance to human and environmental health, has been relatively much less studied. There are likely several reasons for this. The most obvious is that, in contrast to the well-documented contamination of fish and other seafood by marine algal toxins, there are very few recognized cases of acute human or animal intoxication via consumption of bioaccumulated cyanobacterial toxins. It is further proposed that this may be due, in part, to less commercial fishing in freshwater water habitats - and thus consumption of freshwater fish and shellfish - compared to marine fisheries. Indeed, a recent report by the United Nations' Food and Agriculture Organization (FAO) estimated the 2008 global fisheries catch as approximately 90 million tonnes, but it was comprised of only a "record 10 million tonnes from inland waters," compared to more than 80 million tonnes from marine sources (FAO, 2010).

Regardless of the relatively limited focus on cyanobacterial toxins in freshwater fish and shellfish, a growing body of knowledge – summarized in Table 1 – does, in fact, support the occurrence of cyanobacterial toxins in a range of trophic levels, including species with direct potential for human exposure, as well as possible implications for ecosystem health (see *7. Implications for Ecosystem Health*, below). Indeed, a number of thorough reviews on the topic have recently appeared (e.g. Ibelings and Chorus, 2007; Ferrao-Filho et al., 2011; Kozlowsky-Suzuki et al., 2012). Owing to the relatively polar (i.e. water-soluble) nature of the recognized cyanobacterial toxins, it has been generally suggested that bioaccumulation in the food-web will be limited to relatively "low" trophic positions. Indeed, in freshwater food webs, this has included particularly high rates of bioaccumulation of toxins in planktivorous fish, and filter-feeding or other grazing invertebrates (Table 1). Reported concentrations of accumulated cyanobacterial toxins are, at first glance, typically quite low (Table 1). However, levels are obviously expected to vary - as shown in experimental studies (e.g. Osswald et al., 2011) - with concentrations of toxins and/or algal cell density to which animals are exposed. Moreover, it is suggested by various studies that levels may be sufficient for long-term (and consequently difficult to study) health effects, and that these reported data (as discussed further below) may underestimate - due to limitations of typical analytical methodologies, food preparation techniques used and other variables - the possible contribution of these food-borne toxins.

From inspection of the available data on the accumulation of cyanobacterial toxins in fish and shellfish (Table 1), it is clear that MCs are, by far, the most commonly reported. Indeed, MCs are generally considered the most widespread of the freshwater cyanobacterial toxins. Frequently, these data are reported in terms of "MC-LR equivalents," as typical quantitative analyses (e.g. ELISA, LC-MS) use this common variant as a reference standard, despite the fact that as many as ninety variants have been reported (see Welker and von Döhren, 2006). In addition to being among the most commonly detected of the microcystins, MC-LR is also one of the most toxic variants (Zurawell et al., 2005). That said, studies suggest variability in the uptake and detoxification of the variants. Xie et al. (2004), for example, studied MC-LR and MC-RR distribution and depuration in phytoplanktivorous carp, and proposed, based on these findings, a possible preferential uptake of MC-RR, or inhibited uptake of and/or active mechanism to "degrade" MC-LR.

Fish	Toxin(s)[a]	Tissue(s)	Toxin Conc. ($\mu g\ g^{-1}$)[b]	Reference(s)
Silverside (*Odontesthes bonariensis*)	MC-RR	Muscle	0.05 (mean) 0.34 (max)	Cazenave et al., 2005
Silver Carp (*Hypophthalmichthys molitrix*)	MC-LR/RR	Muscle	0.00025-0.097	Chen et al., 2005
	MC-LR (eq)	Muscle	0.0016	Shen et al., 2005
Carp (*Cyprinus carpio*)	MC-LR (eq)	Muscle	0.038	Li et al., 2004
	MC-LR (eq)	Muscle	0.005	Berry et al., 2011a
	ATX-a	Whole (juvenile)	0.005	Osswald et al., 2007 (experimental studies)
Goodea spp.	MC-LR (eq)	Muscle	0.157	Berry et al., 2011a
		Viscera[c]	0.867	
"Charales" (*Chirostoma* sp.)	MC-LR (eq)	Whole[c]	0.0185	Berry et al., 2011a
Redbreast Tilapia (*Tilapia rendalli*)	MC-LR (eq)	Muscle	0.002-0.337	Magalhaes et al., 2001
Nile Tilapia (*Oreochromis niloticus*)	MC-LR (eq)	Muscle	0.102	Mohammed et al., 2003
Blue Tilapia (*Oreochromis aureus*)	CYN	Muscle	0.00009	Berry et al., 2011b
	STX/PSTs	Muscle	0.00003	
Topote (*Dorosoma mexicana*)	CYN	Muscle	0.0008	Berry et al., 2011b
	STX/PSTs		0.0003	
Flounder (*Platichthys flesus*)	NOD	Muscle	0.0005-0.1	Sipia et al., 2006
Roach (*Rutilus rutilus*)	NOD	Muscle	0.0004-0.2	Sipia et al., 2006
Trout (*Oncorhynchus mykiss*)	MC-LR (eq)	Muscle	0.035	Wood et al., 2006
	ATX-a	Whole (juveniles)	3.9-23.6	Osswald et al., 2011 (experimental studies)
Yellow Perch (*Perca flavescens*)	MC-LR (eq)	Muscle	0.0008 (max)[d]	Wilson et al., 2008
Unidentified species	MC-LR (eq)	Muscle	0.04	Magalhaes et al., 2003
	NOD	Muscle	0.0007-0.025	Van Buynder et al, 2001
Shellfish				
Bivalves: Mussels				
Anodonta woodiania	MC-LR (eq)	Muscle/foot Whole[c]	0.009 (mean) 0.026 (max) 0.064	Chen & Xie, 2005a
Anodonta cygnea	STX/PSTs	Whole[c]	2.6	Pereira et al., 2004 (experimental study)
Alathyria condola	STX/PSTs	Whole[c]	57	Negri & Jones, 1995 (experimental study)
Hyriopsis cumingii	MC-LR (eq)	Muscle/foot Whole[c]	0.022 (mean) 0.039 (max) 0.188	Chen & Xie, 2005a
Cristaria plicata	MC-LR (eq)	Muscle/foot Whole[c]	(mean) 0.023 (max) 0.096	Chen & Xie, 2005a

Fish	Toxin(s)[a]	Tissue(s)	Toxin Conc. (μg g^{-1})[b]	Reference(s)
Lamprotula leai	MC-LR (eq)	Muscle/foot	0.021 (mean)	Chen & Xie, 2005a
		Whole[c]	0.058 (max)	
			0.131	
Mytilus galloprovincialis	MC-LR	Whole	1.8 (max)e	Vasconcelos, 1995
	ATX-a	Soft tissue[c]	0.006 (max)	(experimental study)
				Osswald et al., 2008 (experimental study)
Unidentified mussel species	CYN	Whole[c]	0.247	Saker et al., 2004
Unidentified mussel species	NOD	Whole[c]	2.5	Van Buynder et al., 2001
Gastropods: Snails				
Apple Snails (*Pomacea patula*	CYN	Wholec	0.003	Berry and Lind, 2010
catemacensis)	STX/PSTs	Wholec	0.001	
Crustaceans: Shrimp, Crab and Crayfish				
Crayfish (*Procambarus clarkia*)	MC-LR (eq)	Muscle	0.005 (mean)	Chen & Xie, 2005b
			0.010 (max)	
Red Claw Crayfish (*Cherax*	CYN	Muscle	0.18[f] (mean)	Saker & Eaglesham, 1999
quadricarinatus)		Hepato-	0.86[f] (mean)	
		pancreas		
Freshwater Shrimp (*Palaemon*	MC-LR (eq)	Muscle	0.006 (mean)	Chen & Xie, 2005b
modestus)		Whole	0.026 (max)	
			0.0114	
Freshwater Shrimp	MC-LR (eq)	Muscle	0.004 (mean)	Chen & Xie, 2005b
(*Macrobrachium nipponensis*)		Whole	0.012 (max)	
			0.051	
Unidentified crab species	MC-LR (eq)	Muscle	0.103	Magalhaes et al., 2003
Unidentified prawn species	CYN	Muscle	0.205	Saker et al., 2004
	NOD	Muscle	0.005-0.022	Van Buynder et al., 2001

[a] Total MC content frequently reported as MC-LR equivalents ("MC-LR(eq)" in the table).

[b] Toxin concentrations given as either range, or maximum ("max") or mean (if not otherwise indicated).

[c] Fish or shellfish eaten whole including muscle and viscera. In the case of shellfish, shell or exoskeleton/carapace is typically removed, and the inner flesh consumed.

[d] Converted from dry weight to wet weight using conversion factor of 5 as per U.S. EPA recommendation, assuming ~80% water content of fish (Holcomb et al., 1976).

[e] Conversion from dry weight to wet weight using conversion factor of 5.8 as per Ricciardi and Bourget (1998).

[f] Conversion from dry weight to wet weight using conversion factor of approximately 5 as per Headon and Hall (xxx)

Table 1. Measured concentrations of cyanobacterial toxins in freshwater fish and aquatic invertebrates eaten by humans. Adapted, in part, from Ibelings and Chorus (2007).

As shown in Table 1, concentrations of MC in these tissues are generally quite low, and might imply a consequently low concern with respect to human exposure. However, there is evidence – as discussed above - to suggest that chronic expoure to low levels of these toxins may pose concern for long-term health (e.g. increased rates of cancer). Moreover, not shown in this table is the generally higher accumulation of MCs by liver and associated organ systems due to active transport of these toxins to hepatocytes and related cells (as discussed above). Although, in the case of fish, in particular, muscle tissues (i.e. "flesh," e.g. filets, etc.) are most typically eaten, there are exceptions. Berry et al. (2011a), for example, evaluated the MC content (see Table 1) of fish caught from a persistent cyanobacterial bloom in Lake Patzcuaro (Mexico), and specifically reported considerable levels for those fish (i.e. "charales" and *Goodea* spp.) that are locally eaten in their entirety, including muscle and associated viscera. Accordingly, these results suggest that preparation technique can have a key role in assessing the potential for human exposure.

Bioaccumulation, however, is not limited to the MCs, and a growing number of studies (see recent review by Kinnear, 2010) have, for example, also reported variable levels of the hepatotoxic CYN in relevant fish and shellfish species (Table 1). In fact, soon after the identi-fication of CYN as the toxin responsible for the Palm Island Mystery (Ohtani et al., 1992), Saker and Eaglesham (1999) reported quite high levels of the toxin in both fish ("Rainbow Fish," *Melanotaenia eachemensis*) and invertebrate (i.e. "Red Claw Crayfish," *Cherax quadricarinatus*) species. Although, the former is not generally considered edible, the latter is, in fact, extensively aquacultured as freshwater "seafood" commercially. Since that time, the potential for bioac-cumulation CYN has been reported in several field and laboratory studies (Norris et al., 2001; Nogueira et al., 2004; White et al., 2006; White et al., 2007), although most have focused on species not – or rarely (e.g. Swan Mussel, *Anodonta cygnea;* Saker et al., 2004) – eaten by humans, and therefore, not generally relevant to human diet and health. As a notable excep-tion, Seifert et al. (2007) reported CYN from Eel-Tailed Catfish (*Tandanus tandanus*), an omnivorous species of game fish; the toxin, however, was not detected in several other less planktivorous species of fish (e.g. perch, bass). More recently, evaluation of CYN in the endorheic lake system of Lake Catemaco (Mexico) identified the toxin in species of both finfish (Berry et al., 2012) and relevant species of invertebrates (i.e. freshwater snails; Berry and Lind, 2010) consumed in this region.

Although not as well recognized (nor investigated), emerging evidence suggests that cyano-bacterial neurotoxins may also accumulate in relevant freshwater species (Table 1). With regards to human health, STX and related "paralytic shellfish toxins" (PSTs) are – based on their well-described association to intoxication via seafood – perhaps of most obvious concern. STX/PSTs have widely documented as contaminants of marine shellfish, and particularly bivalves, representing a recognized concern for public health (Van Dolah, 2000). More recently, there have been increasing reports of STX/PSTs in fish, and particularly species of "pufferfish" (Family Tetraodontidae), alongside the toxicologically related (i.e. voltage-gated sodium channel blocking) tetrodotoxins that have been well described from these species. Similar to contamination of shellfish, however, it has been recently shown (Landsberg et al., 2006) that marine dinoflagellates (e.g. *Pyrodinium* spp.) are likely the source of STX/PSTs in the case of these typically estuarine fish. That said, studies (Negri and Jones, 1995; Pereira et al., 2004) have shown that – like marine bivalves – freshwater mussels can also accumulate cyanobacterially derived STX/PSTs. Although the mussel species (*Alathyria condola*) examined in these studies (e.g. Negri and Jones, 1995) are not one typically eaten by humans (although frequently by other animal species), more recent studies (Pereira et al., 2004) have measured considerable levels of PSTs (fed via PST-producing *Aphanizomenon issatschenkoi*) in the Swan Mussel (*Anodonta cygnea*) that, as previously mentioned, is occasionally consumed within certain human populations in Europe and elsewhere. Even more recently, while evaluating the apparent bioaccumulation of CYN associated with a bloom of *C. raciborskii* in Lake Catemaco (Mexico), it was found that both edible "tegogolo" snails (Berry and Lind, 2010), and locally consumed species of freshwater finfish (Berry et al., 2012), were found to accumulate STX/PSTs. These studies, furthermore, point to a shared source of CYN and STX/PSTs, and specifically *C. raciborskii* that is abundant in this lake system (Berry et al., 2012).

In addition to STX/PSTs, cyanobacteria are known to produce several other neurotoxic metabolites, including (as discussed above) the toxicologically related ATX-a and anatoxin-a(s). Compared to other cyanotoxins, the neurotoxic ATX-a is generally considered chemically quite labile, and it is generally anticipated that the potential for bioaccumulation of this unstable toxin would be, accordingly, rather low. That said, in experimental studies, it has been shown that both fish – including trout (*Oncorhynchus mykiss*; Osswald et al., 2011) and juvenile carp (*Cyprinus carpio*; Osswald et al, 2007) - and shellfish (e.g. mussel, *Mytilus galloprovincialis*; Osswald et al., 2008) can, in fact, accumulate the toxin presented in either dissolved (added to tank water) or cell-bound form. Moreover, in a recent study (Mejean et al., 2010), bioaccumulation of this toxin in the giant clam (*Tridacna maxima*), frequently consumed in the South Pacific, was evaluated in relation to several "ciguatera-like" intoxication cases reported in the region, and found to contain the potently toxic analog, homoanatoxin-a, as well as possible traces of ATX-a. Though confirmation of these toxins, as the causative agent of these reported poisoning, remains to be made, this study represents of the very few examples of possible acute intoxication by a food-borne cyanobacterial toxin.

Similarly, despite the emerging picture of its biomagnification in terrestrial species (e.g. fruit bats feeding on cycads; see above) over the past several decades, as well as the particularly conspicuous abundance of cyanobacteria in aquatic systems, relatively limited attention has been paid to the possible bioaccumulation of neurotoxic BMAA in aquatic food-webs. Several recent studies (Jonasson et al., 2010; Brand et al., 2010; Mondo et al., 2012), however, have suggested both accumulation, and possible biomagnifications of BMAA in marine systems, including those species (i.e. fish, seafood) directly related to human health. In one very recent case, the fins of several species of sharks, as "apex" marine predators, were examined, and found to be laden with BMAA (Mondo et al, 2012), and consequently proposed to present – via widespread consumption in the form of "sharkfin soup" – a potentially important route of exposure to this toxin, and thus a public health concern, in Asian countries where shark fins are considered a delicacy. Likewise, one of these studies, specifically evaluating BMAA in South Florida waters, and more specifically including Caloosahatchee River, did, in fact, detect this putatively toxic amino acid in both invertebrate (i.e. mussel) and fish species, including those consumed – at least occasionally - by humans (e.g. bass, bowfin, alligator gar) in this freshwater system. Most interestingly perhaps, it was found in this, as well as concurrent studies of marine food-webs, that measured BMAA levels were, in fact, higher in higher trophic levels suggesting the possibility of biomagnifications of this metabolite. As a highly water-soluble amino acid - with a low octanol/water-partitioning coefficient - it is not expected that BMAA would biomagnify by conventional means (i.e. via deposition in fat bodies, etc.); however, alternative mechanisms to this end are proposed (discussed below).

Finally, it bears mention that a growing number of studies have documented apparent uptake of cyanobacterial toxins by various plant species via toxin-contaminated irrigation water. Uptake of cyanobacterial toxins by plants was first suggested in a study by Pflugmacher et al. (2001) that reported both uptake - and associated metabolism - of MC-LR by the water reed (*Phragmites australis*). Subsequently, uptake and metabolism was similarly found to occur in several agriculturally important species including various legumes, maize, wheat and alfalfa (Peuthert et al., 2007). Similarly, it was recently reported that various cruciferous vegetables (e.g. *Brassica* spp., *Sinapsis alba*) are capable of accumulating 10-21% of CYN provided to roots, reaching as high as 49 μg/g (fresh weight) in the leafy components (Kittler et al., 2012). Although not bioaccumulation *per se* (i.e. via trophic transfer), the rather high levels of these compounds found in exposed plants, and specifically several agriculturally important crop plant species, suggest that exposure to cyanotoxins through plant crops may pose a very real public health concern.

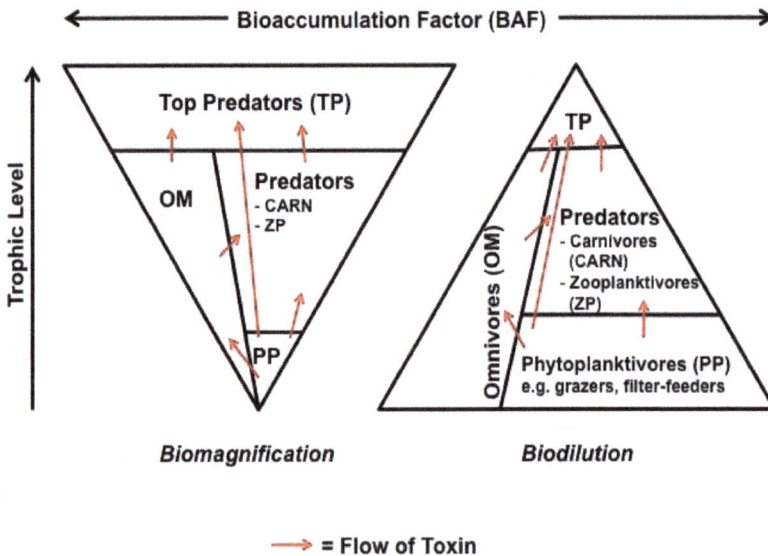

Figure 7. Depiction of biomagnification (left) and biodilution (right) of toxins in food-webs.

4. Trophic transfer and bioavailability of cyanobacterial toxins

Despite emerging evidence to suggest the bioaccumulation of cyanobacterial toxins within food webs (as summarized above; Table 1), relatively little is known regarding the process of trophic transfer, and the subsequent bioavailability of "food-derived" cyanotoxins. For lipophilic contaminants, including recognized anthropogenic pollutants (e.g. PCBs, DDT) and even some HAB toxins (e.g. ciguatoxins), uptake and storage in fat tissues have been largely implicated as a means of trophic transfer. However, there is no clear mechanism for bioaccumulation and/or biomagnification of the most widely recognized and, moreover, typically water-soluble cyanobacterial toxins. Likewise, although growing evidence suggests that cyanobacterial toxins are, in fact, present in relevant components of freshwater food webs (see section 3. *Evidence for bioaccumulation of cyanobacterial toxins in food-webs*, above), a very limited number of studies have investigated whether toxins contained within ingested tissues are, in fact, released, available and/or taken up in the digestive process. The following sections will summarize the current state of knowledge regarding both of these aspects.

4.1. Trophic transfer

As discussed in the previous section, a growing number of studies do, indeed, suggest that cyanobacterial toxins are transferred via dietary/trophic transfer within aquatic food-webs. It has been shown, in particular, that a range of phytoplanktivorous species, including zooplankton, fish, benthic grazers and filter-feeders consume toxin-laden algal cells, and directly accumulate these toxins. Alternatively, it has been shown (Karjalainen et al., 2003) that certain species, specifically including zooplankton, can accumulate, i.e. *bioconcentrate*, dissolved toxins directly from water as might be found, in particular, during algal bloom senescence. However, given the generally water-soluble (i.e. non-lipophilic) nature of the best known cyanobacterial toxins (see 2. *Recognized cyanobacterial toxins: chemistry and toxicology*, above), as well as currently available data on the apparent accumulation of these toxins within food webs (see 3. *Evidence for accumulation of cyanobacterial toxins aquatic food-webs*, above), it has been largely argued that transfer of these toxins follows a trophic pattern of *biodilution* rather than biomagnification (e.g. Ibelings et al., 2005; Ibelings and Chorus, 2007; Kozlowsky-Suzuki et al., 2012; Fig. 7). In a very recent, and particularly thorough, meta-analysis of existing data by Kozlowsky-Suzuki et al. (2012), it was shown that biodilution generally prevails. However, the authors of this study do highlight several exceptions and related caveats with relevant implications for potential exposure to toxins via food webs. Likewise, although concerns regarding human exposure to aquatic toxins – particularly in freshwater systems – are most frequently focused on higher trophic levels (i.e. sport and commercially caught fish species) as sources of toxins, a growing number of studies (Ibelings and Chorus, 2007; Berry and Lind, 2009; Berry et al., 2011; Berry et al., 2012) have documented accumulation of cyanobacterial toxins by species from lower trophic levels (i.e. freshwater shellfish, phytoplanktivorous fish) that are, indeed, consumed by humans, such that lack of biomagnification would not preclude possible human dietary exposure.

The potential for trophic transfer of cyanobacterial toxins is, generally speaking, controlled by three interrelated factors: *selection, chemical availability, toxin uptake* and *detoxification/elimination* (Fig. 8). Chemical availability will be discussed in the next section (*4.2. Bioavailability*). With regard to the former (i.e. selection), this factor would be most likely expected to be limited to initial consumption of toxin-producing algal cells by planktivores (that can subsequently serve as vectors for the toxins). This would be expected since production of toxins by cyanobacteria cells has been suggested to be linked to possible chemical defenses (i.e. feeding deterrency) against potential grazer, and evidence (see below) does, in fact, suggest that toxins may deter potential phytoplanktivorous grazers. As a corollary of this, it is suggested by this avoidance that potential grazers are capable of "detecting" the presence of toxins in algal cells. On the other hand, little or no evidence exists to suggest that toxin subsequent present in animal tissues can be so detected, and thus it is generally assumed that selection further "up the chain" is not a factor in higher trophic transfer. That said, other aspects of feeding behavior, including both general feeding preferences/strategies (e.g. herbivory versus carnivory), and more specific behaviors, particularly including selection of certain tissues by predators (e.g. preference of human consumers toward fish muscle versus other organs/tissues), might be argued to contribute to selection, and consequently the potential for trophic transfer.

A preponderance of evidence, in fact, supports a possible avoidance of toxigenic cyanobacteria by phytoplanktivores. In particular, selectivity with regards to trophic transfer is perhaps best demonstrated by numerous studies that have investigated feeding by zooplankton, and particularly *Daphnia* spp., as a widespread cladoceran micrograzer, in relation to the MCs. Microcystins have been shown to be toxic to *Daphnia* and other micrograzers, and toxicity has been shown to specifically correlate with rate of ingestion of the toxin. However, subsequent studies – specifically using "knock-out" non-toxic strains of *Microcystis* – have also, in contrast, indicated that *Daphnia* may not have the ability to distinguish toxic versus non-toxic algal cells (Rohrlack et al., 2001). Moreover, it has been generally found that interaction between grazers and their cyanobacterial prey are dependent on class of grazer (e.g. micro- versus mesozooplankton), species and even inter-specific genetic differences (Kurmayer and Jüttner, 1999; Davis and Gobler, 2011). More recently, it has been proposed (e.g. Wilson et al., 2005 and 2006; Lemaire et al., 2012) that differences in the observed feeding deterrence, relative to toxin content, may be explained by so-called "genotype x genotype interactions" whereby effects on feeding behavior are determined by the combination of grazer genotype (e.g. tolerance or susceptibility to toxin) and algal genotype (i.e. toxic or non-toxic). Finally, studies have suggested (e.g. Kurmayer and Jüttner, 1999; Reinikainen et al., 2001) that avoidance of potentially toxic cyanobacterial cells may be related to currently unknown, and particularly lipophilic, metabolites rather than recognized toxins (e.g. MCs). Understanding of the role of selection in trophic transfer, therefore, will rely on our increasing knowledge of genetic and chemical variability of both cyanobacteria and their grazers.

Even if toxin-containing items are selected for ingestion, however, several lines of evidence suggest both rather limited uptake of diet-derived toxin, as well as active and passive mechanisms for detoxification and/or elimination of these toxins, which together would be expected to limit the potential for trophic transfer. Understanding the contribution of these factors to trophic transfer, requires knowledge of – and/or means to investigate - the physiological, cellular and possible molecular processes involved in both uptake and potential detoxification/ elimination. In the cases of MCs, for example, it has been suggested by multiple studies that the gastrointestinal tract, and particularly mid-gut wall, of fish may be an important site for toxin absorption (Chen et al., 2007; Dyble et al., 2011). Given the assumption that bioaccumu- lation is generally limited to lower trophic levels, it is not perhaps surprising, however, that most insight in this regard has been, likewise, largely limited to phytoplanktivore models. In order, for example, to evaluate the uptake (and subsequent elimination) of MC-LR by fish, in relation to possible human exposure, specifically using the juvenile yellow perch (*Perca flavescens*) model, Dyble et al. (2011) fed known doses of the toxin to fish orally via diet (i.e. "toxin-doped" pellets), and determined concentration and distribution within relevant tissues (i.e. muscle and liver) over time. Consistent with active transport of MCs to (for subsequent detoxification in) hepatocytes, higher levels were found in fish livers, and kinetically speaking, achieved a maximum level in liver cells (8-10 hours following dosing) prior to a subsequent peak in muscle tissue (12-16 hours post-dosing). Moreover, the concentrations measured represented orders of magnitude lower levels than those expected if the entire dose was assimilated. Moreover, roughly equivalent concentrations were observed for two doses used (5 and 20 µg), suggesting a possible maximum capacity for uptake. Furthermore, studies showed a rapid increase in the toxin concentration (dependent in magnitude on dose) following peak levels measured in the fish tissues (after approximately 10 hours), implying a rather rapid elimination of the toxin by excretion (i.e. urine, feces). These finding support both rather limited uptake, and rapid elimination of the toxin, however, it should be noted that these data also correspond to a single dosing of the fish, whereas in aquatic habitats (i.e. during blooms, or through persistent occurrence of toxic cyanobacteria) it would be expected that possible grazers (and even other higher trophic levels) would be exposed more continuously to toxins, such that the effective "window" of time for trophic transfer would be considerably longer.

As pointed-out, the initial step for trophic transfer (from cyanobacterial cell to grazer) might be expected to represent, in terms of selectivity, uptake and detoxification/elimination, a rather distinct process compared to subsequent uptake by higher trophic levels. To understand this higher-level transfer, therefore, it is necessary to evaluate the role of toxin derived from primary consumer with respect to secondary (and subsequent) consumers. In a particularly elegant example, Karjalainen et al. (2005) experimentally demonstrated uptake of NOD by planktivorous fish larvae (i.e. Northern Pike) and invertebrate (i.e. mysid shrimp, *Neomysis integer*) via pre-exposure of relevant zooplankton prey to the toxin both in pure form, and as cell-free extracts of *N. spumigens* (as would be representative of the toxin released by decaying blooms). Prior studies had shown that zooplankton accumulate NOD directly from water (Karjalainen et al., 2003). In these subsequent studies, equal amounts of NOD (approximately 0.20 ng produced by an individual per 24 h) were detected in fecal pellets of pike larvae - suggesting diet derived uptake and passage of the toxin - fed zooplankton exposed to both pure toxin and NOD-containing extracts. Moreover, the authors of the study utilized radiola- beled NOD (i.e. ^{3}H-dihydronodularin) to quantify the transfer of the toxin from zooplankton to planktivores. Indeed, radiolabel was detected in both *N. integer* and pike larvae fed zooplankton, previously exposed to ^{3}H-NOD, with a maximum calculated accumulation of the toxin at 12 h (0.31 ng/individual) and 48 h (0.47 ng/individual), respectively, for the two species. Levels of NOD calculated based on these studies, however, were quite low (approximately 0.12% and 0.03%, respectively, for shrimp and fish larvae) compared to the amounts predicted based on measured ingestion rate and concentration of toxin in zooplankton. These results are, therefore, generally consistent with a proposed biodilution, rather than biomagnifications, of this toxin within this food-chain. Furthermore, although ingestion rates were quite different (i.e. more than 5-fold higher) for fish larvae compared to shrimp, both accumulated rather similar levels (i.e. concentration per weight or individual) of the toxin. Accordingly, these studies point to both a difference in the type of potential planktivore vector (i.e. fish versus invertebrate systems), as well as a likely role of uptake and/or detoxification (and subsequent elimination) of the toxin in relation to the observed biodilution.

In addition to understanding physiological, cellular and molecular aspects of potential grazers/ predators, uptake and detoxification can also be closely tied to the chemistry of the toxin. Certainly, among the cyanobacterial toxins, the potential for uptake, and subsequent detoxi-fication/elimination, might be expected – due the chemically diverse nature of these com-pounds – to vary considerably with this chemical variability. This is most obviously exemplified by the distinction of so-called "hepatotoxins" (e.g. CYN, MCs) that, as implied by this classification, and unlike other cyanotoxins (e.g. PSTs, ATX-a, BMAA), are actively transported via characterized organic anion transporter (OAT) proteins to hepatocytes for subsequent detoxification/elimination. However, even with toxin families, variability in uptake and elimination has been reported. For example, in studies on the uptake of MCs, Xie et al. (2004) compared relative distribution following dosing with two common variants, namely MC-LR and MC-RR, in phytoplanktivorous silver carp. Interestingly, dietary exposure to MC-LR and MC-RR (in algal cells) resulted in considerably higher levels of the latter distributed in various tissues, but rather limited tissue concentration/distribution of the former, and more toxic, variant (Xie et al., 2004). Moreover, detection of relative amounts of the two variants in gut and feces specifically supported an apparent barrier to uptake of MC-LR, compared to the less toxic MC-RR (Xie et al, 2004). It should be pointed-out, however, that results in this phytoplanktivorous model differ substantially from similar studies in a generally carnivorous fish model, namely rainbow trout, particularly with respect to apparently rapid uptake of MC-LR by the latter species, and consequently suggest a role of both consumer species, and differential species physiology, relative to the potential for uptake (and subse-quent trophic transfer). Finally, uptake (and subsequent trophic transfer) may even be determined, in part, by chemical presentation of the toxin. For example, it has been shown that in a benthic grazer model, namely the snail, *Lymnaea stagnalis,* that MCs are more readily taken-up from ingested cyanobacterial cells compared to dissolved toxin (Lance et al., 2010a). Furthermore, concurrent studies comparing the fate of MC-LR presented in either dissolved or cell-bound form (Lance et al., 2010b) suggested that, whereas no toxin from ambient/ dissolved dosings was found covalently bound in tissues, as much as 67% of cell-derived MCs were accumulated via covalent binding (to targed PPase enzymes) representing a potentially considerable reservoir of the toxin for subsequent trophic transfer (as discussed further below).

The potential for trophic transfer is not likely limited to the most studied cyanobacterial hepatotoxins (i.e. MCs). Although relatively few studies have evaluated their bioaccumulation, the transfer of the neurotoxic STX/PSTs, for example, has been studied with respect to its accumulation in marine animals, and specifically in relation to non-cyanobacterially (i.e. marine dinoflagellate) derived toxin. As a particularly important vector for PSTs, several filter-feeding mollusks are recognized to accumulate toxin-containing algal cells, and represent a possible route for both direct exposure (i.e. "shellfish" consumption), as well as possible indirect exposure to these toxins (i.e. trophic transfer to, and consumption of, secondary consumers/vectors, e.g. fish). There is, in fact, emerging (albeit currently limited) evidence to suggest that these neurotoxins may be transferred, to some extent, from filter-feeding invertebrates to higher trophic levels. In particular, however, these studies suggest that biotransformation via metabolism of PSTs – represented, as a group, by as many as fifty variants (Wiese et al., 2010) - may be a critical consideration. In studies by Kwong et al. (2006), black sea bream were exposed to green-lipped mussels, previously exposed to the PST-producing dinoflagellate, *Alexandrium fundyense*. Through these studies, it was generally found that relatively little PST was transferred to the fish, and that the toxins were rapidly depurated after transferring to toxin-free mussels. Mooreover, toxin profiles suggested considerable biotransformation, and particularly conversion of C2 to C1 variants (see 2.2.2. *Saxitoxins and "Paralytic Shellfish Toxins,"* above). Likewise, subsequent studies (Costa et al., 2010) using white seabream, similarly exposed to PST-contaminated cockles, confirmed the rather low uptake of the toxin, and additionally reported an apparently selective uptake/elimination and/or biotransformation such that only B1 and dcSTX were found in fish. This conversion and/or selective uptake/elimination during trophic transfer would have clear implications for subsequent bioavailability of this neurotoxin, and associated health concerns, as there is considerable variability in the toxicity of the PST congeners. Most generally, these studies point to the importance of the vectors (e.g. fish versus shellfish) for the toxin.

Before moving on, to consider bioavailability, perhaps the one exception to the observed pattern of biodilution, which consequently bears discussion, appears to be the trophic transfer of BMAA. In the limited studies that have investigated BMAA in marine and freshwater foodwebs, it was shown, in fact, that levels of the toxic amino acid were higher for top trophic levels (e.g. predatory fish) compared to lower trophic levels (e.g. Brand et al., 2010; Jonasson et al., 2010). In a recent study, for example, Jonasson et al. (2010) examined BMAA within food webs of the Baltic Sea, and reported a discernible positive correlation between levels of the toxin and trophic level. It seems likely, though, that the pattern is not quite as simple as classic biomagnification. For example, the Jonasson et al. (2010) and other studies (e.g. Brand et al., 2010) also suggest particularly high levels for benthic versus pelagic species (of both vertebrates and invertebrates). These studies also suggest differences in tissue distribution of the toxin with highest levels of BMAA observed in brain compared to, for example, muscle, and, therefore, underscore the importance of feeding ecology within food-webs, as well as the likely important role of subsequent bioavailability (including uptake and metabolism) and tissue distribution of toxins, in regards to trophic transfer.

Detoxification/Elimination

Selection ⟶ Chemical   ↗ Uptake   ↘ Bioaccumulation
             Availability

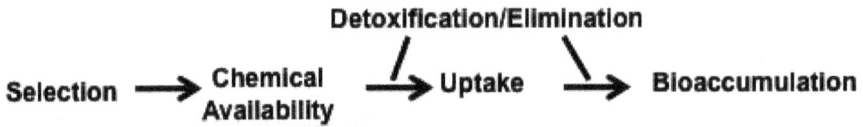

Figure 8. Factors affecting trophic transfer and bioavailabily of cyanobacterial toxins in food webs.

4.2. Bioavailability

Just as selection, chemical availability, uptake and detoxification/elimination would determine trophic transfer of cyanobacterial toxins through food-webs, these factors are, likewise, expected to primarily determine the bioavailability of these toxins to human as would be ostensibly considered – with respect to the current discussion of emerging public health concerns – the "top predator" in this regard. Although not perhaps, strictly speaking, a "bioavailability factor" selectivity with respect to human consumption can certainly contribute to the potential for exposure to food-borne cyanotoxins. In a general sense, several Tiers of selectivity can dictate the likelihood of exposure (in concert with other bioavailability factors) to cyanobacterial toxins in food. As mentioned previously, the generally limited consumption of freshwater fish and shellfish, relative to much more common consumption of fish and other seafood from marine sources, would be expected – given the recognized abundance of cyanobacterial toxins in freshwater systems – to, likewise, generally limit the possible exposure to these toxins. Even within freshwater systems, the relative consumption of fish and shellfish species from lower trophic (i.e. phytoplanktivorous) levels of food webs would similarly contribute to the possible exposure. However, as detailed above (3. *Evidence for bioaccumulation of cyanobacterial toxins in aquatic food-webs*), there are certainly numerous documented cases of toxin bioaccumulation by phytoplanktivorous species of freshwater fish and invertebrates (e.g. snails, bivalves) which are, indeed, consumed by humans. Finally, even with species, and particularly fish species, selectivity of certain tissues/organs can influence possible exposure scenarios. Most notably, with respect to this latter tier, the general preference for fish flesh (i.e. muscle) versus viscera (e.g. toxin-accumulating liver, etc.) has clear implications for the potential for exposure to these toxins. Selectivity aside, however, the real issue of bioavailability is clearly expected to be most closely linked to those biochemical and physiological processes of digestion (i.e. uptake) and possible detoxification/elimination.

Cyanobacterial toxins, as discussed previously (see 2. *Recognized cyanobacterial toxins: chemistry and toxicology*), have been traditionally classified based on their "target" organs. Specifically, the most commonly studied cyanotoxins have been grouped into those targeting either the liver/hepatocytes or brain/CNS, respectively, in the case of the so-called "hepatotoxins" (i.e. MCs, CYN) and "neurotoxins" (i.e. STX/PSTs, ATX-a, BMAA). Based on both evaluation of toxin distribution (e.g. high levels of MC and CYN in livers of exposed animals), and recognized manifestations of toxicity (e.g. neurotoxicity of STX/PSTs and ATX-a), following exposure, effective bioavailability to these organs is largely assumed. In the case of the MCs, however, active transport of the toxin to hepatocytes has actually been shown to be specifically facilitated by a family of organic anion transporter polypeptides (OATPs) that are particularly abundant in these cells (Fischer et al., 2005; Lu et al., 2008; Fischer et al., 2010), and even suggested to play a role in the selective uptake of certain MC congeners by hepatocytes (Fischer et al., 2010). That said, OATPs are, in fact, found in other cell types, and it has been also been suggested, for example, that OATPs in the brain may allow passage of MCs across the blood-brain barrier (Fischer et al., 2005), and they have, accordingly, been linked to oxidative stress in neurons, and subsequent effects on short and long term memory, caused by the toxin in a rat model (Maidana et al., 2006). Although, likewise, considered a hepatotoxin, and found to accumulate primarily in hepatocytes, the mechanism for CYN is not currently known. On the other hand, studies of neurotoxic cyanotoxins have demonstrated the apparent ability of STX/ PSTs, ATX-a and BMAA to cross the blood-brain barrier (BBB) as a fundamentally limiting step for all toxins that affect the CNS. For example, STX - as a representative PST - was detected through brain tissues (from sacrificed animals), and consequently suggested to cross the BBB, following both intravenous (Andrinolo et al., 1999) and intraperitoneal (Cervantes Cianca et al., 2007) in mammalian (i.e. cat, rat) models. In support of the implied passage to - as suggested by its purported toxicity, and measured presence in the brain - studies of BMAA, dating back more than twenty years, and well prior to the recent resurgence of interest in this putative neurotoxin, not only have shown that this unusual amino acid is capable of crossing the BBB, but that transport might be specifically facilitated by large neutral amino acid carriers at the blood-brain interface (Smith et al., 1992).

Although the potential for bioavailability of cyanobacterial toxins to target organs is implied by their patterns of bioaccumulation, and observed toxic effects on certain organ systems, as well as limited number of *in vivo* studies, most studies have focused on either exposure to toxins via water ingestion, or in the case of laboratory studies, have examined fate of the toxin, following intraperitoneal injection, or related forms of administering the toxin. The actual bioavailability, with respect to foodborne toxins, is obviously limited by the prior chemical availability (discussed further below), as determined by release (from food), uptake and detoxification/elimination, prior to transport to target organs. To-date, however, studies on uptake and detoxification/elimination of cyanobacterial toxins derived from foods are essentially non-existent.

Rather, as with other aspects of health concerns regarding cyanobacterial toxins, the very few studies that have considered bioavailablity of these toxins – and implicitly uptake and detoxification/elimination as key factors - have generally relied on data, and subsequent inferences, extrapolated from water-borne cyanotoxins, including dissolved or algal cell-derived toxins. Most notably, several authors have considered World Health Organization (WHO) guidelines regarding acceptable concentrations of MCs - as the clearly most widespread cyanobacterial toxin family - in water, and subsequently derived guideline values for total daily intake (TDI) of this toxin. Values of TDI are generally based on observed *no* or *lowest observable adverse effect levels* (NOAELs and LOAELs, respectively) from very a very limited number of oral exposure studies in mouse and pig models (Falconer et al., 1994; Fawell et al., 1999). Accordingly, acceptable values for lifetime, one-time and occasional TDI have been estimated, respectively, as 0.04, 25 and 0.4 µg per kg body weight

(Fromme et al., 1999; Ibelings and Chorus, 2007). In a particular thorough treatment, Ibelings and Chorus (2007) extrapolated this to proposed guideline values that incorporate exposure via both water and food (and particularly "seafood"). Acknowledging a high variability in the amounts of food consumed, as well as other relevant factors (e.g. body weight), the guidelines estimated in this way ranged greatly from 6 μg/kg for daily lifetime exposures to 1900 μg/kg for acute (i.e. "one-time") exposures for adults, with corresponding lower values for children (i.e. 0.08-250 μg/kg body weight). That said, all such values regarding intake (and, implicitly, the necessary consideration of subsequent uptake and detoxification/elimination) are, as mentioned, solely based on (very limited) estimates derived from oral exposure to a single toxin in water, and out of necessity, ignore bioavailability from a more complex "matrix" of animal tissues. Of course, as more information is obtained with respect to the uptake, and subsequent detoxification/elimination, of toxins from animal-based diet, it is hoped that a more realistic understanding of the potential for food-borne exposure will emerge. In particular, a clearer understanding of these toxins in relation to the dietary matrix, and consequently those factors (e.g. digestion, cellular uptake) that determine fate is still needed.

Aside from considerations of uptake and subsequent detoxification/elimination, as it relates to bioavailablity, it has become clear that, in certain cases, the potential (or lack thereof) for human bioavailability may be considerably affected by *chemical* availability. This has been specifically studied, to-date, in two cases: (1) irreversible, covalent binding of MCs to PPases targets; and (2) erroneous translation and consequent incorporation of BMAA into proteins. In the latter case, for example, it has been suggested that BMAA, as a non-essential amino acid, can be potential incorporated (via faulty translation mechanisms) into growing protein chains. Specifically, investigating this possibility, Murch et al. (2004) analyzed BMAA in cyanobacteria, and brains of patients who died of ALS/Parkinsonism dementia complex (along with cycads and flying foxes from Guam as suggested vectors for the toxin), both with and without prior acid hydrolysis. Measured levels of BMAA were on the order of 10- to 240-fold higher following acid hydrolysis, suggesting an apparent release of this amino acid from proteins in these samples. This finding, therefore, not only supported incorporation of BMAA into proteins as a mechanism of toxicity (see *1. Recognized cyanobacterial toxins: chemistry and toxicology*, above), as well as possible limitations in the analytical methodologies applied to this toxin (discussed further below; see *Methodologies for evaluating cyanobacterial toxins in food-webs*), but furthermore, pointed to an "endogenous reservoir" of the toxin. Such a reservoir would specifically provide a means of "slow release," of the toxin as possible mechanism for BMAA bioavailability, and would correlate with the generally late onset of these diseases. It is, of course, implied from these studies that BMAA bound in proteins in this way would, in fact, be readily available following peptidolytic digestion, however, this remains to be confirmed.

As discussed earlier in the chapter (see *1. Recognized cyanobacterial toxins: chemistry and toxicology*), MCs are known to bind to PPases found ubiquitously in cells of all known organisms. In addition, however, to reversible binding to the active site of PPases, it has been shown (MacKintosh et al., 1995; Pereira et al., 2012) that the toxin, once in the active site, will form covalent bonds (via Michael addition) between the Mdha (present in many MCs) and a cysteine (Cys273) found in the active site of Ser/Thr Type 1/2A PPases. Accordingly, it has been suggested that a portion of all Mdha-containing MCs might become bound in this way (Williams et al., 1997a and 1997b; Yuan et al., 2006; Suchy and Berry, 2012), and indeed, estimates - based on specific analysis of the bound toxin (see 5. *Methodologies for analysis of cyanobacterial toxins in the food web*) - suggest a considerable pool of so bound MCs. In classic studies by Williams et al. (1997a and 1997b), for example, analysis of bound MC demonstrated that as little as 24% of MC administered (via i.p. injection) to salmon could be recovered by conventional solvent extraction and analyses, and likewise that as much as 10,000-fold more of the toxin, measured in Dungeness crab larvae, could be detected in the presumptively "bound form" compared to the "free form." More recently, Hilborn et al. (2007) measured both free and bound MCs in dialysis patients exposed (through improperly treated water) to the toxin, and similarly measured significantly higher levels when total (i.e. free and bound) levels were compared to those of the unbound toxin (i.e. measured by solvent extraction and conventional detection, e.g. ELISA), and specifically that only approximately 8-51% of MCs were measured by the latter method, compared to the former.

A preponderance of evidence continues to suggest that bound MCs do, indeed, represent a considerable pool of the toxin, however, very few studies have investigated whether these bound MCs are, in fact, biologically available. To address this question, Smith et al. (2010) recently investigated the potential for digestive enzymes to release covalently bound MC from PPases. Whereas digestive proteases (e.g. trypsin, chymotrypsin, pepsin) were found, as expected, to effectively hydrolyze a control protein (i.e. angiotensin), they had no effect on the cyclic peptides (i.e. MC-LR and MC-LY). Furthermore, based on the assumption that protein-bound MCs could be partially released by these peptidolytic enzymes, the investigators synthesized four Cys-containing MC-oligopeptide adducts, specifically predicted for hydrolytic digestion of the PPase active site by these enzymes, and subsequently evaluated them for toxicity (i.e. inhibition of protein phosphatase). Although inhibition was reduced (compared to MC-LR alone) to approximately 58% for MC-peptide adducts - composed of the cyclic MC-LR covalently bound, via cysteine, to predicted tetra- and nonomeric peptide fragments - this residual biological activity supports the possible bioavailability of potentially toxic bound MCs following protein hydrolysis in the digestive system. Interestingly, concurrent studies (Zhang et al., 2010) evaluated the effects of cooking as an alternative mechanism for release of covalently bound MCs with respect to potential availability of the toxin. In these studies, it was specifically found that levels of MC-LR in carp (injected intraperitoneally with the toxin) were significantly higher (approximately 4-fold) in both muscle tissue and water following boiling, compared to lyophilization and subsequent solvent extraction only, and it was suggested that elevated levels were due to release of covalently bound toxin from these tissues. Although such studies do point to the possible chemical availability of covalent bound toxins, clearly further studies are needed to fully elucidate the possible bioavailability of these in relation to human exposure.

5. Methodologies for evaluating cyanobacterial toxins in the food-web

Techniques for chemical detection and quantitative analysis of cyanobacterial toxins have evolved alongside recognition of their potential health impacts. The majority of the previously established analytical methods (e.g. HPLC-UV, LC-MS, ELISA) have, therefore, primarily focused on the identification of toxin in algal cells and/or dissolved in water, with water (i.e. contamination of drinking water, recreational exposure) being an established direct route of exposure. As for these applications, analytical techniques applied to measurement of toxins in food webs have, likewise, generally focused on two approaches (Sivonen, 2008; Humpage et al., 2010). The first, and arguably most common - given the complex nature of these biological matrices (discussed further below) - has included a number of so-called "hyphenated meth-ods" in which analytical separation, including liquid chromatography (LC) and capillary electrophoresis (CE), in particular, are coupled to one or more suitable detection/measurement technique, including UV absorbance, fluorescent derivatization/detection (FL), mass spec-trometry (MS) and electrochemical detection. Alternatively, with the relatively recent com-mercial availability of enzyme-linked immunosorbent assay (ELISA) kits for several cyanobacterial toxins, as well as growing understanding of the toxicology of these metabolites - and thus development of several biochemical techniques (e.g. protein phosphatase inhibition assays for MCs) - these bioanalytical techniques have been also applied to the evaluation of cyanobacterial toxin in relation to food-webs and bioaccumulation (e.g. Lance et al., 2006; Berry and Lind, 2010; Berry et al., 2011; Berry et al., 2012). However, unlike detection of several non-cyanobacterial, marine algal toxins as contaminants of fish and seafood for which there are validated analytical techniques, there are presently no validated methods for evaluating cyanobacterial toxins in biological matrices.

Both of the aforementioned approaches present potential limitations, but generally speaking, it would be argued that the two consequently complement one another. In particular, ELISA-based methods have been somewhat criticized (Metcalf et al., 2000; Mountfort et al., 2005) as being potentially susceptible to non-targeted molecules (i.e. matrix components) in samples that may immunologically cross-react with antibodies, or alternatively not being able to distinguish more toxic variants among co-occurring congeners within toxin groups. As antibodies used in ELISAs are typically generated in relation to a particular representative variant of these toxins, relying on chemical similarity and cross-reactivity to detect other variants, they do not enable co-occurring congeners to be distinguished from total toxin concentrations. This latter limitation is perhaps best exemplified by the ELISA-based analysis of MCs. Although commercially available ELISAs for MCs exploit the generally conserved Adda moiety found in most variants (Fig. 2), MC variants lacking (or containing modified versions of) Adda have been reported (Namikoshi et al., 1990 and 1992; Sivonen et al., 1992; Oksanen et al., 2004), and would be missed in these analyses leading to some degree of "false negatives," or at least possible underestimation of MC content. Alternatively, studies have shown that improper use of ELISA kits – as well as factors such as organic solvents, salinity and pH - can contribute to the potential for false positives (Metcalf et al., 2005). Additionally, it is recognized that toxicity of MCs varies with congener, and therefore the inability to distinguish particular variants, with respect to this relative toxicity, does not enable what is essentially a proxy of "total MC" to be evaluated in terms of actual relevance to toxicity (Mountfort et al., 2005). As an alternative, enzyme assays - and particularly the various PPase inhibition assays developed for MCs (Mountfort et al., 2005) – are, in fact, capable of assessing cyanobacterial toxins based on relevant biological activity. However, such assays are typically not as sensitive as, for example, ELISA, and likewise may be susceptible to matrix components, as well as being unable to chemically distinguish particular toxin variants. That said, sensitivity of methods such as ELISA are generally higher than for most other methods, and moreover, although coupling analytical separation to detection (e.g. LC-MS) may enable identification of particular chemical variants, this is only applicable to those variant which are specifically targeted. In other words, even though LC coupled to tandem mass spectrometry (MS/MS) can, for example, selectively detect several common MC variants based on characteristic molecular ions, and subsequent "daughter ions," without prior knowledge of the optimal parameters (i.e. parent/daughter ions, ionization energy, etc.) - and/or availability of suitable analytical standards - to use for other for other less common (or perhaps yet uncharacterized) variants, and their metabolic products, these would be generally missed by such an approach (Mountfort et al., 2005). Accordingly, a strategy which incorporates both approaches and their relative benefits (i.e. highly sensitive detection of "total" MC by ELISA, target-based bioassay and selective analytical separation and detection of individual MC variants) might be expect to provide the most comprehensive toxin profile.

In general, the obvious challenge posed in adapting analytical techniques, originally developed for water (and, to a lesser extent, algal) samples, to bioaccumulation in food webs is the relatively more complex matrix of biological specimens (i.e. animal tissues). Other components of these biological matrices can interfere with analyses by specifically requiring a higher degree of selectivity (to discern the analyte from other components of the matrix), and as well as leading to suppression of the detection response (e.g. suppression of ionization in MS). To some extent, these challenges are inherently addressed when coupling detection to optimized analytical separation (e.g. LC-MS) that essentially isolates components (e.g. as chromatographic *peaks* based on retention time, etc.), but has also been generally supplemented by sample preparation steps prior to analysis. In particular, sample preparation steps have included selective extraction (e.g. Metcalf et al., 2002; Msagati et al., 2006), solid-phase extraction (SPE; e.g. James et al., 1998; Metcalf et al., 2002; McElhiney and Lawton, 2005; Scott et al., 2009) and other so-called "clean-up steps" to remove these potential interfering chemical species. Of course, in the case of less stable toxins (e.g. ATX-a; discussed below), extensive sample work-up can chemically jeopardize the analyte leading to underestimation or even complete non-detection of these compounds; generally speaking though, most approaches require some degree of sample preparation prior to analysis, particularly when dealing with complex bio-matrices.

One of the particular challenges of a biological matrix is due to the lack of specificity of certain detection methods. For example, although none of the recognized cyanobacterial toxins discussed have a particularly specific chromophore, as to enable unambiguous detection, HPLC coupled to UV spectrophotometric detection has been successfully used – specifically based on shortwave UV detection and established chromatographic retention time, and in conjunction with analytical standards – to detect and measure several cyanobacterial toxins in water samples (e.g. Harada et al., 1994; Gugger et al., 2005; McElhiney and Lawton, 2005; Berry and Lind, 2010). However, in more complex bio-matrices, this lack of a distinguishing UV chromophore, and potential for co-eluting non-targeted components of the matrix generally limit this approach. Similarly, although fluorescence derivatization – and subsequent fluorescence detection coupled to chromatography or other analytical separation techniques (e.g. CE) – has been used as a highly sensitive means of detection/measurement of cyanobacterial toxins (e.g. Harada et al., 1997; James et al., 1998), the derivatization chemistry frequently employed in these approaches exploit common functional groups (e.g. amines, carboxylic acids, dienes). As such, non-toxin analytes (e.g. peptides) present in biological matrices can be coincidentally derivatized and, by co-elution and/or simply poor resolution, interfere with identification of the analyte of interest. Possible overlap in analytical response is not limited to these analytical separation/detection techniques, and indeed, it has been suggested that for ELISA, antibody cross-reactivity with chemically related components of the matrix might, likewise, lead to non-selective detection, and erroneous results in analyses.

Even in the case of highly selective detection techniques, interference due to the bio-matrix can arise. This is particularly seen with quantitative analyses based on mass spectrometry, including LC-MS, and particularly the most commonly used (at present) method of electro-spray ionization (LC-ESI-MS). Components of the sample matrix, including inorganic (e.g. pH, salts/ions) and organic (e.g. proteins and other biomolecules) components, can both interfere with ionization; the former can directly interfere with ionization, whereas the latter can indirectly effect ionization of the analyte, particularly through competitive ionization. In the case of MCs, for example, it has been shown that dissolved organic carbon, pH and ionic strength can suppress signal in LC-MS with the latter being the most significant (Li et al., 2010). More notably in relation to the present discussion, Karlsson et al. (2005) investigated the effect of a biological matrix with respect to the LC-MS detection of MCs and NOD in biological tissues, including aquatic invertebrates (i.e. Blue Mussels, *Mytilus edulis*), fish (i.e. Rainbow Trout, *Onchorhyncus mykiss*) and waterfowl (i.e. Common Eider, *Somateria mollissima*). In these studies, it was found that ion signal varied from 16-134% of the expected signal (from spiked toxin), suggesting a good deal of both ionization suppression and enhancement, which varied with toxin variant (i.e. six MC variants and NOD) and biological matrix. In related studies, investigating the use of an MC oxidation product (discussed below) for LC-MS analysis, Ott and Carmichael (2006) reported losses in signal strength of more than 41% for this analyte. More recently, Li et al. (2012) examined the effects of ionization suppression with respect to quantitative analysis of BMAA, as well as its non-toxic isomer, 2,4,-diaminobutyric acid (DAB), by LC-MS/MS. Although considerable matrix effects were observed for DAB, there appeared to be no contribution to the BMAA signal. Notably, however, this optimized method was used to suggest that BMAA was not seemingly present in several cyanobacterial samples evaluated, and to support the growing indication that this putative toxin is not as widespread as previously suggested. Indeed, although matrix effects represent an analytical challenge, the effects of signal suppression (e.g. ion suppression) can generally be addressed by various strategies, including the use of appropriate *internal standards* and techniques of *standard addition* to assess the extent of this effect on quantitation.

	Limitations	Advantages
Biochemical Methods		
ELISA	Cost (~$400-500/plate) No chemical information, e.g. identification of chemical variants No toxicity information	Highly sensitive (< ppb) Rapid/analyze multiple samples at once Easy/little training required Relatively inexpensive instrumentation (i.e plate readers)
"Target-Based" e.g. PPase inhibition	No chemical information, e.g. identification of chemical variants Somewhat lower sensitivity Low selectivity, e.g. false positives	Provides toxicity information Relatively inexpensive (reagents) Rapid/analyze multiple samples at once Easy/little training required Relatively inexpensive instrumentation (i.e plate readers)
Instrumental Analysis (i.e. analytical separation/detection)		
HPLC/CE-UV	Low sensitivity Low selectivity, e.g. false positives Requires training Limited chemical information, e.g. can't identify unknown variants Moderately expensive instrumentation Relatively slow/can't analyze multiple samples at once Requires sample clean-up	Provides some chemical information, e.g. can identify chemical variants (if standards available) Analysis can be automated
HPLC/CE-FL	Requires derivatization Somewhat low selectivity, e.g. false positives Requires training Limited chemical information, e.g. can't identify unknowns Moderately expensive instrumentation Relatively slow/can't analyze multiple samples at once Requires sample clean-up	Highly sensitive Provides some chemical information, e.g. can identify chemical variants (if standards available) Analysis can be automated
HPLC/CE-MS	Requires training Expensive instrumentation Relatively slow/can't analyze multiple samples at once Requires (some) sample clean-up	Provides chemical information, e.g. can identify chemical variants (if standards available), possible information regarding unknowns Analysis can be automated

Table 2. Limitations and advantages of different analytical techniques used for detection/measurement of cyanobacterial toxins.

Aside from issues specifically related to the complex biological matrices encountered in food webs, some of the same general challenges associated with quantitative analysis of cyanobacterial toxins in water are, likewise, associated with analysis of bioaccumulation. A common consideration, in this regard, includes a requirement of selectively to detect, and discern, isomers and chemically related congeners. Indeed, this is exemplified by all of the recognized cyanobacterial toxins. For example, both PSTs and the MCs belong to rather large families of chemically related, but structurally distinct, variants – specifically represented, at present, by as many as fifty, and more than ninety, reported variants, respectively - with equally variable toxicity for each. In both cases, especially toxic and common variants (i.e. STX and MC-LR) are most frequently considered as a proxies for these toxin families, however, it is known that several other congeners from these groups can, in fact, potentially contribute to toxicity, and moreover, due to differential uptake and bioavailability hold, likewise, variable potential with respect to bioaccumulation. This presents, as discussed above, a clear limitation to ELISA-based analyses of the MCs that is unable to distinguish specific contributions of individual congeners. Likewise, although LC-MS and related methods, which employ analytical separation prior to detection, are able (if sufficiently optimized) to chromatographically resolve/separate congeners, the requirement for established molecular ionization and fragmentation parameters to detect these variants (by mass spectrometry) limits which variants will, and will not, be detected. Although considerably less complex, on the other hand, both CYN and ATX-a, likewise, have structurally related congeners and/or structural isomers, including for homoATX-a and 7-epiCYN, respectively, that are found alongside the "primary" toxins. In both of these cases, the congeners are also associated with toxicity, and evaluation of their contribution with respect to food-borne toxins needs to be included. On the other hand, although only BMAA (among several structural isomers) has been reported as potentially toxic, it has been suggested that natural occurrence of numerous possible isomeric congeners, all sharing the same molecular mass (Fig. 9), may greatly confound mass spectrometric analysis of this toxic amino acid (Banack et al., 2010), and specifically it has been suggested that, due to this, the once considered widespread occurrence of this neurotoxin may, in fact, be considerably over-estimated (Jiang et al., 2012; Li et al., 2012).

Although many of the cyanotoxins are generally considered chemically quite stable, and thus persistent in the environment, stability has, likewise, been suggested to limit quantitative analysis in some cases - and particularly ATX-a as perhaps the most chemically labile of the known toxins from cyanobacteria. Indeed, ATX-a has an estimated (Stevens and Krieger, 1991) half-life of only about 1-2 days – or even as low as 4-10 hours - in solutions emulating relevant biological conditions, including sunlight (i.e. photolysis) and pH (i.e. acidification). Degradation products, moreover, are generally not considered toxic (Stevens and Krieger, 1991). This instability poses obvious challenges, and particularly the potential for this toxin being underestimated or even missed in chemical analyses, and may, in fact, contribute to the absence of any reports on its bioaccumulation in food webs. Accordingly, it is generally advised that appropriate precautions regarding sample collection, transport and storage be taken to minimize recognized factors (i.e. light exposure, pH), and methods have been developed to increase speed of analysis (e.g. Smith and Lewis, 1987), to minimize this factor in assessing the possible role of ATX-a in relation to food-borne health concerns.

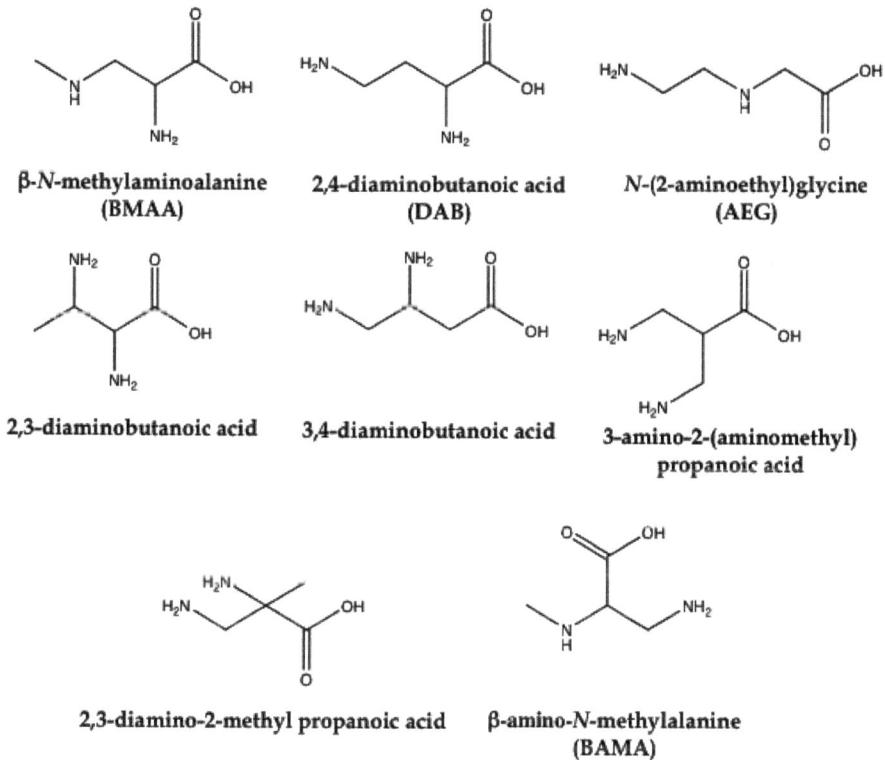

Figure 9. Isomers of the toxic amino acid, BMAA, suggested to potentially confound MS analysis.

As we learn more about the fate of cyanobacterial toxins in food webs, it is becoming increasingly recognized that at least two of the recognized cyanotoxins, namely MCs and BMAA, may present specific analytical challenges due to their specific chemical toxicology. As previously discussed (see 4.2 *Bioavailability*), in addition to reversible binding of the MCs to "targeted" PPases, covalent and thus effectively irreversible binding of these toxins, specifically via Mdha (Fig. 10), may lead to considerable underestimation of the total MC content as quantitative chemical analyses based on solvent extraction, and subsequent detection of the non-bound molecule, would generally miss these bound-forms of the toxin. Indeed, it has been estimated that more than 75% of MC-LR (as representative Mdha-containing variant) in exposed fish, and as much as 99.9% in exposed invertebrates (e.g. mussels), is effectively "tied up" by covalent, irreversible binding (Williams et al., 1997a and 1997b). Similarly, as also discussed previously, one of the proposed mechanisms of toxicity for BMAA is erroneous incorporation into proteins, leading to aberrant protein aggregates which are hallmarks of neurodegenerative disease (e.g. ALS, Alzheimers' Disease) linked to this toxic amino acid. Accordingly, this bound pool of the amino acid would not be immediately available to subsequent analyses relying solely on solvent extraction from the biological matrix. Considering this, several recent developments have focused on analytical strategies for including these "bound-forms" of the toxins in the overall assessment of their contribution to food-web bioaccumulation.

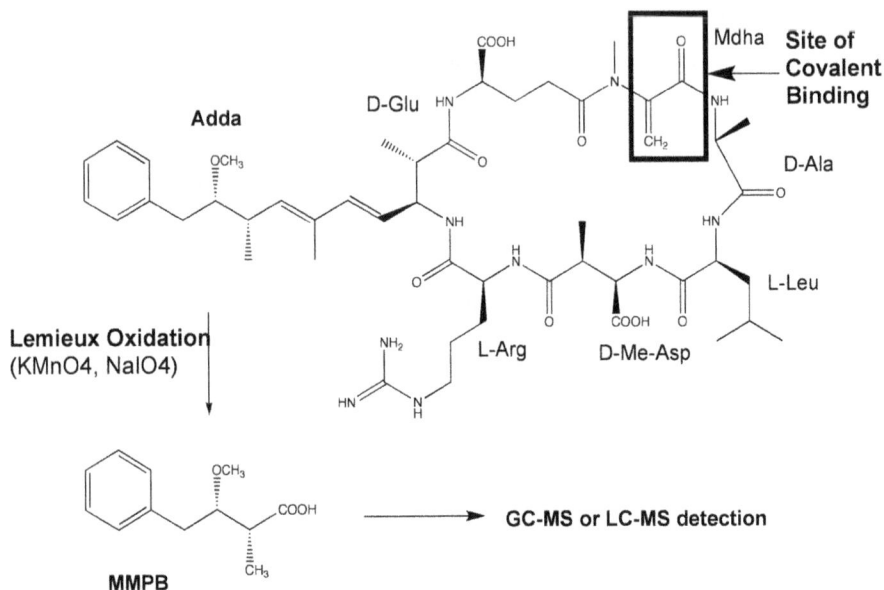

Figure 10. Lemieux oxidation of MC-LR, and detection of product (MMPB) as a surrogate for total MCs.

Perhaps the most elegant of these has been the development of the so-called "MMPB method," based on detection of the Adda oxidative cleavage product, 3-methyl-4-methoxy-phenylbu-tanoic acid (MMPB), as a proxy for total (i.e. bound and unbound) microcystins. As stated previously, Adda is both a key component of the MCs with respect to their toxicity, and is, indeed, conserved in the vast majority of variants (Fig. 2). Taking advantage of this conserved moiety, Sano et al. (1992) developed an analytical technique, specifically based on *Lemieux oxidation* that utilizes permanganate/periodate oxidation to cleave MMPB from the pendant Adda of microcystins (Fig. 10). This analyte can be subsequently quantified by several techniques, including GC-MS (Sano et al., 1992; Williams et al., 1997a and Williams et al., 1997b; Suchy and Berry, 2012) and LC-MS (e.g. Ott and Carmichael, 2006; Yuan et al., 2006). As Adda is distal to the Mdha, and site of covalent linkage to the PPase active site, the liberated MMPB can be used as a proxy – with no otherwise known naturally occurring counterpart – for both bound and free MCs. In fact, when subsequently applied to a range of fish and invertebrates, it became clear both that a the vast majority of MCs in exposed animals are not detected by analytical methods based on solvent extraction of the free toxin (suggesting a considerable loss of the exposure dose), and that significantly more of the toxin were detectable by the MMPB method (suggesting covalent binding as a likely "sink" for this lost toxin). Williams et al. (1997a and 1997b) most famously applied this method to the analysis of experimentally (i.e. intraperitoneally) exposed salmon, as well as samples of Dungeness crab larvae and mussels (*Mytilus edulis*). In these studies it was found, for example, that while nearly 100% of exposure dose (from *Microcystis* cells) could be recovered by the MMPB method, only approximately 0.1% of MC of the expected levels were detected by McOH extraction coupled to a PPase inhibition assay (Williams et al., 1997a). Likewise, for i.p.-exposed salmon, approximately 34% recovery of MC by Lemieux oxidation, specifically coupled to GC-MS, was reported, compared to approximately 8% recovery for MeOH extraction and PPase inhibition assay, and similarly more than 10,000-fold higher MC was detected by the MMPB method compared to extraction/PPase inhibition in populations of crab larvae (Williams et al., 1997b). More recently, the modified MMPB method (i.e. SPME-GC-MS detection of MMPB) was applied to evaluation of MCs in several fish species, including those consumed by humans, from various freshwater lake systems, and it was similarly found that this approach measured significantly higher levels of the toxin (5- to 40-fold higher) than those detected by ELISA (Suchy and Berry, 2012). Since initial development of the technique, the MMPB has been further refined to include improvements In the sample preparation steps, including SPE (Ott and Carmichael, 2006) and solid-phase microextraction (SPME; Suchy and Berry, 2012), as well as subsequent detection methods (e.g. LC-MS, and LC-MS/MS, versus GC-MS; Ott and Carmichael, 2006; Yuan et al., 2006; Neffling et al., 2010), and It has been applied to a range of matrices including assessment of human exposure (e.g. Yuan et al., 2006). Accordingly, the MMPB method represents a tremendous advancement to both our understanding of trophic transfer/bioavailability of this toxin, as well as our ability to assess its role in food webs and bioaccumulation with respect to public health.

Similar to the covalent binding of MCs to PPase targets, the possible incorporation of BMAA into proteins, and consequent potential for underestimation, has been addressed in recent – albeit much fewer - studies. Incorporation of BMAA into proteins, with respect to both analytical challenges, and its possible role in bioavailability and trophic transfer of the toxin, was first reported by Murch et al. (2004). In this study, acid hydrolysis (i.e. 24 h boiling in 6 M HCl) – to digest proteins, and release BMAA - coupled to subsequent HPLC-FL analysis measured levels of the toxin in cycad flours exceeding those previously measured, following simple solvent extraction (i.e. presumptively unbound BMAA), by as much as 90-fold. In the same study, BMAA in brain tissues from patients who had died of Alzheimer's Disease were, likewise, analyzed following acid digestion, and similarly showed levels of the toxin that were 60- to 130-fold great than those measured following solvent extraction (i.e. "free BMAA" only). The presence of this bound pool of BMAA in proteins was accordingly suggested to represent a previously unrecognized reservoir of the toxin available for both trophic transfer (i.e. following proteolytic enzyme digestion), and as a slowly released form of the toxin with respect to the recurrent damage and "latency period" observed in the onset of these neurodegenerative diseases (Murch et al., 2004). Moreover, these results point to a limitation in the prior analytical approach, and specifically a likely underestimation of the toxin in food webs. Accordingly, subsequent studies (Rosen and Hellenäs, 2008; Baptista et al., 2011; Cervantes Cianca et al., 2012) have undertaken development and validation – as well as application - of various analytical techniques (e.g. HPLC-FL, LC-MS/MS and CE-UV) that incorporate acid hydrolysis a means of characterizing "total BMAA" content. As these methods are validated, they will no doubt provide a key tool for evaluating both the ecology (e.g. trophic transfer within food-webs) and toxicology of this cyanobacterial metabolite, and clarify its possible role in human health.

6. Other cyanobacterial toxins and their bioaccumulation

A rather limited number of secondary metabolites produced by cyanobacteria – as discussed throughout this chapter (i.e. MCs, CYN, STX/PSTs, ATX-a and BMAA) – are generally considered, specifically based on association with documented intoxication events, as "toxins." However, the blue-green algae are, in fact, widely recognized to produce a myriad of biolog- ically active metabolites (Gerwick et al., 2001; Tan, 2007; Tan, 2010). Rather than toxins though, the majority of these chemically diverse, bioactive compounds have been identified as part of "drug discovery" efforts (Tan, 2007). That said, many of the biological systems used to prospect for potential pharmaceuticals – most notably perhaps including cytotoxicity as a means of identifying anticancer drugs – could clearly be extended to include those compounds (i.e. "cytotoxins") which may have negative impacts on human health, as toxins, rather than, or in addition to, their intended therapeutic targets. Indeed, it has been argued (e.g. Berry et al., 2008) that many (or perhaps even most) of the bioactive secondary metabolites from cyano- bacteria – including several investigated as drug leads - are likely produced as *allelochemi- cals*, serving a role as chemical agents for deterrence, specifically through their "toxicity," toward other organisms.

Although limited to no literature exists, due to the nature of their discovery (as drug candi- dates), on either the potential for either toxicity or bioaccumulation of these many previously identified bioactive metabolites, indirect evidence suggests that as-of-yet unidentified metabolites do, indeed, contribute to toxicity of the cyanobacteria. Specifically, several studies (e.g. Pietsch et al., 2001; Kurmayer and Jüttner, 2009) have compared relative toxicity of pure cyanobacterial toxins to crude extracts, and consistently found higher degrees of biological activity for the latter suggesting an additive or even synergistic role of congeners in these mixtures, including both chemically related (i.e. variants within a toxin family) and/or potentially unrelated, and likely uncharacterized, metabolites. These finding, therefore, generally point to the higher toxicity of metabolic mixtures, and specifically suggest the possibility of unknown toxins which might be relevant to bioaccumulation – and, thus, consequent health concerns - within food-webs. Identification of these additional toxic metabolites will, therefore, be essential to a holistic understanding of the health effects of cyanobacterial toxins, including their potential contribution to food-borne toxicity.

Due, perhaps in part, to the nature of the biological assays used (e.g. cytotoxicity assays, enzyme inhibition assays) that rely on water-solubility of test compounds, the majority of the bioactive metabolites identified from blue-green algae as potential drug candidates have typically focused on rather water-soluble or polar compounds, and particularly the diverse non-ribosomal peptides (NRPs) characteristic of the cyanobacteria (Welker and Von Döhren, 2006). Indeed, a few such NRPs have, in fact, been identified alongside recognized toxins, specifically based on potential relevance to chemical ecology. A particularly notable example is the identification of several chemically related, and apparently quite widespread, peptides – isolated, alongside MCs, from *Microcystis* - as protease inhibitors (e.g. microviridin J, aeruginosin) with demonstrated ability to serve as feeding deterrents to the zooplankton, *Daphnia* (Harada et al., 1993; Martin et al., 1993; Okino et al., 1993; Tsukamoto et al., 1993; Rohrlack et al., 2004; von Elert et al., 2005). As for MCs, very recent studies suggest a genotype x genotype interaction between toxin and grazer, and consequent development of tolerance to these protease inhibitors (Schwarzenberger et al., 2012; von Elert et al., 2012). Accordingly, these latter findings would open up the door to possible bioaccumulation, and possible human exposure, although to-date there have not been any studies to investigate this aspect within freshwater food-webs.

In marine environments, a particularly salient example is lyngbyatoxin, and severally chemically related cyclic peptides (e.g. aplysiatoxin, debromoaplysiatoxin), isolated from marine species of the genus, *Lyngbya*, a well known producer of several known cyanobacterial toxins (i.e. MCs, CYN, STX/PSTs). Although these former peptide toxins, specifically acting as activators of protein kinase C, have been associated with direct human exposure (i.e. dermatotoxins) as well as being investigated with respect to possible pharmacological potential – the toxins, found in filamentous cyanobacteria in marine shallows, have also been reported to be incidentally grazed by marine animals, including invertebrates – and particularly various species of gastropods that accumulate the toxin (Capper et al., 2005) - and vertebrates, most notably including sea turtles (Yasumoto et al., 1998; Arthur et al., 2008). Given the recognized toxicity to mammals (e.g. Ito et al., 2002), it is suggested that possible bioaccumulation, and subsequent consumption, could represent a route of human exposure and toxicity. In fact, as one of the few examples of acute toxicosis possibly associated with foodborne cyanotoxins, the presence of these toxins in turtle meat has been linked (Yasumoto et al., 1998) to several cases of human intoxication in the South Pacific and Madagascar (Hashimoto et al., 1967; Champetier et al., 1998) specifically characterized by ulceration of mucosal membranes, as well as apparent neurotoxic effects. It is also worth noting that these toxins have been hypothesized (Arthur et al., 2008) to explain chronic health effects – and specifically promotion of tumors associated with fibropapillomatosis – in exposed turtles, and these results, therefore, underscore the largely unstudied, possible contribution of these toxins to similar human health concerns associated with long-term, food-borne exposure.

Although the vast majority of bioactive secondary metabolites identified have, for reasons stated above, particularly included a number of peptides and other hydrophilic compounds, the cyanobacteria are known to produce a variety of lipophilic metabolites as well. In support of a possible role of these metabolites in relation to food webs, when evaluating the effects of toxic metabolites from the recognized toxigenic cyanobacterial species, *Planktothrix rubescens*, Kurmayer and Jüttner (1999) observed that lipophilic extraction reduced feeding deterrence of the cyanobacterial cells with respect to zooplankton grazers, and pointed to an uncharacterized lipophilic metabolite in this species. In more recent studies, Berry et al. (2009) evaluated non-polar extracts of the CYN-producing species, *Aphanizomenon ovalisporum* and *Cylindrospermopsis raciborskii*, specifically using the zebra-fish embryo model, and identified apparent lipophilic toxins, chemically unrelated to CYN or other water-soluble toxins produced by these species. It is not, therefore, surprising that considerable research in this area has identified numerous lipophilic metabolites ranging from alkaloids to lipopeptides (Orjala et al., 1995; Wu et al., 2000; Li et al., 2001; Edwards et al., 2004) to fatty acids (e.g. polyunsaturated fatty acid [PUFAs], Reinikainen et al., 2001) and seemingly simple hydrocarbons (Jaja-Chimedza et al., 2012).

Although much of the chemistry behind these observations remains to be characterized, one particularly well-studied group of lipophilic metabolites is a diverse family of indole alkaloids produced by members of the relatively widespread, but otherwise understudied, Stigonema-taceae (e.g. Raveh and Carmeli, 2007; Mo et al., 2010; Kim et al., 2012; and many more). Although this chemically diverse, and taxonomically restricted, group of metabolites have been generally identified based on antimicrobial activity (e.g. Raveh and Carmeli, 2007; Mo et al., 2012), and in fact, have been linked to possible allelopathy (i.e. inhibition of photosynthetic microbial competitors) in their natural environment, several biological activities supporting animal toxicity have also been reported (e.g. inhibition of RNA polymerase; Doan et al., 2001). This finding, and their seemingly widespread occurrence, raises the question as to whether these quite lipophilic metabolites may contribution to toxicity within food webs, including perhaps human health concerns.

Similarly, considerable work over the past 15 years or more has identified a diversity of lipopeptides, particularly isolated from the widespread marine cyanobacterial species, *Lyngbya majuscula* (Orjala et al., 1995; Orjala et al., 1996; Li et al., 2001; Nogle et al., 2001; Edwards et al., 2004; Choi et al., 2010) and others (e.g. *Anabaena;* Kaya et al., 2002). Although bioactivity associated with these metabolites runs the gamut from inhibition of specific enzymes to cytotoxicity in mammalian cells to toxicity in a range of organisms (e.g. antifungal, molluscicidal, ichthyotoxicity), potent neurotoxicity has, in particular, been associated with a number of these (e.g. Li et al., 2001; Nogle et al., 2001; Edwards et al., 2004; Choi et al., 2010). However, although a wealth of information regarding toxicity has emerged alongside their chemical discovery, essentially no insight as to possible bioaccumulation – despite the global abundance of these taxa, e.g. *Lyngbya*, in marine and freshwater habitats – currently exists.

More recently – following-up on prior studies (Berry et al., 2009; as discussed briefly above) – an apparently widespread group of toxic, lipophilic metabolites have been identified from several species of otherwise toxigenic cyanobacteria. Utilizing the zebrafish (*Danio rerio*) embryo as a vertebrate model of so-called developmental toxicity, and specifically as a means of *bioassay-guided fractionation*, Jaja-Chimedza et al. (2012), in very recent studies, identified a family of isotactic polymethoxy-1-alkenes (PMAs) from *Aphanizomenon ovalisporum*, specifi-cally as lipophilic inhibitors of developmental pathways in this model system. Both this species, and the genus (i.e. *Aphanizomenon)*, more generally, are recognized producers of CYN (genus/species; e.g. Preussel et al., 2006), as well as the neurotoxic STX/PSTs and ATX-a (species; e.g. Mahmood and Carmichael, 1986 and Ballot et al, 2010, respectively). The identification of PMAs as lipophilic metabolites in this species, including CYN-producing strains (Berry et al., 2009), suggests that they may contribute to the overall toxicity of this widely distributed species, as well as - given the highly lipid-soluble nature of these compounds - the potential for their bioaccumulation, and even biomagnfication, within food-webs. Moreover, prior studies have identified the same or similar PMAs from a wide range of cyanobacteria (e.g. Mynderse and Moore, 1979; Mori et al., 1991), although previous studies did not originally link their presence to potential toxicity (but rather identified them based on chemical characterization), and subsequent studies (Jaja-Chimedza et al., forthcoming), using the same toxicity, have identified them in otherwise recognized toxigenic species (e.g. *C. raciborskii, M. aeruginosa*). These emerging findings suggest that this group of metabolites may be widespread, and further underscore the potential role in food-derived toxicity. In fact, identification of closely related metabolites in marine sponges (Rama and Faulkner, 2002) has been attributed to a cyanobacterial biosynthetic origin/source (likely via filter-feeding of algal cells), and further support the potential for their uptake and accumulation in higher trophic levels. To-date, however, studies on their bioaccumulation (beyond this example) in food-webs remains to be addressed.

7. Implications for ecosystem health

Finally, although beyond the scope of this chapter (and volume), it is worthwhile to consider – before concluding our discussion with respect to public health implications of cyanobacterial toxins in food webs – the apparent contribution of cyanobacterial toxins in food webs with respect to animal and ecosystem health. Obviously, understanding the impacts of these toxins on animal health with respect to ecosystems is essential to understanding the potential for trophic transfer of these toxins. Moreover, insights regarding the potential for human health concerns of food-borne toxins – especially as contaminants of shared food-webs - can be often studied indirectly, and to some extent extrapolated, by understanding the role of these toxins in non-human animals. Indeed, with regards to the toxicity of cyanobacterial metabolites, the first reported case of intoxication by a cyanobacterial bloom was made based on animal health, and specifically reported livestock poisonings associated with pond scums (later identified as cyanobacteria) in a so-called "poisonous lake," famously detailed in the pioneering works by George Francis in the late 19th century (Francis, 1878).

Given that current evidence generally suggests limited trophic transfer of most of the known cyanobacterial toxins, and consequent restriction of foodborne cyanobacterial toxins to lower trophic levels in food-webs, it is not surprising that toxicity to animals has particularly focused on those vertebrate (i.e. fish) and invertebrates which are exposed either directly (through phytoplanktivory), or through "single vector" (e.g. zooplanktivory), transfer. For example, the previously discussed studies of Karjalainen et al. (2005), not only demonstrated that pre-exposure of zooplankton to cell-free, NOD-containing extracts of *N. spumigens* – representative of the toxin released during blooms –resulted in subsequent bioaccumulation of this toxin in zooplanktivorous, larval fish predators, but also decreased (compared to unexposed controls) ingestion, growth rate and fecal production of the experimentally fed zooplanktivorous larvae of Northern Pike (*Esox lucius*), suggesting a possible toxic effect to these predators without direct exposure to the toxin-containing water or algal cells. Interestingly enough, no such statistically significant effects was observed for larvae fed zooplankton which were pre-exposed to pure NOD, suggesting a possible contribution of other, currently unknown, toxins (Karjalainen et al., 2005).

Numerous studies, encompassing essentially all of the other known cyanotoxins, as well as yet uncharacterized, but apparently toxic, metabolites, likewise, have demonstrated the potential toxic effects to various aquatic species exposed at this lower end of the trophic scale. At the level of zooplanktivorous grazers, numerous studies have documented the apparent toxic effects of, not only MCs (as discussed above), but also other cyanobacterial toxins, including CYN (Nogueira et al., 2004), STX/PSTs (Filho et al., 2008) and ATX-a (Sieroslawska et al., 2010) - as well as perhaps other unidentified metabolites (present in extracts) - on *Daphnia*, and various other species. Likewise, biochemical and histopathologic analyses of both benthic grazers, particularly including snail species (Lance et al., 2010), and filter-feeding bivalves (Puerto et al., 2011; Sabatini et al., 2011), exposed to cell-bound toxins, including MCs and CYN, as well as unidentified toxic metabolites, demonstrate toxicity – along with apparent bioaccumulation – corresponding to uptake and transport pathways from the digestive system. Similarly, toxicity of several cyanobacterial metabolites to fish – and particularly several, representative phytoplanktivorous species (e.g. carp, tilapia) - exposed to dietary sources of these toxins has been well documented (e.g. Jos et al., 2005; Osswald et al., 2007; El Ghazali et al., 2010; Qiao et al., 2012).

On the other hand, relatively fewer studies to-date have clearly documented toxic effects of subsequent predation on toxin-laden invertebrates (e.g. zooplankton, benthic invertebrates), or phytoplanktivorous fish. However, the limited studies that have do generally point to the potential for toxicity – along with toxin transfer – to higher trophic levels. In one particularly notable study, Qiu et al. (2007) examined – using biochemical and histopathological ap-proaches - four trophic levels, comprised of a phytoplanktivorous, omnivorous and carnivo-rous fish species in a Chinese lake in relation to a MC-producing bloom. Surprisingly in this case, the most pronounced histopathological signs of toxicity were observed for carnivorous fish, whereas the largest biochemical response (i.e. particularly the production of several antioxidant enzymes/pathway, e.g. superoxide disumutase, catalase, glutathione, glutathione peroxidase), were measured for phytoplanktivorous species. These results suggest not only that carnivores can be exposed to cyanobacterial metabolites, and toxic effects via food webs, but that grazers of cyanobacteria (i.e. phytoplanktivores) may, as such, be specifically adapted to the direct exposure to these toxins.

The toxic effects of cyanobacterial metabolites on higher trophic levels, aside from fish, in aquatic food webs remain quite scarce, despite the fact that numerous taxa, including bird and mammalian species, are recognized as frequent "top consumers" in these systems. However, examples are beginning to emerge in the literature. In an especially insightful example, Miller et al. (2010) recently reported on the apparent toxic effects - including several animal deaths among - among southern sea otters, along the Pacific coast of the U.S., exposed to MCs bioaccumulated by bivalves (i.e. clams, mussels and oysters) consumed by these carnivorous predators. Following an unusually high number of sea otters deaths in the Monterey Bay, and surrounding coastal areas, particularly during the period of 2005-2008, necropsy on these stranded animals was performed. Based on the detection of relatively high levels (up to 348 ppb) of several variants of microcystins, including MC-RR, -LR and -desmethyl LR, in livers of sea otters, along with gross and microscopic pathological indications - particularly in livers of the animals - consistent with MC intoxication, it was concluded that animals had, indeed, died from exposure to this cyanobacterial toxin. The source of the toxin was ultimately traced to outflow from the nearby Pinto Lake into the marine waters of Monterey Bay, and subsequent bioaccumulation of the toxin by mollusks, consumed by sea otters, in the Bay. Characterized as a "super-bloom" of cyanobacteria, levels of MC in Pinto Lake, during this time, were measured as high as 2,100 ppm (more than six orders of magnitude higher than the WHO limit of 1 ppb), and use of Solid Phase Adsorption Toxin Tracking (SPATT) samples enabled tracking of the toxin from the lake toward the Bay. Subsequent laboratory studies confirmed the bioaccumulation of MC - at levels as high 1,324 ppb - by various bivalve (i.e. clam, mussel, oyster) species that make up a primary component of the sea otters' diet. Indeed, this case is particularly revealing as it not only supports hypothesis that higher trophic levels – including mammalian carnivores - can, in fact, be exposed to toxic (and even lethal) levels of cyanobacterial toxins through food-webs, but also that toxins can transfer not only within ecocystems, but between (in this case, freshwater and marine) systems. Moroever, although levels of MCs, in this case, were exceptionally high, this study further provides – through quantificationof the toxin in (livers of) exposed animals – a first estimation of relevant (i.e. lethal) exposure doses for mammalian consumers in relation to environmental concentration both in water, and vectors (i.e. bioaccumulation in bivalves) of the toxin.

8. Conclusions

Cyanobacteria are prolific producers of toxic, and otherwise biologically (i.e. pharmacologically) active, metabolites. Although ubiquitous in the environment, the cyanobacteria are arguably most conspicuous, and generally more abundant, in aquatic systems, particularly in association with so-called "harmful algal blooms." As such, exposure to several cyanobacterial toxins through contamination of drinking water, and related routes, has been clearly linked to both acute toxicoses, including human and animal mortalities, as well as being increasingly tied to several long-term health effects (e.g. cancer, neurodegenerative disease). Consequently, waterborne cyanotoxins are widely acknowledged as a global health concern.

Given this particularly widespread occurrence of the "blue-green algae" in marine and freshwater ecosystems, it is not, therefore, surprising, that bioaccumulation of nearly all of the "recognized" cyanobacterial toxins within relevant species of aquatic food webs has been reported. In light of the enormous human reliance on the world's oceans and freshwater systems, particularly as a source of food (i.e. fish, seafood), as well as culminating evidence to suggest that global climate change is fueling an apparently rapid increase in cyanobacterial abundance, bloom frequency and perhaps even toxigenicity in aquatic systems, cyanobacterial toxins in food webs, likewise, represent a clearly important human health issue.

As an emerging concern, however, clearly more questions than answers remain, at present, regarding the potential role of cyanobacterial toxins in food webs, particularly in terms of possible human and environmental health concerns. Although a preponderance of evidence indicates that diverse taxa of aquatic animal species do, in fact, accumulate cyanotoxins, the biochemical, physiological and ecological processes that control trophic transfer within food-webs remains to be clarified. Likewise, although trophic transfer of the largely water-soluble "known" cyanobacterial toxins appears to follow a pattern of biodilution, rather than biomagnification to top consumers, a growing number cases indicate that species, known to be consumed as part of human diets, do bioaccumulate significant quantities of these toxins, yet the potential implications for human health remains to be elucidated. This, it is argued is due, in part, to the lack of information regarding bioavailability, as well as limitations and challenges in current analytical methodologies used to assess this contribution.

Although the scientific evidence that does exist strongly suggests a potential (and, in fact, high probability) for human exposure to, and consequent health concerns associated with, food-borne cyanobacterial toxins, the implications with respect to public health policy remains almost entirely to be addressed. Indeed, while our scientific understanding of the bioaccumulation of cyanobacterial toxins in relation to human health currently remains rather limited - particularly relative to many other environmental health concerns – the public health implications, including relevance to policy makers and stakeholders, lags even more so. And, in fact, it is asserted that it is many of the same gaps in knowledge that limit our scientific understanding which, likewise, limit public health policy with regards to food-borne cyanotoxins, and thus addressing these gaps will be critical in this regard. First, and perhaps foremost, is the preeminent need to understand the toxicology of food-borne cyanotoxins, including both laboratory and (currently non-existent) epidemiological studies to elucidate what (if any) health effects exist, and which groups are most likely affected. Similarly, clarifying the actual health effects, including relevant doses, mechanisms of action, bioavailability, etc., will be fudnamental to developing effective regulatory guidelines. Although, as described above, attempts have been made (e.g. Ibelings and Chorus, 2007) to extrapolate current (albeit limited) toxicological knowledge in this regard to possible acceptable levels for food-borne cyanotoxins, these are based entirely on data from water-borne toxins, and are not likely to be accurate in terms of exposure through food. Furthermore, even the provisional guidelines that exist for cyanobacterial toxins in water are only recommendations, and policy will not only need to clarify acceptable levels, but also address monitoring and enforcement of these guidelines. As such, improvements, validation and standardization of methods for chemical analysis of cyanobacterial toxins – toward effective monitoring and enforcement - in food will be key. Continued investigations in these areas will, therefore be of the crucial toward developing a comprehensive picture of this emerging public health concern.

Author details

John Berry*

Department of Chemistry and Biochemistry, Florida International University, U.S.A.

References

[1] Andrinolo, D, Michea, L. F, & Lago, N. (1999). Toxic effects, pharmacokinetics and clearance of saxitoxin, a component of paralytic shellfish poison (PSP) in cats. *Toxicon*, , 37, 447-464.

[2] Aráoz, R, & Molgó, J. Tandeau de Marsac, N. ((2010). Neurotoxic cyanobacterial toxins. *Toxicon*, , 56, 813-828.

[3] Arthur, K, Limpus, C, Balazs, G, Capper, A, Udy, J, Shaw, G, Keuper-bennet, U, & Bennet, P. (2008). The exposure of green turtles (*Chelonia mydas*) to tumour promoting compounds produced by the cyanobacterium *Lyngbya majuscula* and their potential role in the aetiology of fibropapillomatosis. *Harmful Algae*, , 7, 114-125.

[4] Ballot, A, Fastner, J, Lentz, M, & Weidner, C. (2010). First report of anatoxin-a-producing cyanobacterium *Aphanizomenon issatschenkoi* in northeastern Germany. *Toxicon*, , 56, 964-971.

[5] Banack, S. A, Downing, T. G, Spacil, Z, Purdie, E. L, Metcalf, J. S, Downing, S, Esterhulzen, M, Codd, G. A, & Cox, P. A. (2010). Distinguishing the cyanobacterial neurotoxin beta=N-methylamino alanine (BMAA) from its structural isomer 2,4-diaminobutyric acid (DAB). *Toxicon*, 56, 868-879., 2(4)

[6] Banker, R. S, Carmeli, O, Hadas, B, Teltsch, R, Porat, R, & Sukenik, A. (1997). Identification of cylindrospermopsin in *Aphanizomenon ovalisporum* isolated from Lake Kinneret, Israel. *Journal of Phycology*, , 35, 613-616.

[7] Banker, R. S, Carmeli, S, Werman, M, Teltsch, B, Porat, R, & Sukenik, A. (2001). Uracil moiety is required for toxicity of the cyanobacterial hepatotoxin cylindrospermopsin. *Journal of Toxicology and Environmental Health, Part A*, , 62, 281-288.

[8] Baptista, M. S, Cianca, R. C, Lopes, V. R, Almeida, C. M, & Vasconcelos, V. M. (2011). Determination of the non protein amino acid β-N-methylamino-L-alanine in estuarine caynobacteria by capillary electrophoresis. *Toxicon*, , 58, 410-414.

[9] Bazin, E, Huet, S, & Jarry, G. Le Hegarat, L.; Munday, J. S.; Humpage, A. R. & Fessard, Cytotoxic and genotoxic effects of cylindrospermopsin in mice treated by gavage or intraperitoneal injection. *Environmental Toxicology*, 27, 277-284., 2012

[10] Beltran, E. C, & Neilan, B. A. (2000). Geographical separation of the neurotoxin-producing cyanobacterium *Anabaena circinalis*. *Applied Environmental Microbiology*, , 66, 4468-4474.

[11] Berry, J. P, Gantar, M, Perez, M. H, Berry, G, & Noriega, F. G. (2008). Cyanobacterial toxins as allelochemicals with potential applications as algaecides, herbicides and insecticides. *Marine Drugs*, , 6, 117-146.

[12] Berry, J. P, Gibbs, P. D, Schmale, M. C, & Saker, M. L. (2009). Toxicity of cylindrospermopsin, and other apparent metabolites from *Cylindrospermopsis raciborskii* and *Aphanizomenon ovalisporum*, to the zebrafish (*Danio rerio*) embryo. *Toxicon*, , 52, 289-299.

[13] Berry, J. P, & Lind, O. (2010). First evidence of "paralytic shellfish toxins" and cylindrospermopsin in a Mexican freshwater system, Lago Catemaco, and apparent bioaccumulation of the toxins in "tegogolo" snails (*Pomacaee patula catemacensis*). *Toxicon*, , 55, 930-938.

[14] Berry, J. P, Lee, E, Walton, K, Wilson, A. E, & Bernal-brooks, F. (2011). Bioaccumulation of microcystins by fish associated with a persistent cyanobacterial bloom in Lago de Patzcuaro (Michoacan, Mexico). *Environmental Toxicology and Chemistry*, , 30, 1621-1628.

[15] Berry, J. P, Jaja-chimedza, A, Davalos-lind, L, & Lind, O. (2012). Apparent bioaccumulation of cylindrospermopsin and paralytic shellfish toxins by finfish in Lake Catemaco (Veracruz, Mexico). *Food Additives and Contaminants Part A*, , 29, 314-321.

[16] Bourke, A. T. C, Hawes, R. B, Neilson, A, & Stallman, N. D. (1983). An outbreak of hepato-enteritis (the Palm Island mystery disease) possibly caused by algal intoxication. *Toxicon*, , 3, 45-48.

[17] Brand, L. E, Pablo, J, Compton, A, Hammerschlag, N, & Mash, D. (2010). Cyanobacterial blooms and the occurrence of the neurotoxin beta-N-methylamino-L-alanine (BMAA) in South Florida aquatic food webs. *Harmful Algae*, , 9, 620-635.

[18] CallerT. A; Doolin, J. W.; Haney, J. F.; Murby, A. J.; West, K. G.; Farrar, H. E.; Ball, A.; Harris, B. T. & Stommel, E. W. ((2009). A cluster of amyotrophic lateral sclerosis in New Hampshire: a possible role for toxic cyanobacteria blooms. *Amyotrophic Lateral Sclerosis*, 10 Suppl. , 2, 101-108.

[19] Capper, A, Tibbets, I. R, Neil, O, & Shaw, J. M. G. R. ((2005). The fate of *Lyngbya majuscula* toxins in three potential consumers. *Journal of Chemical Ecology*, , 31, 1595-1606.

[20] Carmichael, W. W, Evans, W. R, Yin, Q. Q, Bell, P, & Mosczydlowski, E. (1997). Evidence for paralytic shellfish poisons in the freshwater cyanobacterium *Lyngbya wollei*. *Applied Environmental Microbiology*, , 63, 3104-3110.

[21] Carpenter, E. J, & Romans, K. (1991). Major role of the cyanobacterium *Trichodesmium* in nutrient cycling in the North-Atlantic Ocean. *Science*, , 254, 1356-1358.

[22] Cervantes CiancaR. C.; Pallares, M. A.; Barbosa, D. R.; Adan, V. L.; J. M. L. Martins; Gago-Martinez, A. ((2007). Application of precolumn oxidation HPLC method with fluorescence detection to evaluate saxitoxin levels in discrete brain regions of the brain. *Toxicon,* , 49, 89-99.

[23] Cervantes Cianca., R. C.; Baptista, M. S.; Pinto da Silva, L.; Lopes, V. R. & Vasconce-los, V. M. ((2012). Reversed-phase HPLC/FD method for the quantitative analysis of the neurotoxin BMAA (β-N-methylamino-L-alanine) in cyanobacteria. *Toxicon,* , 59, 379-384.

[24] ChampetierR. G; Ranaivoson, G.; Ravaonindrina, N.; Rakotonjabelo, A. L.; Rasolofo-nirina, N.; Roux, J. F. & Yasumoto, T. ((1998). Un probléma de santé publique réé-mergent á Madagascar: les intoxications collectives par consommation d'animaux marins. *Arch. Inst. Pasteur Madagascar,* , 64, 71-76.

[25] Chen, J, Xie, P, Zhang, D, & Lei, H. (2007). In situ studies on the distribution patterns and dynamics of microcystins in a biomanipulation fish- bighead carp (*Aristichthys nobilis*). *Environmental Pollution,* , 147, 150-157.

[26] Choi, H, Pereira, A. R, Cao, Z, Shuman, C. F, Engene, N, Byrum, T, Matainaho, T, Murray, T. F, Mangoni, A, & Gerwick, W. H. (2010). The holamides, structurally in-triguing neurotoxic lipopeptides from Papua New Guinea marine cyanobacteria. *Journal of Natural Products,* , 73, 1411-1421.

[27] Costa, P. R, Lage, S, Barata, M, & Pousão-ferreira, P. (2011). Uptake, transformation, and elimination kinetics of paralytic shellfish toxins in white seabream (*Diplodus sar-gus*). *Marine Biology,* , 158, 2805-2811.

[28] Cox, P. A, Banack, S. A, & Murch, S. J. (2003). Biomagnification of cyanobacterial neurotoxins and neurodegenerative disease among the Chamorro people of Guam. *Proceedings of the National Academy of Sciences U.S.A.,* , 100, 13380-13383.

[29] Cox, P. A, Banack, S. A, Murch, S. J, Rasmussen, U, Tien, G, Bidigaire, R. R, & Met-calf, J. S. (2005). Diverse taxa of cyanobacteria produce beta-N-methylamino-L-ala-nine, a neurotoxic amino acid. *Proceedings of the National Academy of Sciences U.S.A.,* , 102, 5074-5078.

[30] Cox, P. A, Richer, R, Metcalf, J. S, Banack, S. A, Codd, G. A, & Bradley, W. G. (2009). Cyanobacteria and BMAA exposure from desert dust: a possible link to sporadic ALS among Gulf War veterans. *Amyotrophic Lateral Sclerosis,* 10 Suppl. , 2, 109-117.

[31] Craig, M, Luu, H. A, Mccready, T. L, Williams, D, Andersen, R. J, & Holmes, C. F. (1997). Molecular mechanisms underlying the interaction of motuporin and micro-cystins with type-1 and type-2A protein phosphatases. *Biochemical and Cellular Biolo-gy,* , 74, 569-578.

[32] Cucchiaroni, M. L, Viscomi, M. T, Bernardi, G, Molinari, M, Guatteo, E, & Mercuri, N. B. (2010). Metabotropic glutamate receptor 1 mediates electrophysiological and

toxic actions of the cycad derivative beta-N-methylamino-L-alanine on substantia nigra pars compacta dopinergic neurons. *The Journal of Neuroscience*, , 30, 5176-5188.

[33] Davis, T. W, & Gobler, C. J. (2011). Grazing by mesozooplankton and microzoolankton on toxic and non-toxic strains of *Microcystis* in the Transquaking River, a tributary of Chesapeake Bay. *Journal of Plankton Research*, 33, 415-430.

[34] Doan, N. T, Stewart, P. R, & Smith, G. D. (2001). Inhibition of bacterial RNA polymerase by the cyanobacterial metabolites 12-epi-hapalindole E isonitrile and calothrixin A. *FEMS Microbiology Letters*, , 196, 135-139.

[35] Dyble, J, Gossiaux, D, Landrum, P, Kashian, D. R, & Pothoven, S. (2011). A kinetic study of accumulation and elimination of microcystin-LR in Yellow Perch (*Perca flavescens*) tissue and implications for human fish consumption. *Marine Drugs*, , 9, 2553-2571.

[36] Edwards, D. J, Marquez, B. L, Nogle, L. M, Mcphail, K, Goeger, D. E, Roberts, M. A, & Gerwick, W. H. (2004). Structure and biosynthesis of the jamaicamides, new mixed polyketide-peptide neurotoxins from the marine cyanobacterium *Lyngbya majuscula*. *Chemical Biology*, , 11, 817-833.

[37] El Ghazali, I, Sagrane, S, & Carvalho, A. P. Ouahid, Y; Del Campo, F. F.; Vasconcelos, V & Oudra, B. ((2010). Effects of mirocystin profile of a cyanobacterial bloom on growth and toxin accumulation in common carp *Cyprinus carpio* larvae. *Journal of Fish Biology*, , 76, 1415-1430.

[38] Etheridge, S. M. (2010). Paralytic shellfish poisoning: seafood safety and human health perspectives. *Toxicon*, , 56, 108-122.

[39] Eriksson, J, Jonasson, S, Papaefthimiou, D, Rasmussen, U, & Bergman, B. (2009). Improving deriviatization efficiency of BMAA utilizing AccQ-taq in a complex cyanobacterial matrix. *Amino Acids*, , 36, 43-48.

[40] Falconer, I. R, Burch, M. D, Steffensen, D. A, Choice, M, & Coverdale, O. R. (1994). Toxicity of the blue-green alga (cyanobacterium) *Microcystis aeruginosa* in drinking water to growing pigs, as an animal model for human injury and risk assessment. *Environmental Toxicology and Water Quality*, , 9, 131-139.

[41] FAO Fisheries and Aquaculture Department ((2010). The state of world fisheries and aquaculture 2010United Nations Food and Agriculture Organization, Rome, 2010.

[42] Fawell, J. K, Mitchell, R. E, Everett, D. J, & Hill, R. E. (1999). The toxicity of cyanobacterial toxins in the mouse. I: Microcystin-LR. *Human and Experimental Toxicology*, , 18, 162-167.

[43] Ferrao-filho, A. S, & Kozlowsky-suzuki, B. (2011). Cyanotoxins: bioaccumulation and effects on aquatic organisms. *Marine Drugs*, , 9, 2729-2772.

[44] Filho, A. S. da Costa, S. M.; Ribeiro, M. G. & Azevedo, S. M. ((2008). Effects of a saxi-toxin-producer strain of *Cylindrospermopsis raciborskii* (cyanobacteria) on the swimming movements of cladocerans. *Environmental Toxicology*, , 23, 161-168.

[45] Fischer, W. J, Altheimer, S, Cattori, V, Meier, P. J, Dietrich, D. R, & Hagenbuch, B. (2005). Organic anion transporting polypeptides in liver and brain mediate uptake of microcystin. *Toxicology and Applied Pharmacology*, , 203, 257-263.

[46] Fischer, A, Hoeger, S. J, Stemmer, K, Feurstein, D. J, Knobeloch, D, Nussler, A, & Dietrich, D. R. (2010). The role of organic anion transporting polypeptides (OATP/ SLCOs) in the toxicity of different microcystin congeners *in vitro*: a comparison of primary human hepatocytes and OATP-transfected HEK293 cells. *Toxicology and Applied Pharmacology*, , 245, 9-20.

[47] Francis, G. (1878). Poisonous Australian lake. *Nature*, , 18, 11-12.

[48] Fromme, H, Kohler, A, Krause, R, & Fuhrling, D. (2000). Occurrence of cyanobacterial toxins- microcystins and anatoxin-a- in Berlin water bodies with implications to human health and regulations. *Environmental Toxicology*, , 15, 120-130.

[49] Froscio, S. M, Humpage, A. R, Burcham, P. C, & Falconer, I. R. (2001). Cell-free protein sysnthesis inhibition assay for cyanobacterial toxin cylindrospermopsin. *Environmental Toxicology*, , 16, 408-412.

[50] Funari, E, & Testai, E. (2008). Human health risk assessment related to cyanotoxins exposure. *Critical Reviews in Toxicology*, , 38, 97-135.

[51] Gerwick, W. H, Tan, L. T, & Sitachitta, N. (2001). Nitrogen-containing metabolites from marine cyanobacteria. *The Alkaloids: Chemistry and Biology*, , 57, 75-184.

[52] Griffiths, D. J, & Saker, M. L. (2003). The Palm Island Mystery Disease 20 years on: a review of research on the cyanotoxin cylindrospermopsin. *Environmental Toxicology*, , 18, 78-93.

[53] Gulledge, B. M, Aggen, J. B, Eng, H, Sweimeh, K, & Chamberlin, A. R. (2003). Microcystin analogues comprised of only Adda and a single additional amino acid retain moderate activity as PP2A inhibitors. *Biorganic and Medicinal Chemistry Letters*, 13, 2907-2911., 1.

[54] Gugger, M, Lenoir, S, Berger, C, Ledreux, A, Druart, J. C, Humbert, J. F, Guette, C, & Bernard, C. (2005). First report in a river in France of the benthic cyanobacterium *Phormidium favosum* producing anatoxin-a associated with dog neurotoxicosis. *Toxicon*, , 45, 919-928.

[55] Harada, K. I, Ohtani, I, Iwamoto, K, Suzuki, M, Watanabe, M. F, Watanabe, M, & Terao, K. (1994). Isolation of cylindrospermopsin from a cyanobacterium *Umezakia natans* and its screening method. *Toxicon*, , 32, 73-84.

[56] Harada, K, Oshikata, M, Shimada, T, Nagata, A, Ishikawa, N, Suzuki, M, Kondo, F, Shimizu, M, & Yamada, S. (1997). High-performance liquid chromatographic separa-

tion of microcystins derivatized with a highly fluorescent dienophile. *Natural Toxins, ,* 5, 201-207.

[57] Hashimoto, Y, Ko-nosu, S, & Yasumoto, T. (1967). Epidemiological research of poisoining caused by sea turtles in Okinawa.

[58] Hawkins, P. R, Runnegar, M. T. C, Jackson, A. R. B, & Falconer, I. R. (1985). Severe hepatotoxicity caused by the tropical cyanobacterium *Cylindrospermopsis raciborskii* isolated from a domestic water supply reservoir. *Applied and Environmental Microbiology, ,* 50, 1291-1295.

[59] Heintzelman, G, Fang, W, Keen, K, Wallace, S. P, & Weinreb, G. A. S. M. ((2001). Stereoselective total synthesis of the cyanobacterial hepatotoxin 7-epicylindrospermopsin: revision of the stereochemistry of cylindrospermopsin. *Journal of the American Chemical Society, ,* 123, 8851-8853.

[60] Hilborn, E. D, Carmichael, W. W, Soares, R. M, Yuan, M, Servaites, J. C, Barton, H. A, & Azevedo, S. M. (2007). Serologic evaluation of human microcystin exposure. *Environmental Toxicology, ,* 22, 459-463.

[61] Holcombe, G. W, Benoit, D. A, Leonard, E. N, & Mckim, J. M. (1976). Long-term effects of lead exposure on three generations of Brook Trout (*Salvenius fontinalis*). *Journal of Fisheries Research Board of Canada, ,* 33, 1731-1741.

[62] Humpage, A. R, Rositano, J, Bretag, A. H, Brown, R, Baker, P. D, Nicholson, B. C, & Steffensen, D. A. (1994). Paralytic shellfish poisons from Australian cyanobacterial blooms. *Australian Journal of Marine and Freshwater Research, ,* 45, 761-771.

[63] Humpage, A. R, & Falconer, I. R. (2003). Oral toxicity of the cyanobacterial toxin cylindrospermopsin in male Swiss albino mice: determination of no observed adverse effect level for deriving drinking water guideline value. *Environmental Toxicology, ,* 18, 94-103.

[64] Humpage, A. R, Fontaine, F, Froscio, S, Burcham, P, & Falconer, I. R. (2005). Cylindrospermopsin genotoxicity and cytotoxicity: role of cytochrome and oxidative stress. *Journal of Toxicology and Environmental Health A,* 68, 739-753., 450.

[65] Humpage, A. R, Magalhaes, V. F, & Froscio, S. M. (2010). Comparison of analytical tools and biological assays for detection of paralytic shellfish poisoning toxins. *Analytical and Bioanalytical Chemistry, ,* 397, 1655-1671.

[66] Ibelings, B. W, Bruning, K, De Jonge, J, Wolfstein, K, Pires, L. M, Postma, J, & Burger, T. (2005). Distribution of microcystins in a lake foodweb: no evidence for biomagnification. *Microbial Ecology, ,* 49, 487-500.

[67] Ibelings, B. W, & Chorus, I. (2007). Accumulation of cyanobacterial toxins in freshwater "seafood" and its consequences for public health: a review. *Environmental Pollution, ,* 150, 177-192.

[68] Jackim, E, & Gentile, J. (1968). Toxins of a blue-green alga: similarity to saxitoxin. *Science*, , 162, 915-916.

[69] Jaja-chimedza, A, Gantar, M, Gibbs, P. D. L, Schmale, M. C, & Berry, J. P. (2012). Polymethoxy-1-alkenes from *Aphanizomenon ovalisporum* inhibit vertebrate development in the zebrafish (*Danio rerio*) embryo model. *Marine Drugs*, , 10, 2322-2336.

[70] James, K, J, Furey, A, Sherlock, I. R, Stack, M. A, Twohig, M, Caudwell, F. B, & Skulberg, O. M. (1998). Sensitive determination of anatoxin-a, homoanatoxin-a and their degradation products by liquid chromatography with fluorometric detection. *Journal of Chromatography*, , 798, 147-157.

[71] Jiang, L, Aigret, B, De Borggraeve, W. M, Spacil, Z, & Ilag, L. L. MS method for the identification of BMAA from its isomers in biological samples. *Analytical and Bioanalytical Chemistry*, , 403, 1719-1730.

[72] Jonasson, S, Eriksson, J, Berntzon, L, Spacil, Z, Ilag, L. L, Ronnevi, L. O, Rasmussen, U, & Bergman, B. (2010). Transfer of a cyanobacterial neurotoxin within a temperate aquatic ecosytem suggests a pathway for human exposure. *Proceedings of the National Academy of Science U. S. A.,* , 107, 9252-9257.

[73] Jos, A, Pichardo, S, Prieto, A, Repetto, G, Vazquez, C. M, Moreno, I, & Camean, A. M (2005). Toxic cyanobacterial cells containing microcystins induce oxidative stress in exposed tilapia fish (*Oreochromis* sp.) under laboratory conditions. *Aquatic Toxicology*, , 72, 261-271.

[74] Karjalainen, M, Reinkainen, M, Lindvall, F, Spoof, L, & Meriluoto, J. A. (2003). Uptake and accumulation of dissolved, radiolabeled nodularin in Baltic Sea zooplankton. *Environmental Toxicology*, , 18, 52-60.

[75] Karjalainen, M, Reinikainen, M, Spoof, L, Meriluoto, J. A, Sivonen, K, & Viitasalo, M. (2005). Trophic transfer of cyanobacterial toxins from zooplankton to planktivores: consequences for pike larvae and mysid shrimps. *Environmental Toxicology*, , 20, 354-362.

[76] Karlsson, K. M, Spoof, L. E, & Meriluoto, J. A. (2005). Quantitative LC-ESI-MS analyses of microcystins and nodularin-R in animal tissue- matrix effects and method validation. *Environmental Toxicology*, , 20, 381-390.

[77] Kaya, K, & Mahakhant, A. Keovara, L; Sano, T.; Kubo, T. & Takagi, H. ((2002). Spiroidesin, a novel lipopeptide from the cyanobacterium *Anabaena spiroides* that inhibits cell growth of the cyanobacterium *Microcystis aeruginosa*. *Journal of Natural Products*, , 65, 920-921.

[78] Kim, H, Lantvit, D, Hwang, C. H, Kroll, D. J, Swanson, S. M, Franzblau, S. G, & Orjala, J. (2012). Indole alkaloids from two cultured cyanobacteria, *Westiellopsis* sp. and *Fischerella muscicola*. *Bioorganic and Medicinal Chemistry*, , 20, 5290-5295.

[79] Kinnear, S. (2010). Cylindrospermopsin: a decade of progress on bioaccumulation research. *Marine Drugs,* , 8, 542-564.

[80] Kittler, K, Schreiner, M, Krumbein, A, Manzei, S, Matthias, K, Sascha, R, & Maul, R. (2012). Uptake of the cyanobacterial toxin cylindrospermopsin in *Brassica* vegetables. *Food Chemistry,* , 133, 875-879.

[81] Kozlowsky-suzuki, B, Wilson, A. E, & Ferrao-filho, A. (2012). Biomagnification or biodilution of microcystins in aquatic food-webs? Meta-analyses of laboratory and field studies. *Harmful Algae,* , 18, 47-55.

[82] Kurmayer, R, & Jüttner, F. (1999). Strategies for co-existence of zooplankton with the toxic cyanobacterium *Planktothrix rubescens* in Lake Zürich. *Journal of Plankton Research,* , 21, 659-683.

[83] Kwong, R. W. M, Wang, W, Lam, X, & Yu, P. K. S. P. K. N. ((2006). The uptake, distribution and elimination of paralytic shellfish toxins in mussels and fish exposed to toxic dinoflagellates. *Aquatic Toxicology,* , 80, 82-91.

[84] Lagos, N, Onodera, H, Zagatto, P. A, Andrinolo, D, Azevedo, M. F. Q, & Oshima, Y. (1999). The first evidence of paralytic shellfish toxins in the freshwater cyanobacterium *Cylindrospermopsis raciborskii* isolated from Brazil. *Toxicon,* , 37, 1359-1373.

[85] Lance, E, Neffling, M. R, Gerard, C, Meriluto, J, & Bormans, M. (2010a). Accumulation of free and covalently bound microcystins in tissues of *Lymnaea stagnalis* following toxic cyanobacteria or dissolved microcystin-LR exposure. *Environmental Pollution,* , 158, 674-680.

[86] Lance, E, Josso, C, Dietrich, D, Ernst, B, Paty, C, Senger, F, Bormans, M, & Gerard, C. and microcystin distribution in *Lymnaea stagnalis* following toxic cyanobacterial or dissolved microcysti-LR exposure. *Aquatic Toxicology,* , 98, 211-220.

[87] Landsberg, J. H, Hall, S, Johannessen, J. N, White, K. D, Conrad, S. M, Abbott, J. P, Flewelling, L. J, Richardson, R. W, Dickey, R. W, Jester, E. L, Etheridge, S. M, Deeds, J. R, Van Dolah, F. M, Leighfield, T. A, Zou, Y, Beaudry, C. G, Benner, R. A, Rogers, P. L, Scott, P. S, Kawabata, K, Wolny, J. L, & Steidinger, K. A. (2006). Saxitoxin puffer fish poisoning in the United States, with the first report of *Pyrodinium bahamense* as the putative toxin source. *Environmental Health Perspectives,* , 114, 1502-1507.

[88] Lemaire, V, Brusciotti, S, Van Gremberghe, I, Vyverman, W, Vanoverbeke, J, & De Meester, L. (2012). Genotype x genotype interactions between the toxic cyanobacterium *Microcystis* and its grazer, the waterflea *Daphnia. Evolutionary Applications,* , 5, 168-182.

[89] Li, A, Fan, H, Ma, F, Mccarron, P, Thomas, K, Tan, X, & Quilliam, M. A. (2012). Elucidation of matrix effects and performance of solid-phase extraction for LC-MS/MS analysis of β-N-methylamino-L-alanine (BMAA) and diaminobutyric acid (DAB) neurotoxins in cyanobacteria. *Analyst,* 137, 1210-1219., 2(4)

[90] Li, W, Duan, J, Niu, C, Qiang, N, & Mulcahy, D. (2010). Determination of microcystin-LR in drinking water using UPLC tandem mass spectrometry- matrix effects and measurement. *Journal of Chromatographic Science*, , 49, 665-670.

[91] Li, W. I, Berman, F. W, Okino, T, Yokokawa, F, Shioiri, T, Gerwick, W. H, & Murray, T. F. (2001). Antillatoxin is a marine cyanobacterial toxin that potently activates voltage-gated sodium channels. *Proceedings of the National Academy of Sciences U.S.A.* , 98, 7599-7604.

[92] Lobner, D, Piana, P. M, Salous, A. K, & Peoples, R. W. (2007). Beta-N-methylamino-L-alanine enhances neurotoxicity through multiple mechanisms. *Neurobiological Disease*, , 25, 360-366.

[93] Lu, H, Choudhuri, S, Ogura, K, Csanaky, I. L, Lei, X, Cheng, X, Song, P. Z, & Klaassen, C. D. (2008). Characterization of organic anion transporting polypeptide 1b2-null mice: essential role in hepatic uptake/toxicity of phalloidin and microcystin-LR. *Toxicological Science*, , 103, 35-45.

[94] MacKintoshR. W.; Dalby, K. N.; Campbell, D. G.; Cohen, P. T.; Cohen, P. & MacKintosh, C. ((1995). The cyanobacterial toxin microcystin binds covalently to cystein-273 on protein phosphatase 1. *FEBS Letters*, , 371, 236-240.

[95] Mahmood, N. A, & Carmichael, W. W. (1986). Paralytic shellfish poisons produced by the freshwater cyanobacterium *Aphanizomenon flos-aquae*). *Toxicon*, , 24, 175-186.

[96] Maidana, M, Carlis, V, Galhardi, F. G, Yunes, J. S, Geracitano, L. A, Monserrat, J. M, & Barros, D. M. (2006). Effects of microcystins over short- and long-term memory and oxidative stress generation in hippocampus of rats. *Chemico-Biological Interactions*, , 159, 223-234.

[97] Martin, C, Oberer, L, Ino, T, König, W. A, Busch, M, & Weckesser, J. (1993). Cyanopeptolins, new depsipeptides from the cyanobacterium *Microcystis* sp. PCC 7806. *Journal of Antibiotics* (Tokyo), , 46, 1550-1556.

[98] Mcelhiney, J, & Lawton, L. A. (2005). Detection of the cyanobacterial hepatotoxins microcystins. *Toxicology and Applied Pharmacology*, , 203, 219-230.

[99] Mejean, A, Peyraud-thomas, C, Kerbrat, A. S, Golubic, S, Pauillac, S, Chinain, M, & Laurent, D. (2010). First identification of the neurotoxin homoanatoxin-a from mats of *Hydrocoleum lyngbyaceum* (marine cyanobacterium) possibly linked to giant clam poisoning in New Caledonia. *Toxicon*, , 56, 829-835.

[100] Metcalf, J. S, Hyenstrand, P, Beattie, K. A, & Codd, G. A. (2000). Effects of physico-chemical variables and cyanobacterial extracts on the immunoassay of microcystin-LR by two ELISA kits. *Journal of Applied Microbiology*, , 89, 532-538.

[101] Metcalf, J. S, Beattie, K. A, Saker, M. L, & Codd, G. A. (2002). Effects of organic solvents on the high performance liquid chromatographic analysis of the cyanobacterial

toxin cylindrospermopsin, and its recovery from environmental eutrophic waters by solid-phase extraction. *FEMS Microbiology Letters*, , 216, 159-164.

[102] Miller, M. A, Kudela, R. M, Mekebri, A, Crane, D, Oates, S. C, Tinker, M. T, Staedler, M, Miller, W. A, Toy-choutka, S, Dominik, C, Hardin, D, Langlois, G, Murray, M, Ward, K, & Jessup, D. A. (2010). Evidence for a novel marine harmful algal bloom: cyanotoxin (microcystin) transfer from land to sea otters. *PLoS One*, 5, e12576.

[103] Mo, S, Krunic, A, Chlipala, G, & Orjala, J. (2009). Antimicrobial ambiguine isonitriles from the cyanobacterium *Fischerella ambigua*. *Journal of Natural Products*, , 72, 894-899.

[104] Mondo, K, Hammerschlag, N, Basile, M, Pablo, J, Banack, S. A, & Mash, D. C. (2012). Cyanobacterial neurotoxin beta-N-methylamino-L-alanine (BMAA) in shark fins. *Marine Drugs*, , 10, 509-520.

[105] Mori, Y, Kohchi, Y, Suzuki, M, Carmeli, S, Moore, R. E, & Patterson, G. M. L. (1991). Isotactic polymethoxy 1-alkenes from the blue-green algae. Synthesis and absolute stereochemistry. *Journal of Organic Chemistry*, , 56, 631-637.

[106] Mountfort, D. O, Holland, P, & Sprosen, J. (2005). Method for detecting classes of microcystins by combination of protein phosphatase inhibition assay and ELISA: comparison with LC-MS. *Toxicon*, , 45, 199-206.

[107] Msagati, T. A, Siame, B. A, & Shushu, D. D. (2006). Evaluation of methods for the isolation, detection and quantification of caynobacterial hepatotoxins. *Aquatic Toxicology*, , 78, 382-397.

[108] Murch, S. J, Cox, P. A, & Banack, S. A. (2004). A mechanism for slow release of biomagnified cyanobacterial neurotoxins and neurodegenerative disease in Guam. *Proceedings of the National Academy of Science U.S.A.*, , 101, 12228-12231.

[109] Mynderse, J. S, & Moore, R. E. (1979). Isotactic polymethoxy-1-alkene from the blue-green alga *Tolypothrix conglutinata* var. *Chlorata*. *Phytochemistry*, , 18, 1181-1183.

[110] Namikoshi, M, Rinehart, K. L, Sakai, R, Sivonen, K, & Carmichael, W. W. (1990). Structures of three new cyclic hepatotoxins produced by the cyanobacterium (blue-green alga) *Nostoc* sp. strain 152. *Journal of Organic Chemistry*, , 55, 6135-6139.

[111] Namikoshi, M, Rinehart, K. L, Sakai, R, Stotts, R. R, Dahlem, A. M, Beasley, C. R, Carmichael, W. W, & Evans, A. M. (1992). Identification of 12 hepatotoxins from Homer lake bloom of the cyanobacterium *Microcystis aeruginosa*, *Microcystis viridis*, and *Microcystis wesenbergii*: nine new microcystins. *Journal of Organic Chemistry*, , 57, 866-872.

[112] Nakamura, M, Oshima, Y, & Yasumoto, T. (1984). Occurrence of saxitoxin in puffer fish. *Toxicon*, , 22, 381-385.

[113] Negri, A. P, Jones, G. J, & Hindmarsh, M. (1995). Sheep mortality associated with paralytic shellfish poisons from the cyanobacterium *Anabaena circinalis*. *Toxicon*, , 33, 1321-1329.

[114] Nishiwaki-matsushima, R, Nishiwaki, S, Ohta, T, Yoshizawa, S, Suganuma, M, Harada, K, Watanabe, M. F, & Fujiki, H. (1991). Structure-function relationships of microcystins, liver tumor promoters, in interaction with protein phosphatases. *Japanese Journal of Cancer Research*, , 82, 993-996.

[115] Nogle, L. M, Okino, T, & Gerwick, W. H. a neurotoxic lipopeptide from the marine cyanobacterium *Lyngbya majuscula*. *Journal of Natural Products*, , 65, 983-985.

[116] Nogueira, I. C, Saker, M. L, Pflugmacher, S, Wiegand, C, & Vasconcelos, V. M. (2004). Toxicity of the cyanobacterium *Cylindrospermopsis raciborskii* to *Daphnia magna*. *Environmental Toxicology*, , 19, 453-459.

[117] Norris, R. L, Seawright, A. A, Shaw, G. R, Smith, M. J, Chiswell, R. K, & Moore, M. R. (2001). Distribution of 14C cylindrospermopsin in vivo in the mouse. *Environmental Toxicology*, , 16, 498-505.

[118] Ohtani, I, Moore, R. E, & Runnegar, M. T. C. (1992). Cylindrospermopsin: a potent hepatotoxin from the blue-green alga *Cylindrospermopsis raciborskii*. *Journal of the American Chemical Society*, , 114, 7942-7944.

[119] Okino, T, Murakami, M, Haraguchi, R, Munetata, H, Matsuda, H, & Yamaguchi, K. and trypsin inhibitors from the blue-gren alga *Microcystis aeruginosa*. *Tetrahedron Letters*, , 34, 8131-8134.

[120] Oksanen, I, Jokela, J, Fewer, D. P, Wahlsten, M, Rikkinen, J, & Sivonen, K. (2004). Discovery of rare and highly toxic microcystins from lichen-associated cyanobacterium *Nostoc* sp strain IO-102-I. *Applied and Environmental Microbiology*, , 70, 5756-5763.

[121] Orjala, J, Nagle, D. G, Hsu, V, & Gerwick, W. H. (1995). Antillatoxin: an exceptionally ichthyotoxic cyclic lipopeptide from the tropical cyanobacterium *Lyngbya majuscula*. *Journal of the American Chemical Society*, , 117, 8281-8282.

[122] Osborne, N. J, & Shaw, G. R. (2008). Dermatitis associated with exposure to a marine cyanobacterum during recreational water exposure. *BMC Dermatology*, 8, 5.

[123] Osswald, J, Rellan, S, Carvalho, A. P, Gago, A, & Vasconcelos, V. (2007). Acute effects of an anatoxin-a producing cyanobacterium on juvenile fish- *Cyprinus carpio*. *Toxicon*, , 49, 693-698.

[124] Osswald, J. A, Vasconcelos, V, & Guilhermino, L. (2011). Experimental determination of bioconcentration factors for anatoxin-a in juvenile rainbow trout (*Oncorhynchus mykiss*). *Proceedings of the International Academy of Ecology and Environmental Sciences*, 1, 77-86.

[125] Osswald, J, Rellan, S, Gago, A, & Vasconcelos, V. (2008). Uptake and depuration of anatoxin-a by the mussel *Mytilus galloprovincialis* under laboratory conditions. *Chemosphere*, , 72, 1235-1241.

[126] Ott, J. L, & Carmichael, W. W. MS method development for the analysis of hepatotoxic cyclic peptide microcystin in animal tissues. *Toxicon*, , 47, 734-741.

[127] Pablo, J, Banack, S. A, Cox, P. A, Johnson, T. E, Papapetropoulos, S, Bradley, W. G,
Buck, A, & Mash, D. C. (2009). Cyanobacterial neurotoxin BMAA in ALS and Alzheimer's disease. *Acta Neurological Scandinavica*, , 120, 216-225.

[128] Paerl, H, & Huisman, J. (2009). Climate change: a catalyst for global expansion of
harmful cyanobacterial blooms. *Environmental Microbiology Reports*, , 1, 27-37.

[129] Pereira, P, Dias, E, Franca, S, Pereira, E, Carolino, M, & Vasconcelos, V. (2004). Accumulation and depuration of cyanobacterial paralytic shellfish toxins by the freshwater mussel *Anodonta cygnea*. *Aquatic Toxicology*, , 68, 339-350.

[130] Pereira, S. R, Vasconcelos, V. M, & Antunes, A. (2012). Computational study of the
covalent bonding of microcystins to cystein residues- a reaction involved in the inhibition of the PPP family of protein phosphatases. *FEBS Journal*, in press.

[131] Peuthert, A, Chakrabarti, S, & Pflugmacher, S. (2007). Uptake of microcystins-LR
and-LF (cyanobacterial toxins) in seedlings of several important agricultural plant
species and the correlation with cellular damage (lipid peroxidation). *Environmental
Toxicology*, , 22, 436-442.

[132] Pflugmacher, S, Wiegand, C, Beattie, K. A, Krause, E, Steinberg, C. E, & Codd, G. A.
(2001). Uptake, effects, and metabolism of cyanobacterial toxins in the emergent reed
plant *Phragmites australis*, *Environmental Toxicology and Chemistry*, , 20, 846-852.

[133] Pietsch, C, Wiegand, C, Ame, M. V, Nicklisch, A, Wunderlin, D, & Pflugmacher, S.
(2001). The effects of cyanobacterial crude extract on different aquatic organisms: evidence for cyanobacterial toxin modulating factors. *Environmental Toxicology*, , 16,
535-542.

[134] Pomati, F, Sacchi, S, Rossetti, C, Giovannardi, S, Onodera, H, Oshima, Y, & Neilan, B.
A. (2000). The freshwater cyanobacterium *Planktothrix* sp. FP1: molecular identification and detection of paralytic shellfish poisoning toxins. *Journal of Phycology*, , 36,
553-562.

[135] Preu, K, Stüken, A, Wiedner, C, Chorus, I, & Fastner, J. (2006). First report on cylindrospermopsin producing *Aphanizomenon flos-aquae* (Cyanobacteria) isolated from
two German Lakes. *Toxicon*, , 47, 156-162.

[136] Proksh, P, Edrada, R. A, & Ebel, R. (2002). Drugs from the seas- current status and
microbiological implications. *Applied Microbiology and Technology*, , 59, 125-134.

[137] Puerto, M, Campos, A, Prieto, A, & Camean, A. da Almeida, A. M.; Coelho, A. V. &
Vasconcelos, Differential protein expression in two bivalve species: *Mytilus gallopro-
vincalis* and *Corbicula fluminea*, exposed to *Cylindrospermopsis raciborskii* cells. *Aquatic
Toxicology*, 101, 109-116., 2011

[138] Qiao, Q, Liang, H, & Zhang, X. (2012). Effect of cyanobacteria on immune function of crucian carp (*Carassius auratus*) via chronic exposure in diet. *Chemosphere*, in press.

[139] Qiu, T, Xie, P, Ke, Z, & Guo, L. (2007). In situ studies on physiological and biochemical respones in four fishes with different trophic levels to toxic cyanobacterial blooms in a large Chinese lake. *Toxicon*, , 50, 365-376.

[140] Rama, R. M, & Faulkner, D. J. (2002). Isotactic polymethoxydienes from the Philippines sponge *Myriastra clavosa*. *Journal of Natural Products*, , 65, 1201-1203.

[141] Rao, P. V, Gupta, N, Bhaskar, A. S, & Jayaraj, R. (2002). Toxins and bioactive compounds from cyanobacteria and their implications on human health. *Journal of Environmental Biology*, , 23, 215-224.

[142] Rao, S. D, Banack, S. A, Cox, P. A, & Weiss, J. H. (2006). BMAA selectively injures motor neurons via AMPA/kainite receptor activation. *Experimental Neurology*, , 201, 244-252.

[143] Raveh, A, & Carmeli, S. (2007). Antimicrobial ambigues from the cyanobacterium *Fischerella* sp. collected in Israel. *Journal of Natural Product*, , 70, 196-201.

[144] Reinikainen, M, Meriluoto, J. A. O, Spoof, L, & Harada, K. (2001). The toxicities of a polyunsaturated fatty acid and a microcystin to *Daphnia magna*. *Environmental Toxicology*, , 16, 444-448.

[145] Ricciardi, A, & Bourget, E. (1998). Weight-to-weight conversion factors for marine benthic macroinvertebrates. *Marine Ecology Progress Series*, , 163, 245-251.

[146] Rogers, E. H, Zehr, R. D, Gage, M. I, Humpage, A. R, Falconer, I. R, Marr, M, & Chernoff, N. (2007). The cyanobacterial toxin, cylindrospermopsin, induces fetal toxicity in the mouse after exposure late in gestation. *Toxicon*, , 49, 855-864.

[147] Rohrlack, T, Dittman, E, Börner, T, & Christoffersen, K. (2001). Effects of cell-bound microcystins on survival and feeding of *Daphnia* spp. *Applied and Environmental Microbiology*, , 67, 3523-3529.

[148] Rohrlack, T, Christoffersen, K, Kaebernick, M, & Neilan, B. A. (2004). Cyanobacterial protease inhibitor microviridin J causes lethal molting disruption in *Daphnia pulicaria*. *Applied Environmental Microbiology*, , 70, 5047-5050.

[149] Rosen, J, & Hellenäs, K. E. Determination of the neurotoxin BMAA (beta-N-methylamino-L-alanine) in cycad seed and cyanobacteria by LC-MS/MS (liquid chromatography tandem mass spectrometry). *Analyst*, , 133, 1785-1789.

[150] Runnegar, M. T. C, Kong, S. M, Zhong, Y. Z, Ge, J. L, & Lu, S. C. (1994). The role of glutathione in the toxicity of a novel cyanobacterial alkaloid cylindrospermopsin in cultured rat hepatocytes. *Biochemistry and Biophysics Research Communication*, , 201, 235-241.

[151] Runnegar, M. T. C, Kong, C. M, Zhong, Y. Z, & Lu, S. (1995). Inhbition of reduced glutathione synthesis by cyanobacterial alkaloid cylindrospermopsin in cultured rat hepatocytes. *Biochemical Pharmacology*, , 49, 219-225.

[152] Sabitini, S. E, Brena, B. M, & Luquet, C. M. San Julian, M.; Pirez, M. & Carmen Rios de Molina, M. D. ((2011). Microcystin accumulation and antioxidant responses in the freshwater clam *Diplodon chilensis patagonicus* upon subchronic exposure to toxic *Microcystis aeruginosa*. *Ecotoxicology and Environmental Safety*, , 74, 1188-1194.

[153] Saker, M. L, & Eaglesham, G. K. (1999). The accumulation of cylindrospermopsin from the cyanobacterium *Cylindrospermopsis raciborskii* in tissues of the Redclaw crayfish (*Cherax quadricarinatus*). *Toxicon*, , 37, 1065-1077.

[154] Sano, T, Nohara, K, Shiraishi, F, & Kaya, K. (1992). A method for micro-determination of total microcystin content in waterblooms of cyanobacteria (blue-green algae). *International Journal of Environmental Analytical Chemistry*, , 49, 163-170.

[155] Schwarzenberger, A, Kuster, C. J, & Von Elert, E. (2012). Molecular mechanisms of tolerance to cyanobacterial protease inhibitors revealed by clonal differences in *Daphnia magna*. *Molecular Ecology*, in press.

[156] Scott, P. M, Niedzwladek, B, Rawn, D. F, & Lau, B. P. (2009). Liquid chromatographic determination of the cyanobacterial toxin beta-n-methylamino-L-alanine in algae food supplements, freshwater fish, and bottled water. *Journal of Food Protection*, , 72, 1769-1773.

[157] Seifert, M. (2007). The ecological effects of the cyanobacterial toxin cylindrospermopsin. Dissertation, The University of Queensland, Brisbane, Australia.

[158] Shaw, G. R, Seawright, A. A, Moore, M. R, & Lam, P. K. S. (2000). Cylindrospermopsin, a cyanobacterial alkaloid: evaluation of its toxicological activity. *Therapeutic Drug Monitoring*, , 22, 89-92.

[159] Shen, X, Lam, P. K. S, Shaw, G. R, & Wikramsinghe, W. (2002). Genotoxicity investigation of a cyanobacterial toxin, cylindrospermopsin. *Toxicon*, , 40, 1499-1501.

[160] Sieroslawska, A, Rymuszka, A, Kalinowska, R, Skowronski, T, Bownik, A, & Pawlik-skowronska, B. (2010). Toxicity of cyanobacterial bloom in the eutrophic dam reservoir (Southeast Poland). *Environmental and Toxicological Chemistry*, , 29, 556-560.

[161] Simmons, T. L, Coates, R. C, Clark, B. R, Engene, N, Gonzalez, D, Esquenazi, E, Correstein, P. C, & Gerwick, W. H. (2008). Biosynthetic origin of natural products isolated from marine microorganism-invertebrate assemblages. *Proceedings of the National Academy of Sciences*, , 105, 4587-4594.

[162] Sivonen, K, Namikoshi, M, Evans, W. R, Fardig, M, Carmichael, W. W, & Rinehart, K. L. (1992). Three new microcystins, cyclic heptapeptide hepatotoxins, from *Nostoc* sp. strain 152. *Chemical Research in Toxicology*, , 5, 464-469.

[163] Sivonen, K. (2008). Emerging high throughput analyses of cyanobacterial toxins and toxic cyanobacteria. *Advances in Experimental Medicine and Biology*, , 619, 539-557.

[164] Smith, F. M, Wood, S. A, Van Ginkel, R, Broady, P. A, & Gaw, S. (2011). First report of saxitoxin production by a species of the freshwater benthic cyanobacterium, *Scytonema. Toxicon*, , 57, 566-573.

[165] Smith, J. L, Schulz, K. L, Zimba, P. V, & Boyer, G. L. (2010). Possible mechanism for the foodweb transfer of covalently bound microcystins. *Ecotoxicology and Environmental Safety*, , 73, 757-761.

[166] Smith, Q. R, Nagura, H, Takada, Y, & Duncan, M. W. (1992). Facilitated transport of the neurotoxin, beta-N-methylamino-L-alanine, across the blood brain barrier. *Journal of Neurochemistry*, , 58, 1330-1337.

[167] Smith, R. A, & Lewis, D. (1987). A rapid analysis of water for anatoxin a, the unstable toxic alkaloid from *Anabaena flos-aquae*, the stable non-toxic alkaloids left after bioreduction and a related amine which may be nature's precursor to anatoxin a. *Veterinary and Human Toxicology*, , 29, 153-154.

[168] Spencer, P. S, Nunn, P. B, Hugon, J, Ludolph, A. C, Ross, S. M, Roy, D. N, & Robertson, R. C. (1987). Guam amyotrophic lateral sclerosis-parkinsonism-dementia linked to a plant excitant neurotoxin. *Science*, , 237, 517-522.

[169] SpoofL; Berg, K. A.; Rapala, J.; Lahti, K.; Lepistö, L.; Metcalf, J. S.; Codd, G. A. & Meriluoto, J. ((2006). First observation of cylindrospermopsin in *Anabaena lapponica* isolated from the boreal environment (Finland). *Environmental Toxicology*, 21, 552-560.

[170] Staton, P. C, & Bristow, D. R. (1997). The dietary excitotoxins beta-N-methylamino-L-alanine and beta-N-oxalylamino-L-alanin induce necrotic and apoptotic-like cell death of rat cerebellar granule cells. *Journal of Neurochemistry*, , 69, 1508-1518.

[171] Stevens, D. K, & Krieger, R. I. (1991). Stability studies on the cyanobacterial nicotinic alkaloid anatoxin-a. *Toxicon*, , 29, 167-179.

[172] Stevens, M, Peigneur, S, & Tytgat, J. (2011). Neurotoxins and their binding areas on voltage-gated sodium channels. *Frontiers in Pharmacology*, 2, 71.

[173] Stewart, I, Webb, P. M, Schluter, P. J, & Shaw, G. R. (2006). Recreational and occupational field exposure to freshwater cyanobacteria- a review of anecdotal and case reports, epidemiological studies and the challenges for epidemiologic assessment. *Environmental Health*, 5, 6.

[174] Suchy, P, & Berry, J. (2012). Detection of total microcystin in fish tissues based on lemieux oxidation and recovery of 2-methyl-3-methoxy-4-phenylbutanoic acid (MMPB) by solid-phase microextraction gas chromatography-mass spectrometry (SPME-GC/MS). *International Journal of Environmental Analytical Chemistry*, , 92, 1443-1456.

[175] Sukenik, A, Reisner, M, Carmeli, S, & Werman, M. (2006). Oral toxicity of the cyano-bacterial toxin cylindrospermopsin in mice: long-term exposure to low doses. *Environmental Toxicology*, , 21, 575-582.

[176] Tan, L. T. (2007). Bioactive natural products from marine cyanobacteria for drug discovery. *Phytochemistry*, , 68, 954-979.

[177] Tan, L. T. (2010). Filamentous tropical marine cyanobacteria: a rich source of natural products for anticancer drug discovery. *Journal of Applied Phycology*, , 22, 659-676.

[178] Terao, K, Ohmori, S, Igarashi, K, Ohtani, I, Watanabe, M. F, Harada, K. I, Ito, E, & Watanabe, M. (1994). Electron microscopic studies on experimental poisoning in mice induced by cylindrospermopsin isolated from blue-green alga *Uzmekia natans*. *Toxicon*, , 32, 833-843.

[179] Ting, C. S, Rocap, G, King, J, & Chisholm, S. W. (2002). Cyanobacterial photosynthesis in the oceans: the origins and significance of divergent light-harvesting strategies. *Trends in Microbiology*, , 10, 134-142.

[180] Tsukamoto, S, Painuly, P, Young, K. A, Yang, X, Shimizu, Y, & Cornell, L. a novel cell differentiation-promoting depsipeptide from *Microcystis aeruginosa Journal of the American Chemical Society*, , 115(15-1840), 11046-11047.

[181] Ueno, Y, Nagata, S, Tsutsumi, T, Hasegawa, A, Watanabe, M. F, Park, H, Chen, D, Chen, G. -C, & Yu, G. S.-Z. ((1996). Detection of microcystsins, a blue-green algal hepatotoxin, in drinking water sampled in Haimen and Fusui, endemic areas of primary liver cancer in China, by highly sensitive immunoassay. *Carcinogenesis*, , 17, 1317-1321.

[182] Van Dolah, F. M. (2000). Marine algal toxins: origins, health effects, and their increased occurrence. *Environmental Health Perspectives*, , 108, 133-141.

[183] Vega, A, & Bell, E. A. (1967). amino-β-methylaminopropionic acid, a new amino acid from seeds of *Cycas circinalis*. *Phytochemistry*, , 6, 759-762.

[184] Von Elert, E, Oberer, L, Merkel, P, Huhn, T, & Blom, J. F. (2005). Cyanopeptolin 954, a chlorine-containing chymotrypsin inhibitor of *Microcystis aeruginosa* NIVA Cya 43. *Journal of Natural Products*, , 68, 1324-1327.

[185] Von Elert, E, & Zitt, A. Schwarzenberger ((2012). Inducible tolerance to dietary protease inhibitors in *Daphnia magna*. *Journal of Experimental Biology*, , 215, 2051-2059.

[186] Xie, L, Xie, P, Ozawa, K, Honma, T, Yokoyama, A, & Park, H. D. (2004). Dynamics of microcystins-LR and-RR in the phytoplanktivorous silver carp in a sub-chronic toxicity experiment. *Environmental Pollution*, , 127, 431-439.

[187] Welker, M, & Von Döhren, H. (2006). Cyanobacterial peptides- nature's own combinatorial biosynthesis. *FEMS Microbiology Reviews*, , 30, 530-563.

[188]   White, S. H, Duivenvoorden, L. J, Fabbro, L. D, & Eaglesham, G. K. (2006). Influence of intracellular toxin concentrations on cylindrospermopsin bioaccumulation in a freshwater gastropod (*Melanoides tuberculata*). *Toxicon*, , 47, 497-509.

[189]   White, S. H, Duivenvoorden, L. J, Fabbro, L. D, & Eaglesham, G. K. (2007). Mortality and toxin bioaccumulation in *Bufo marinus* following exposure to *Cylindrospermopsis raciborskii* cell extracts and live cultures. *Environmental Pollution*, , 147, 158-167.

[190]   Williams, D. E, Dawe, S. C, Kent, M. L, Andersen, R. J, Craig, M, & Holmes, C. F. and clearance of microcystins from salt water mussels, *Mytilus edulis*, and in vivo evidence for covalently bound microcystins in mussel tissues. *Toxicon*, , 35, 1617-1625.

[191]   Williams, D. E, & Craig, M. McCready; Dawe, S. C.; Kent, M. L.; Holmes, C. F. & Andersen, R. J. ((1997b). Evidence for covalently bound form of microcystin-LR in salmon liver and Dungeness crab larvae. *Chemical Research in Toxicology*, , 10, 463-469.

[192]   Wilson, A. E, Sarnelle, O, Neilan, B. A, Salmon, T. P, Gehringer, M. M, & Hay, M. E. (2005). Genetic variation of the bloom-forming cyanobacterium *Microcystis aeruginosa* within and among lakes: implications for harmful algal blooms. *Applied and Environmental Microbiology*, , 71, 6126-6133.

[193]   Wilson, A. E, Wilson, W. A, & Hay, M. E. (2006). Interspecific variation in growth and morphology of the bloom forming cyanobacterium *Microcystis aeruginosa*. *Applied and Environmental Microbiology*, , 72, 7386-7389.

[194]   Wu, M, Okino, T, Nogle, L. M, Marquez, B. L, Williamson, R. T, Sitachitta, N, Berman, F. W, Murray, T. F, Mcgough, K, Jacobs, R, Colsen, K, Asano, T, Yokokawa, F, Shioiri, T, & Gerwick, W. H. (2000). Structure, synthesis, and biological properties of Kalkitoxin, a novel neurotoxin from the marine cyanobacterium *Lyngbya majuscula*. *Journal of the American Chemical Society*, , 122, 12041-12042.

[195]   Yasumoto, T. (1998). Fish poisonings due to toxins due to microalgal origins in the Pacific. *Toxicon*, , 36, 1515-1518.

[196]   Yu, S. Z. ((1995). Primary prevention of hepatocellular carcinoma. *Journal of Gastroenterology and Hepatology*, , 10, 674-682.

[197]   Yu, S, Zhao, N, & Zi, X. (2001). The relationship between cyanotoxin (microcystin, MC) in pond-ditch water and primary liver cancer in China. *Zhonghua Zhong Liu Za Zhi*, , 23, 96-99.

[198]   Yuan, M, Carmichael, W. W, & Hilborn, E. D. (2006). Microcystin analysis in human sera and liver from human fatalities in Caruaru, Brazil 1996. *Toxicon*, , 48, 627-640.

[199]   Zhang, D, Xie, P, & Chen, J. (2010). Effects of temperature on the stability of microcystins in muscle of fish and its consequences for food safety. *Bulletin of Environmental Contamination and Toxicology*, , 84, 202-207.

[200] Zurawell, R. W, Chen, H, Burke, J. M, & Prepas, E. E. (2005). Hepatotoxic cyanobacte-
       ria: a review of the biological importance of microcystins in freshwater environ-
       ments. *Journal of Toxicology and Environmental Health B Critical Reviews, ,* 8, 1-37.

Chapter 6

Atmospheric Nanoparticles and Their Impacts on Public Health

Klara Slezakova, Simone Morais and
Maria do Carmo Pereira

Additional information is available at the end of the chapter

1. Introduction

The World Health Organization (WHO) estimates that every year around two million people die annually due to the effects of atmospheric pollution (Tranfield & Walker, 2012). These estimates are based on epidemiological studies that showed associations between air pollution exposure and respiratory and cardiovascular illnesses and deaths. Special efforts thus have been made in order to reduce air pollution on a global level (Slezakova et al., 2012) and, more importantly, aiming to reduce the adverse impacts of atmospheric pollutants. Although these efforts have been leading to a reduction of risks and effects, air pollution is still a matter of great concern, mainly to relative impacts on human health.

Air pollution is a mixture of various gases such as ozone, carbon monoxide, sulphur dioxide, and nitrogen dioxide combined with airborne particles in sizes range of few nanometers to hundreds of micrometers. According to the WHO, these particles are one of the most important pollutants of present times and their presence in the atmosphere has harmful effects both on human health and environment. Nanosized particles (i.e. smaller than 100 nm) are a subgroup of atmospheric particles. Though humans have been exposed to nanosized particles throughout their evolutionary stages, the respective exposure has dramatically increased over the last century due to contribution from various anthropogenic sources. In addition, the rapidly developing field of nanotechnology is likely to become another source of these particles through increased use of engineered nanomaterials. Thus information about safety and potential hazards is urgently needed. Apart from their role for possible adverse health effects (Hoek et al., 2010; Knol et al., 2009), nanoparticles are important precursors for the formation of coarser particles that are known to strongly influence global climate (Intergovernmental Panel on Climate Change [IPCC], 2007; Strawa et al., 2010) and urban visibility (Horvath, 1994). They may also influence the atmospheric chemistry in general as their chemical composition and reactivity are different from coarser particles, thus opening novel chemical transformation pathways in the atmosphere (Anastasio & Martin, 2001).

This chapter focuses specifically on airborne nanosized particles and their importance to public health. Various aspects are discussed in the following sections including sources, levels, chemical compositions, regulations, and health and environmental impacts.

2. Characteristics of atmospheric particles

2.1. Particle sizes

The size of particles in the atmosphere ranges from few nanometers up to hundred micrometers. There is no doubt that the particle size is an important parameter. It controls much of the dynamic behavior of particles as well as their chemical and physical impacts upon the environment. It is also certainly an important parameter for the health consequences of the respective human exposure as particle size determines: (i) the deposition of particles within human respiratory system; (ii) the amount of surface area that can contact tissues; and (iii) the rate of particle clearance from lungs (Oberdörster et al., 2005). Particles have many irregular shapes so their aerodynamic behavior is expressed in terms of the diameter of an idealized sphere (i.e. aerodynamic diameter), which is usually simply referred to as "particle size". Up to this date various terminologies in relation to particle size are used to describe atmospheric particles. Medical sciences use terms such as inhalable or respirable particles that derived from particles classification according to the entrance into various compartments of the respiratory system (WHO, 2000). Toxicologists typically describe particles as ultrafine, fine and coarse whereas regulatory agencies, namely WHO, US Environmental Protection Agency (USEPA) and European Union (EU) use terms such as PM_x where PM stands for particulate matter and the subscripts identifies the upper 50% cutpoint. The aerosol science uses classification of particles into the modes based on the particles diameter. Each mode has distinctive size range, formation mechanisms, sources, chemical composition and deposition pathways (Hinds, 1999).

Typically, the mass-based size distribution of atmospheric particles is bimodal, with a minimum point that generally occurs in the size range of 1000–3000 nm (i.e. 1–3 µm; Sioutas et al., 2005), which distinguishes the coarse and fine modes (Fig. 1). By convention, the coarse mode consists of particles larger than 2500 nm in aerodynamic diameter. Based on their size, the coarse mode particles can be further subdivided into supercoarse and coarse particles. The coarse particles have diameter between 2500 nm and 10000 nm (Fig. 1). These particles are usually produced by mechanical processes such wind erosion. Particles from sea salt sprays, pollen and spores also belong to this mode as do coarse particles from plant fibers and leaves. As coarse particles are large, they settle out of the atmosphere typically within few hours of formation. Coarse particles deposit in the upper airways of the human respiratory system and they are cleared from human body through nose or by coughing or swallowing. The supercoarse particles are those with aerodynamic diameter bigger than 10000 nm (i.e. 10 μm; USEPA, 2012a). As these particles are too large to enter human respiratory system they are not considered as relevant from the health point of view. However, due to their possible environmental impacts, supercoarse particles are partly assessed when evaluating total suspended particulate matter (TSP) which includes particles of size range up to 30000 nm (i.e. 30 μm).

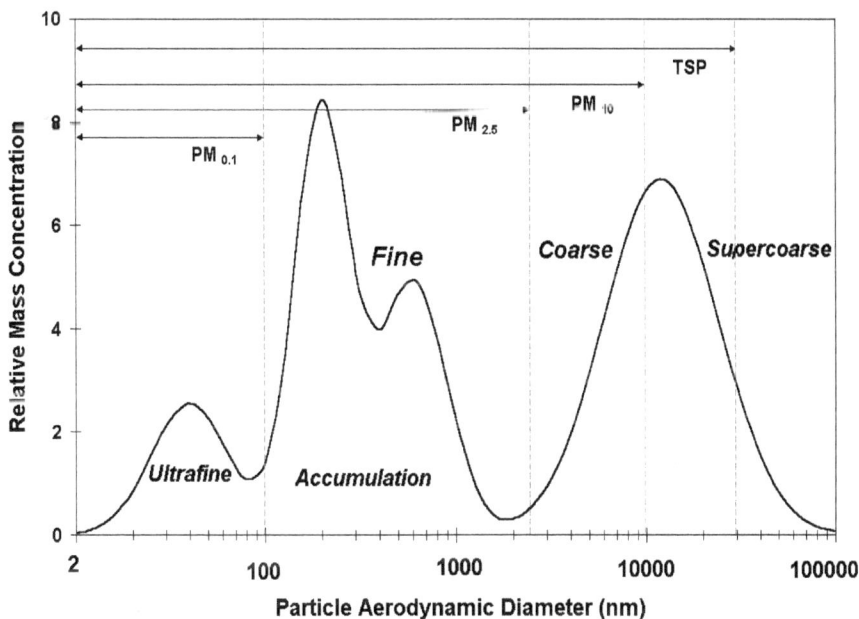

Figure 1. Schematic representation of the size distribution of atmospheric particles.

Fine mode is composed of particles with aerodynamic diameter smaller than 2500 nm (Fig. 1). Typically, these particles are generated by anthropogenic sources. The small sizes of the particles make them less susceptible to the gravitational settling resulting in atmospheric lifetimes in range of days up to weeks and the ability to travel over very long distances in the atmosphere (Anastasio & Martin, 2001). When inhaled fine particles deposit in the conducting airways of the lungs but some of them can penetrate beyond conducting airways into the alveolar region. Based on the formation mechanisms fine mode particles are further subdivide into accumulation and nuclei modes. Accumulation mode consists of particles with aerodynamic diameter between 100-1000 nm. They result from anthropogenic sources (combustions of engine fuel and lubricant oil by diesel-fuelled or direct injection petrol-fuelled vehicles; Kumar et al., 2010, 2011) but can be formed by natural formations, i.e. by coagulation of nuclei-mode particles or by condensation of gas or vapor molecules on the surface of existing particles.

Coagulation is most efficient for large numbers of particles, and condensation is most efficient for large surface areas. Thus the efficiency of both coagulation and condensation decreases as the particle size increases which produces an upper limit of approximately 1000 nm beyond which particles do not grow by these processes. Particles in the range of 100-1000 nm are important because they can represent a significant fraction of the particulate emissions from some types of industrial processes. In addition, sizes of particles in accumulation mode are comparable with the wavelengths of visible light, and hence they account for much of the anthropogenic visibility impairment problem in many urban areas (Seinfeld & Pandis, 2006).

Nuclei mode consist of particles smaller than 100 nm that are also called as ultrafine particles or nanoparticles. In the atmosphere these particles are formed through nucleation, i.e. condensation of low-vapor-pressure substances formed by high temperature vaporization or by chemical reactions in the atmosphere to form new particles (nuclei). These particles are traditionally considered as fresh emissions that yet have to undergo chemical reactions or modification processes. They are mostly composed of nitrates, sulphates, ammonium, organic compounds as well as trace metals when formed from combustion processes (Sioutas et al., 2005; Seinfeld & Pandis, 2006). Nucleation mode particles accounts for the greatest number of atmospheric particles and are found in high number concentrations near their sources. Their concentration in air is most commonly measured and expressed in terms of number concentrations of particles per unit volume of air (in contrast larger particles are measured in terms of mass concentration) (Kumar et al., 2011). Due to their small sizes and large surface area, they are highly chemically reactive. Collisions with each other and with particles in the accumulation mode are largely responsible for their relatively short atmospheric life time (few minutes up to hours). When inhaled these particles are deposited on the alveolar surface (Naga et al., 2005; West, 2008), thereafter, they can transport through the bloodstream or lymphatic system to vital organs (Oberdörster et al., 2004). In addition to their great efficiency to penetrate deep into the lungs, the large surface area may also account for their negative impacts on human health; the scientific evidence indicates that the larger the superficial area the greater the health impacts of particles (Tranfield & Walker, 2012).

The first research studies used the term *ultrafine particles* (Granqvist et al., 1976, 1977). Nowadays this term is still being predominantly used in aerosol and environmental sciences. However, in 1990's the term *nanoparticles* became vastly popular as substitution of ultrafine particles and quickly became adopted in many fields, such as in medicine, material sciences and engineering. Both terms constitute a somewhat arbitrary classification of particles in terms of their size, indicating the significant role of this physical characteristic on particle fate in the air. Theoretically, nanoparticle is any particle with size range in nanometer scale (i.e. bellow 1000 nm; Anastasio & Martin, 2001; Kumar et al., 2010). British Standards Institution (BSI, 2005) defined nanoparticles as those that have one or more dimensions in the order of 100 nm or less. However in current scientific works, the size range definitions for nanoparticles differ significantly. The term nanoparticles was used for atmospheric particles in size ranges such as below 100 nm, 50 nm, 10 nm or occasionally even for particles smaller than 1 μm (Anastasio & Martin, 2001; British Standards Institution, 2005; Morawska et al., 2008). It is worth mentioning that Kumar et al. (2010) recently defined atmospheric nanoparticles as those bellow

300 nm (Fig. 2). Though this size range represents an overlap between particles from nuclei and accumulation mode, authors rationalized that the respective range includes more than 99% of the total number concentration of particles in the ambient atmospheric environments (Kumar et al., 2008a, 2008b, 2009, 2011), being potentially relevant for future regulations.

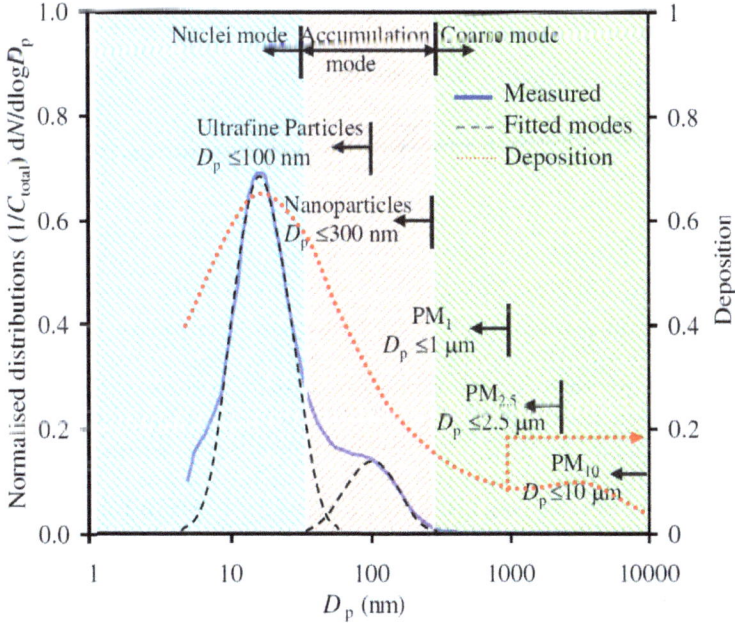

Figure 2. Distribution of atmospheric particles in street canyon in Cambridge, UK (Kumar et al., 2008); Dp, is particle diameter. Definitions of atmospheric particles and their size dependent deposition in alveolar and trancheo-bronchial regions are also shown. Adapted from Kumar et al. (2010).

Therefore, when using the term nanoparticles it is necessary to define the size range of the particles in question. For the purposes of this chapter the term nanoparticles includes ambient nanosized particles < 100 nm (Oberdörster et al., 2005).

2.2. Sources and levels of nanoparticles

The major natural sources of atmospheric nanoparticles (Table 1) are atmospheric formations, vegetation and sea sprays. Volcanic eruptions or forest fires also produce, though sporadically, a large number of atmospheric nanoparticles (Kumar et al., 2011; Oberdörster et al., 2005).

The atmospheric formations of the particles include condensation of semi-volatile organic aerosols, photochemically induced nucleation, and/or nucleation through gas-to particle conversion (Holmes, 2007). Concerning the latter, different nucleation mechanisms have been assumed for the formation of atmospheric nanoparticles (Kumala et al., 2004): (i) binary nucleation of sulphuric acid and water; or (ii) ternary nucleation involving a third molecule, most likely is ammonia that is abundant in the troposphere and has been shown to enhance nucleation rates of sulphuric acid.

Natural sources	Anthropogenic sources	
Atmospheric formations	Engine combustions	Vehicles (petrol-, diesel-, alternative fuels)
Sea spray		Trains, ships, airplanes
Vegetation		Power plants
Forest fires	Industrial emissions	Incinerators
Volcanoes (hot lava)		Various processes (smelting,
Viruses		heating, welding)
	Commercial productions	

Table 1. Sources of nanoparticles (Buseck & Adachi, 2008; Kumar et al., 2011; Oberdörster et al., 2005)

In remote sites, the formation of new particles is preceded by an increase in the atmospheric concentration of sulphuric acid (Holmes, 2007). Various studies reported an increase in particles number occurring about 1–2 h after an increase in sulphuric acid (Weber et al., 1996), being followed by a relatively small particle growth rate (between 1 and 2 nm h^{-1}; Birmili & Wiedensohler, 2000a; Weber et al., 1996, 1997). These findings point towards a linear relationship between the number of newly formed particles and the production rate of sulphuric acid. It is still not clear though whether at these environments the binary nucleation (i.e. water–sulphuric acid nucleation) is solely responsible for the formation of new particles or if a third specie, such as ammonia or an organic compound, is involved (i.e. ternary nucleation). In forests the mechanisms responsible for the formation and growth of atmospheric nanoparticles are not completely understood. Although sulphuric acid is one of the most likely candidates that might be responsible for the formation of the initial nanometre-sized particles (Riipinen et al., 2007), sulphur chemistry does not sustain enough sulphuric acid in the atmosphere to explain more than a small fraction of the observed particle size growth rate (Morawska et al., 2008). Several forest studies have concluded that particle formation can commonly occur from biogenic precursors (O'Dowd et al., 2002), some of them suggesting a direct relation between emissions of monoterpenes and gas-to-particle formation in regions substantially lacking in anthropogenic aerosol sources (Tunved et al., 2006). In addition the authors also estimated that forests provide an aerosol population of $1–2\times10^3$ cm^{-3} of climatically active particles (during the period of late spring to early autumn) thus representing a considerable source of global importance. In the marine environments the possible particle formation mechanisms are (Morawska et al., 2008): seawater bubble-burst process (Clarke et al., 2006; O'Dowd et al., 2004), ternary nucleation producing a reservoir of undetectable particles upon which vapours can condense (Kulmala et al., 2000, 2004), free tropospheric production with mixing down to the boundary layer (Raes, 1995), and generation of coastal iodine particles from macroalgal iodocarbon emissions (Kulmala et al., 2000; O'Dowd et al., 2004; O'Dowd & Hoffmann, 2005). Whereas the iodine-containing particles are not likely to play an important role globally, wind produced bubble-burst particles containing salt are ubiquitous in the marine environments. Clarke et al. (2006) have shown that sea salt aerosols produced by breaking waves are a significant constituent of particles with sizes as small as 10 nm, with 60% of the particles smaller than 100 nm in diameter. The authors estimated that in marine regions between 5% and 90% of the nuclei particles orig inate from the sea salt flux.

The implication of the above referred text is that nanoparticles are formed in the environments due to natural processes. Therefore, they are always present at some concentration levels even in the atmosphere of environments free from the immediate influence of anthropogenic activities. These concentrations should be considered as "natural background". In addition, because the rates of formation and growth of nanoparticles differ significantly between various natural environments, there are significant variations in number concentrations of atmospheric particles. Whereas in marine environments particle number concentrations typically range between 10^2 and 10^3 particles cm^{-3} (O'Dowd et al., 2004; Seinfeld & Pandis, 2006), the usual ranges in forests and rural continental regions are 10^3-10^4 (Birmili & Wiedensohler, 2000b; O'Dowd et al., 2002; Riipinen et al., 2007), though occurrence of forest fires may temporally increased these levels. Meteorological parameters, such as wind speed, precipitation, relative humidity and temperature also influence particle concentrations. Therefore, when evaluating particle concentrations in urban environments it is important to assess the respective background levels and to compare them with concentrations in urban environments in order to correctly estimate the magnitude of the anthropogenic impacts.

The number concentrations of nanoparticles in the atmosphere can vary by up to five or more orders of magnitude (from 10^2 to 10^7 particles cm^{-3}) depending on environmental conditions and source strengths (Kumar et al., 2010) but typically, in natural environments the particle number concentrations are approximately to 1-2 orders of magnitude smaller than those in urban areas (Kumar et al., 2010). Morawska et al. (2008) analysed concentration levels of 71 studies performed on nanoparticles in various environments, including those from clean background and rural background sites (Table 2). The authors found (Morawska et al., 2008), respectively, the mean concentrations of 2.6×10^3 and 4.8×10^3 particles cm^{-3} for clean background and rural background sites compared to 42.1×10^3 and 48.2×10^3 particles cm^{-3} for urban and street canyons; in urban areas anthropogenic sources, such as vehicular emissions are strong contributors of nanoparticles, thus much higher particle concentration levels were observed (Table 2). Road tunnels (167.7×10^3 particles cm^{-3}) account for the highest concentrations. They can act as a trap for pollutants from vehicular emissions that is enhanced by the surrounding built-up environment that limits the dispersion of exhaust emissions (Van Dingenen et al., 2004).

There is no doubt that anthropogenic emissions constitute the major source of atmospheric nanoparticles in urban environments (Table 2). With respect to urban sites various studies have concluded that vehicle exhaust emissions represent a primary source of nanoparticle pollution in urban environments (Harrison et al., 1999; Shi & Harrison, 1999; Shi et al., 2001; Wåhlin et al., 2001) that might be responsible up to 86% of total particle number concentrations (Pey et al., 2009). The vehicle emissions depend on many factors such as type of engines, fuels, lubricating oil, after-treatment or driving conditions. Typically particles emitted from diesel engines are in the size range 20–130 nm (Kittelson, 1998; Harris & Maricq, 2001). Diesel-fuelled vehicles make by far the greatest contributions to total number concentrations (Kumar et al., 2010) although in most of European countries their proportion is lower. In 2009 passenger diesel-fuelled cars in Europe accounted for to 9-10% (Sweden and Cyprus) to 62% (Luxemburg) but in 16 out of 21 European countries (where data is available) their proportion was less than 50% (EU, 2011). Large part of nanoparticles is also produce by heavy duty diesel vehicles (trucks, buses) that exhibit particle number emission factors one to two orders of magnitude larger than a typical petrol car (Ristovski et al., 2005, 2006). In comparison, particles from petrol-fuelled vehicles are in the size range 20–60 nm (Harris & Maricq, 2001; Ristovski et al., 2006), and their emissions vary significantly depending on the engine operating conditions; Graskow et al. (1998) reported that when driven at higher speed (~120 km h^{-1}) or during acceleration, the particle number emissions from petrol vehicles were similar to those observed from diesel vehicles.

Site	Number of analyzed studies	Estimated concentration × 10^3 (particles cm^{-3})	
		Mean	Median
Clean background	5	2.6	3.2
Rural background	8	4.8	2.9
Urban background	4	7.3	8.1
Urban	24	10.8	8.8
Street canyon	7	42.1	39.3
Roadside	18	48.2	34.6
On-road	2	71.5	47.0
Tunnel	3	167.7	99.1

Table 2. Particle number concentrations in different environments (Morawska et al., 2008)

In general particles from vehicle exhaust may be divided into two main categories. Primary particles are directly emitted from the engines. These particles are mostly submicrometer agglomerates (30-500 nm) of solid phase carbonaceous material containing metallic ash (from lubricating oil additives and engine wear) and adsorbed or condensed hydrocarbons and sulphur compounds (Morawska et al., 2008). Secondary particles are formed in the atmosphere when hot exhaust gases are expelled from vehicle tailpipe; as they cool and condensate they form nuclei mode particles (typically smaller than 30 nm) that consists mainly of hydrocarbons and hydrated sulphuric acid (Morawska et al., 2008). On-roads studies (e.g. when a vehicle is being followed by a mobile laboratory; Kittelson et al., 2004, 2006; Casati et al., 2007) and those performed near busy roads (Harrison et al., 1999; Ntziachristos et al., 2007; Rosenbohm et al., 2005; Westerdahl et al., 2005) reported large number of these particles.

The interactions between vehicle tyres and road can also generate particles of submicron sizes, although it was generally believed that tyre wear on the road contributes mainly to larger size (> 2.5 μm). Some more recent studies report (Gustafsson et al., 2008; Dahl et al., 2006) that considerable emissions of nanoparticles might be generated from road and tyre interactions, depending on surface, vehicle and driving conditions. As this source could be a significant contributor to particle number emissions, more research on this topic is needed.

The industrial sources of atmospheric nanoparticles include power plants, incinerators, or various industrial processes such as smelting or welding, heating operations (Oberdörster et al., 2005). Compared to vehicle exhaust emissions, their contribution to atmospheric nanoparticles is though much lower. In a study performed in Barcelona, Spain, Pey et al. (2009) investigated source apportionment of atmospheric particles in size range 13-800 nm (i.e. nuclei and accumulation mode) at an urban background site. The authors identified vehicular exhaust emissions (65%) and regional/urban background (24%) as the largest contributors to total particle number concentrations (mean of 17×10^3 particles cm^{-3}); industrial emissions accounted only for 2% of the total particle number. The levels of this contribution were similar in the study (Pey et al. (2009) to: photochemically induced nucleation (3%), sea spray (2%), and mineral dust (1%); unidentified sources accounted for 3%.

In the last decade nanoscience has been a dynamically developing field of scientific interest in the entire world (Aguar-Fernandez & Hullmann, 2007). Small size and relatively large reactive surface area of nanoparticles led to their increased use in a variety of fields such as in medicine, material sciences, electronics or energy storage (Helland et al., 2007). Thus engineered (i.e. manufactured) nanoparticles have become (apart from vehicle exhaust and industrial emissions) another important anthropogenic source of atmospheric nanoparticles. These nanoparticles are not intentionally released into the environment, though some release may occur during production, use and disposal phases of nanomaterial-integrated products (Bystrzejewska-Piotrowska et al., 2009). Their characteristics (sources, composition, homogeneity or heterogeneity, oxidant potential, exposure and emissions) differ from other atmospheric nanoparticles (Oberdörster et al., 2005). The engineered nanoparticles are nowadays incorporated into many products of daily use (pharmaceuticals, lubricants, cosmetics, pharmaceuticals, fillers, catalysts, electronic devices or other domestic appliances; Nel et al., 2006). The widespread use of manufactured nanoparticles in consumer products may dramatically increase potential environmental, occupational, and public exposures to these particles that may result in adverse health effects if they are not appropriately controlled. In addition, as nanotechnology has being nowadays used in various industries, it becomes responsible for the production of waste containing residue of nanomaterials; considering the unprecedented application of nanoparticles in various products, significant amounts of new-generation-waste will be certainly created in the near future (Bystrzejewska-Piotrowska et al., 2009).

In view of the comprehensive utilizations of nanotechnological applications, concerns regarding the potential health effects of engineered nanoparticles have been raised (Helland et al.,

2005). The available toxicological studies indicate (Nel et al., 2006; Oberdörster et al., 2005) that toxicity of engineered nanoparticles depends on specific physiochemical and environmental factors, implying that toxic potential of each type of nanoparticle has to be evaluated individually (Helland et al., 2007). Due to the great variability in used materials (e.g. titanium dioxide, silver, carbon, gold, cadmium and heavy metals; Kumar et al., 2010) it is thus not possible to generalize the toxicological impacts of the engineered nanoparticles. In addition size, shape, surface characteristics, inner structure and chemical composition may also play an important role in determining toxicity and reactivity (Maynard & Aitken, 2007; Nel et al., 2006).

2.3. Chemical composition of nanoparticles

The composition of atmospheric nanoparticles is highly variable. The source and formations influence their chemical composition and nanoparticles include components such as inorganic compounds (sulphates, nitrates, ammonium, chloride, trace metals), elemental and organic carbon, crystal materials, biological components (viruses), and volatile and semivolatile organic compounds (Oberdörster et al., 2005). They can carry toxic compounds such as heavy metals, dioxins, hydrocarbons and other organic chemicals (some of which are potentially carcinogenic) adhered to their surfaces which then increase their toxicity (Terzano et al., 2010). Apart the source-specificity, composition of nanoparticles also depends on geographical and meteorological parameters which in general lead to great differences in physicochemical properties among nanoparticles.

Several studies including a number of recent ones (Chen et al., 2010; Kim et al., 2011; Klems et al., 2011; Kudo et al., 2011) have evaluated the composition of atmospheric nanoparticles. However, at present, the knowledge on nanoparticles composition is far from comprehensive. The existent scientific studies are conducted at different ways, sample particles in a different size range, use different samplers, and focus on different aspects of particle chemical composition. Thus the reported data are not completely comparable across the studies. In their attempt to improve the current knowledge, Chow & Watson (2007) review and summarized the results of the existent studies. The authors analyzed 25 studies performed at various environments (rural, urban, industrial, coastal, roadside, traffic, city-centre, urban background, and etc.) and in various regions: two studies were conducted in Europe (Finland), four in Japan, three in Asia (one in China, two in Taiwan) and sixteen in USA; eleven US studies were performed in California, eight of them were from different locations within the Los Angeles metropolitan area. Concerning the chemical composition the authors concluded that organic material including polycyclic aromatic hydrocarbons was the most abundant portion of atmospheric nanoparticles in most, but not all environments. High elemental concentrations were found in nanoparticles from industrial sites with potassium, calcium and iron as important elements. Potassium originates from biomass burning, and calcium is used as an oil additive; condensed iron vapors are often found in industrial processes. Much of the nanoparticles appeared to be semi-volatile, consistent with being comprised of organic materials such as hopanes from engine oils or condensed secondary organic aerosol such as organic acids. However, authors emphasize the necessity to conduct more studies on particle chemical composition in to order to provide a more complete understanding on the chemistry of atmospheric nanoparticles and local variations.

3. Regulatory aspects

During last two decades the exponentially growing interdisciplinary research on air quality and health has clearly demonstrated increased incidence and the prevalence of respiratory diseases along with increased air pollution. Particles have emerged as the most dangerous pollutants due their adverse health effects going far beyond the simple toxicity to the lung. The results of the conducted epidemiology studies were so relevant that USEPA and EU have implemented strategies to protect public health which resulted in establishment of regulatory limits of atmospheric particles (PM_{10}). As the ongoing research emphasized the importance of smaller (i.e. fine) particles the new $PM_{2.5}$ standards were proposed and implemented in most of developed countries (Table 3). However, the reduction of atmospheric particulate emissions is nowadays required especially in rapidly developing countries, such as Brazil, China or India but they are only slowly moving towards implementation of these standards (Slezakova et al., 2012); there are still a number of countries, such as Pakistan where any regulatory limits for atmospheric particles have not been proposed yet.

Country	Pollutant	Targeted limit	Note	Reference
European Union	PM_{10}	24h mean: 40 µg/m³	Not to be exceeded more than 35 times per calendar year	Directive 2008/50/EC
		Annual mean: 50 µg/m³		
	$PM_{2.5}$	Annual mean: 25 µg/m³	(in force from 2015)	
USA	PM_{10}	24h mean: 150 µg/m³		
	$PM_{2.5}$	24h mean: 35 µg/m³		USEPA, 2006
		Annual mean : 15 µg/m³		
Canada	$PM_{2.5}$	24h mean : 30 µg/m³		Canadian Council of Ministries of Environment, 2003
Australia	PM_{10}	24h mean: 50 µg/m³		Australian Government, 2012
	$PM_{2.5}$	24h mean: 25 µg/m³		
		Annual mean: 8 µg/m³		
Japan	PM_{10}	24 h mean: 100 µg/m³		Government of Japan, 2012
	$PM_{2.5}$	24h mean: 35 µg/m³		
		Annual mean: 15 µg/m³		

Table 3. Air quality standards for atmospheric particles in selected countries

Unlike fine or coarse particles, the regulatory aspect of nanoparticles has not been addressed yet. The difficulty lies as to which metric of nanoparticles would be the most adequate. Several generic and specific characteristics of particles such as chemical composition, size, geometry or surface area have been discussed (Kumar et al., 2010, 2011) but no conclusion has been reached yet. The mass-based paradigm of PM_{10} and $PM_{2.5}$ regulator limits is not applicable to nanoparticles as their distribution is not dominated by mass but particle number. Some studies have suggested that the particle number concentrations of ultrafine particles (i.e. smaller than 100 nm) are an important parameter as size range comprises the major proportion (about 80%) of the total number concentration of ambient nanoparticles, but negligible mass concentration. Reliable characterization of nanoparticles in the air is thus vital for developing a regulatory framework. At national levels air quality agencies should be encouraged to integrate nanoparticle measurements in their monitoring networks (number and size distributions measurements). Such initiatives might provide comprehensive data and information necessary to correctly address regulatory aspects of atmospheric nanoparticles in order to prevent the public exposures.

4. Health impacts

Due to intensive research, there is an emerging evidence that exposure to nanoparticles may adversely affect human health (Stölzel et al., 2007). The nanoparticles enter human body through the skin, lung and gastrointestinal tract (Nel et al., 2006). When they are inhaled, their behavior differs from coarse particles. Their small size allows them to be breathed deeply into the lungs where they are able to penetrate alveolar epithelium and enter the pulmonary interstitium and vascular space to be absorbed directly into the blood stream (Terzano et al., 2010). They may also translocate within the body to the central nerve system, the brain, into the systemic circulation and to organs like the liver (Helland et al., 2007; Figure 3). They are more reactive and toxic due to the larger surface areas, leading to detrimental health effects such as oxidation stress, pulmonary inflammation and cardiovascular events (Buseck & Adachi, 2008; Nel et al., 2006).

Though the toxicological studies have provided evidence of the toxicity of nanoparticles, epidemiological evidence of the health effects is limited. Currently, there is also no quantitative summary of concentration-response functions for these particles that could be used in health impact assessment (Hoek et al., 2010). Unlike for coarse and fine particles there are relatively few epidemiological studies on the health effects of atmospheric nanoparticles. The first conducted studies on atmospheric nanoparticles have been panel studies, which generally showed associations between short-term exposure to nanosized particles and occurrence of acute respiratory symptoms and lung function (Ibald-Mulli et al., 2002; Peters et al., 1997; Penttinen et al., 2001a, 2001b). Some of these studies have suggested that nanoparticles might be even more strongly associated with adverse respiratory outcomes than fine particles (Peters et al., 1997; Penttinen et al., 2001a) whereas other studies found similar associations in health outcomes of nano and fine particles (von Klot et al., 2002; Pekkannen et al., 1997, Penttinen et al., 2001b).

Up to this date, only few epidemiological studies have assessed more severe end points such as daily, and cause specific mortality and hospital admissions (Stölzel, et al., 2007; Wichman et al., 2000); there are no epidemiological studies on long-term exposure to atmospheric nanoparticles.

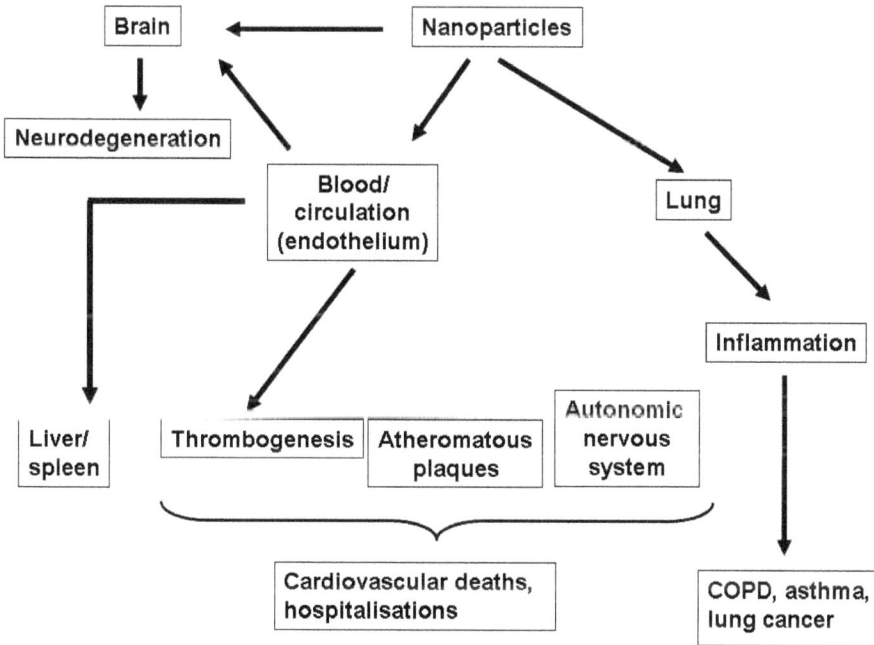

Figure 3. Systemic health effects of atmospheric nanoparticles. Adapted from Terzano et al. (2010).

Although lungs are the primary target of nanoparicles, cardiovascular detrimental consequences due exposure to nanoparticles have been also observed in some epidemiological studies (Kettunen, et al., 2007; Rückerl et al., 2007). Specifically, the "Exposure and Risk Assessment for Fine and Ultrafine Particles in Ambient Air" (i.e. ULTRA) study investigated the health effects of nanoparticles in three European cities (Amsterdam, Erfurt, Helsinki), where daily number concentrations levels of nanoparticles in air were similar (Ruuskanen et al., 2001). The authors followed a cohort of 131 patients aged 40-84 with established coronary heart disease with biweekly submaximal exercise tests over a 6-months period. It was observed that the risk of developing ischemia during exercise was significantly elevated at 2 days after exposure to increased environmental levels of nanoparticles (Pekkanen et al., 2002). The importance of this observation is that it highlights myocardial ischemia as a significant potential mechanism responsible for the adverse cardiac outcomes associated with poor air quality (Terzano et al., 2010). In addition particulate pollution including nanoparticles was associated with decrease in blood pressure (Ibald-Mulli et al., 2004). The study thus started to provide an understanding of how nanoparticles may affect cardiovascular health.

5. Environmental impacts

5.1. Visibility impairment

Impairment of the visibility involves degrading of the ability to perceive the environment. Atmospheric suspended particles are the most important factor in the visibility reduction (Boubel et al., 1994). The reduction of visibility is caused by build-up of the atmospheric particles that absorb or scatter light from the sun (Horvath, 2008); though light scattering by particles is the most important phenomenon responsible for impairment of visibility. The size of particles plays a crucial role for the interaction with light, but so far the existent links between visibility impairment and mass concentrations have been established for larger particles (Boubel et al., 1994; Strawa et al., 2010). Shape and composition of particles are also relevant for visibility reduction; carbon particles may contribute 5–40% of overall visibility reduction through light absorption in polluted areas, whereas particles containing sulphate, organic carbon and nitrate species may cause 60-95% of visibility reduction (Kumar at al., 2010). Finally, visibility impairment is affected by meteorological parameters; it increases with relative humidity and atmospheric pressure and decreases with temperature and wind speed (Kim et al., 2002; Tsai, 2005). In general the role of nanoparticles in visibility impairment is still unclear. However, diesel vehicles emit large number of sulphate and carbonaceous nanoparticles. Particles of these compositions reduce visibility which suggests that nanoparticles might be relevant for visibility impairment. Therefore, deeper understanding of nanoparticles role in visibility impairment is necessary.

5.2. Climate change

Climate system, atmospheric chemistry and even life on the Earth are dependent on solar radiation (Boubel et al., 1994). Approximately 30% of the incoming solar energy is reflected back to space. The remaining 70% is absorbed by the surface–atmosphere system of the Earth. This energy heats the planet and the atmosphere. As the surface and the atmosphere become warm, they release the energy in form of infrared radiation. This process continues until the incoming solar energy and the outgoing heat radiation are in balance. This radiation energy balance provides a powerful constraint for the global average temperature of the planet (Ramanathan & Feng, 2009). Atmospheric greenhouse gases (such as like carbon dioxide and methane) and particles affect the climate by altering the incoming solar and outgoing thermal radiations. In other words changing the atmospheric abundance or properties of these gases and particles can lead to a warming or cooling of the climate system. The influence of a factor (pollutant) that cause change of climate system are typically evaluated in terms of its radiative forcing, which is an estimate of how the energy balance of the Earth-atmosphere system is influenced when the factor in question is altered (IPCC, 2007).

Atmospheric nanosized particles are the main precursors of larger particles. They promote their growth and modify the optical properties thus affecting the radiative properties of the atmosphere. It was generally believed that particles reflect sunlight back to
space before it reaches the surface, and thus contribute to a cooling of the surface (i.e.
negative radiative forcing; Monks et al., 2009). During time as the concentrations of particles increased (along with greenhouse gases) their cooling effect has masked some of
the greenhouse warming (Ramanathan & Feng, 2009). This masking effect could be relative large considering that estimated negative radiative forcing of particles is -1.2 W m^{-2}
compared with $+2.63$ W m^{-2} for greenhouse gases ($+1.66$ W m^{-2} for carbon dioxide, $+0.48$
W m for methane and $+0.16$ W m^{-2} for nitrous oxide, $+0.34$ W m^{-2} for halocarbons; IPCC,
2007). However, in the last years the view of particle role in climate change has deep-
ened. It was found that atmospheric particles may also enhance scattering and absorption of solar radiation thus causing direct warm-up (i.e. positive radiation; IPPC, 2007).
Especially, carbonaceous particles are considered as one of the major contributors to
global warming (i.e. $+0.34$ W m^{-2}); if they are coated with sulphate or organic compounds their radiative forcing can increase up to about $+0.6$ W m^{-2} (Kumar et al., 2010).

Indirectly nanoparticles can also cause a negative radiative forcing through changes in cloud
formations and properties (IPCC, 2007). They can act as cloud condensation nuclei and modify
size and number concentrations of cloud droplets. In clean air, clouds are composed of a relatively small number of large droplets. As a consequence, the clouds are somewhat dark and
translucent. In polluted air with high concentrations of particles (such as urban areas) water
can easily condense on the particles, creating a large number of small droplets. These clouds
are dense, very reflective, and bright white. Due to the decrease of the size of water droplets
these clouds are less efficient at releasing precipitation. They cause large reductions in the
amount of solar radiation reaching Earth's surface, a corresponding increase in atmospheric
solar heating, changes in atmospheric thermal structure, surface cooling, disruption of regional
circulation systems such as the monsoons, suppression of rainfall, and less efficient removal
of pollutants (Ramanathan & Feng, 2009). In general the indirect effects of particles are only
partially understood. The interactions between aerosol particles (natural and anthropogenic
in origin) and clouds are complex and most instruments cannot measure aerosols within the
clouds. Climatologists thus consider the role of clouds to be the largest single uncertainty in
climate prediction.

The close relation between climate and air quality also reflects on the impacts of climate change
on air pollution levels. For example particle pollution levels are strongly influenced by shifts
in the weather (e.g., heat waves or droughts; EEA, 2012a). While closely related, climate change
and air pollution have mostly been treated as separate problems. At the international level,
various efforts have helped to reduce air pollution levels. The largest reductions have been
achieved for emissions of sulphur dioxide which decreased in Europe by 82% between 1990
and 2010 (EEA, 2012b). The implementation of EU regulation limits setting levels of sulphur
dioxide in urban areas and various political actions to control urban atmospheric emissions
(i.e. sulfur abatement technologies in industrial facilities, EEA, 2011; introduction of fuels with
reduced levels of sulfur, Directive 98/70/EC; EN 590/2004) have contributed to these reduc-

tions. In addition, significant reductions were also obtained for emissions of air pollutants that are primarily responsible for formation of harmful ground-level ozone: non-methane volatile organic compounds (56% reduction) and nitrogen oxides (47% reduction; EEA, 2012b). However, based on the future climate scenarios (and in the absence of additional emissions reductions) the IPCC still projected declining air quality in cities into the future as a result of climate change (USEPA, 2012b). In agreement, USEPA has concluded that climate change could have various negative impacts on national air quality levels that included both increases and decreases in particle pollution (USEPA, 2009). Thus in order to protect human health and environment, joined efforts to control air pollution and mitigate climate change have to be done in future: air pollution abatement measures may help protect the regional and global climate whilst taking certain climate change measures may yield additional benefits through improved local and regional air quality.

6. Conclusion

Atmospheric nanoparticles represent an area of growing health concern. Although our understanding of the ambient nanoparticles and their behavior has increased considerably in recent years, the magnitude of the impacts of nanoparticles on human health and the environment has still not been fully understood. Lack of answers from epidemiological studies in relation to atmospheric nanoparticles and the absence of the exposure-response relationships also mean that currently it is not possible to develop health guidelines, a basis for national regulations. Thus, a multidisciplinary approach including atmospheric scientists, nanomaterial engineers, epidemiologists, clinicians and toxicologists is necessary to further investigate sources, generation, physicochemical characteristics and potential harmful effects of nanoparticles. This knowledge would allow better understanding of the potential impacts of the particles on the environment and health and would provide scientific foundation for development of strategies to protect public health.

The knowledge on the characteristics of engineered nanoparticles is in general very limited. Though these nanoparticles appear in smaller concentrations than other atmospheric nanoparticles they may pose much larger health risks (Oberdörster et al., 2005). Therefore, the future studies need to consider the specificity of these nanoparticles and the new kinds of environmental and health impacts resulting from the release of these nanoparticles.

Acknowledgements

The authors would like to thank to Fundação para Ciência e Tecnologia for the financial support through grants number PEst-C/EQB/LA0006/2011 and PEst-C/EQB/UI0511/2011, and fellowship SFRH/BPD/65722/2009.

Author details

Klara Slezakova[1,2], Simone Morais[2] and Maria do Carmo Pereira[1]

1 LEPAE, Departamento de Engenharia Química, Faculdade de Engenharia, Universidade do Porto, Portugal

2 REQUIMTE, Instituto Superior de Engenharia do Porto, Instituto Politécnico do Porto, Portugal

References

[1] Aguar-Fernandez, M.A. & Hullmann, A. (2007). A boost for safer nanotechnology. *Nano Today*, Vol. 2, No. 1, (February 2007), pp. 56, ISSN 1748-0132

[2] Anastasio, C. & Martin, S.T. (2001). Atmospheric nanoparticles, In: *Nanoparticles and the Environment*, J.F. Banfield, A. Navrotsky (Eds.), pp. 293–349, Mineralogical Society of America, ISBN 0-939950-56-1, Washington, DC.

[3] Australian Government, National Environment Protection Council. (2012). *Ambient Air Quality Standards*, August 2012, available from <http://www.environment.gov.au/atmosphere/airquality/standards.html>

[4] Birmili, W. & Wiedensohler, A. (2000a). Evolution of newly formed aerosol particles in the continental boundary layer: a case study including OH and H2SO4 measurements. *Geophysical Research Letters*, Vol. 27, No. 15, (August 2000), pp. 2205–2208, ISSN 0094-8276

[5] Birmili, W. & Wiedensohler, A. (2000b). New particle formation in the continental boundary layer: meteorological and gas phase parameter influence. *Geophysical Research Letter*, Vol. 27, No. 20, (October 2000), pp. 3325-3328, ISSN 0094-8276

[6] Boubel, R.W., Fox, D.L., Turner, D.B. & Stern, A.C. (1994). *Fundamentals of Air Pollution* (3rd edition), Academic Press, ISBN 0-12-118930-0, London, United Kingdom

[7] British Standards Institution. (2005). *Vocabulary — Nanoparticles*. British Standards Institution, ISBN 0 580 45925 X, London, United Kingdom

[8] Buseck, P.R. & Adachi, K. (2008). Nanogeoscience: nanoparticles in the atmosphere. *Elements*, Vol. 4, No. 6, (December 2008), pp. 389-394, ISSN 1811-5209

[9] Bystrzejewska-Piotrowska, G., Golimowski, J. & Urban, P.L. (2009). Nanoparticles: their potential toxicity, waste and environmental management. *Waste Management*, Vol. 29, No. 9, (September 2009), pp. 2587–2595, ISSN 0956053X

[10] Canadian Council of Ministries of Environment. (2000). *Canada-wide Standards for Particulate Matter (PM) and Ozone.* CCME Council of Ministers, Quebec City, August 2012, available from < http://www.ccme.ca/assets/pdf/pmozone_standard_e.pdf>

[11] Casati, R., Scheer, V., Vogt, R. & Benter, T. (2007). Measurement of nucleation and soot mode particle emission from a diesel passenger car in real world and laboratory in situ dilution. *Atmospheric Environment,* Vol. 41, No. 10, (March 2007), pp. 2125–2135, ISSN 1352-2310

[12] Chen, S.-C., Tsai, C.-J., Chou, C.C.-K., Roam, G.-D., Cheng, S.-S. & Wang, Y.-N. (2010). Ultrafine particles at three different sampling locations in Taiwan. *Atmospheric Environment,* Vol. 44, No. 4, (February 2010), pp. 533-540, ISSN 1352-2310

[13] Chow, J.C. & Watson, J.G. (2007). Review of measurement methods and Compositions for ultrafine particles. *Aerosol and Air Quality Research,* Vol. 7, No. 2, (June 2007), pp. 121-173, ISSN 2071-1409

[14] Clarke, A.D., Owens, S.R. & Zhou, J. (2006). An ultrafine sea-salt flux from breaking waves: implications for cloud condensation nuclei in the remote marine atmosphere. *Journal of Geophysical Research D: Atmospheres,* Vol. 111, No. D6, (March 2006), pp. 1–2, ISSN 0148-0227

[15] Dahl, A., Gharibi, A., Swietlicki, E., Gudmundsson, A., Bohgard, M., Ljungman, A., Blomqvist, G. & Gustafsson, M. (2006). Traffic-generated emissions of ultrafine particles from pavement-tire interface. *Atmospheric Environment,* Vol. 40, No. 7, (March 2006), pp. 1314-1323, ISSN 1352-2310

[16] Directive 2008/50/EC. (2008). Directive of the European Parliament and of the Council on Ambient Air Quality and Cleaner Air for Europe. *Official Journal of the European Union,* L152, (June 2006), pp. 1-44

[17] Directive 98/70/EC. (1998). Directive of the European Parliament and of the Council Relating to the Quality of Petrol and Diesel Fuels. *Official Journal of the European Communities,* L350, (December 1998), pp. 58–68

[18] EN Standard 590/2004. (2004). *Automotive Fuels. Diesel. Requirements and Test methods,* European Committee for Standardization, ISBN 05-8044-119-9, Brussels, Belgium

[19] Environmental European Agency (EEA). (2011). *European Union Emission Inventory Report 1990–2009 under the UNECE Convention on Long-range Transboundary Air Pollution (LRTAP).* EEA Technical report No. 9/2011, Office for Official Publications of the European Union, ISBN 978-92-9213-216-3, Luxemburg

[20] Environmental European Agency (EEA). (2012a). *Evaluation of progress under the EU National Emission Ceilings Directive.* EEA Technical report No. 14/2012, Publication Office of the European Union, ISBN 978-92-9213-336-8, Luxemburg

[21] Environmental European Agency (EEA). (2012b). *Urban adaptation to climate change in Europe*. EEA Report No. 2/2012, Office for Official Publications of the European Union, ISBN 978-92-9213-308-5, Luxemburg

[22] European Union (EU). (2011). *Energy, Transport, and Environmental Indicators* (2011 ed.), European Union, ISBN 978-92-79-21384-7, Luxemburg

[23] Government of Japan, Ministry of Environment. (2012). *Environmental Quality Standards in Japan - Air quality*, August 2012, available from <http://www.env.go.jp/en/air/aq/aq.html>

[24] Granqvist, C.G., Buhrman, R.A., Wyns, J. & Sievers, A.J. (1976). Far-infrared absorption in ultrafine Al particles. *Physical Review Letters*, Vol. 37, No. 10, (September 1976), pp. 625–629, ISSN 0031-9007

[25] Granqvist, C.G., Buhrman, R.A., Wyns, J. & Sievers, A.J. (1977). Far-infrared absorption in ultrafine Al particles: Drude model versus Gor'kov-Eliashberg theory. *Journal de Physique Colloque*, Vol.38, pp. C2 93–96, DOI: 10.1051/jphyscol:1977219

[26] Graskow, B.R., Kittelson, D.B., Abdul-Khaleek, I.S., Ahmadi, M.R. & Morris, J.E. (1998). Characterization of exhaust particulate emissions from a spark ignition engine. *SAE Special Publications*, Vol. 1326, (February 1998), pp. 155 165

[27] Gustafsson, M., Blomqvist, G., Gudmundsson, A., Dahl, A., Swietlicki, E., Bohgard, M., Lindbom, J. & Ljungman, A. (2008). Properties and toxicological effects of particles from the interaction between tyres, road pavement and winter traction material. *Science of The Total Environment*, Vol. 393, No. 2-3, (April 2008), pp. 226-240, ISSN 0048-9697

[28] Harris, S.J. & Maricq, M.M. (2001). Signature size distributions for diesel and gasoline engine exhaust particulate matter. *Journal of Aerosol Science*, Vol. 32, No. 6, (June 2001), pp. 749–764, ISSN 0021-8502

[29] Harrison, R., Jones, M. & Collins, G. (1999). Measurements of the physical properties of particles in the urban atmosphere. *Atmospheric Environment*, Vol. 33, No. 2, (January 1999), pp. 309–321, ISSN 1352-2310

[30] Helland, A., Kastenholz, H., Thidell, A., Arnfalk, P. & Deppert, K. (2006). Nanoparticulate materials and regulatory policy in Europe: an analysis of stakeholder perspectives. *Journal of Nanoparticle Research*, Vol. 8, No. 5, (October 2006), pp. 709–719, ISSN 1388-0764

[31] Helland, A., Wick, P., Koehler, A., Schmid, K. & Som, C. (2007). Reviewing the environmental and human health knowledge base of carbon nanotubes. *Environmental Health Perspectives*, Vol. 115, No. 8, (August 2007), pp. 1125-1131, ISSN 0091-6765

[32] Hinds, W.C. (1999). *Aerosol Technology: Properties, Behaviour and Measurement of Airborne Particles*, John Wiley & Sons, ISBN 978-0-471-19410-1, Hoboken, USA

[33] Hoek, G., Boogaard, H., Knol, A., de Hartog, J., Slottje, P., Ayres, J.G., Borm, P., Brunekreef, B., Donaldson, K., Forastiere, F., Holgate, S., Kreyling, W.G., Nemery, B.,
Pekkanen, J., Stone, V., Wichmann, H.E. & van der Sluijs, J. (2010). Concentration response functions for ultrafine particles and all-cause mortality and hospital admissions: results of a European expert panel elicitation. *Environmental Science and
Technology*, Vol. 44, No. 1, (January 2010), pp. 476-482, ISSN 0013-936X

[34] Holmes, N.S. (2007). A review of particle formation events and growth in the atmosphere in the various environments and discussion of mechanistic implications. *Atmospheric Environment*, Vol. 41, No. 10, (March 2007), pp. 2183-2201, ISSN 1352-2310

[35] Horvath, H. (1994). Atmospheric aerosols, atmospheric optics visibility. *Journal of
Aerosol Science*, Vol. 25, Suppl. 1, (May 1994), pp. 23-24, ISSN 0021-8502

[36] Horvath, H. (2008). Conference on visibility, aerosols, and atmospheric optics, Vienna, September 3–6, 2006. *Atmospheric Environment*, Vol. 42, No. 11, (April 2008), pp.
2569-2570, ISSN 1352-2310

[37] Ibald-Mulli, A., Timonen, K.L., Peters, A., Heinrich, J., Wölke, G., Lanki, T., Buzorius,
G., Kreyling, W.G., de Hartog, J., Hoek, G., ten Brink, H.M. & Pekkanen, J. (2004). Effects of particulate air pollution on blood pressure and heart rate in subjects with cardiovascular disease: A multicenter approach. *Environmental Health Perspectives*, Vol.
112, No. 3, (March 2004), pp. 369-37, ISSN 0091-6765

[38] Ibald-Mulli, A., Wichmann, H.E., Kreyling, W. & Peters, A. (2002). Epidemiological
evidence on health effects of ultrafine particles. *Journal of Aerosol Medicine: Deposition,
Clearance, and Effects in the Lung*, Vol. 15, No. 2, (June 2002), pp. 189–201, ISSN
0894-2684

[39] Intergovernmental Panel on Climate Change (IPCC). 2007. *Climate Change 2007: The
Physical Science Basis. Contribution of Working Group I to the Fourth Assessment Report of
the Intergovernmental Panel on Climate Change*, Cambridge University Press, ISBN
978-0-521-88009-1, Cambridge, United Kingdom

[40] Kettunen, J., Lanki, T., Tiittanen, P., Aalto, P.P., Koskentalo, T., Kulmala, M., Salo-
maa, V. & Pekkanen, J. (2007). Associations of fine and ultrafine particulate air pollution with stroke mortality in an area of low air pollution levels. *Stroke*, Vol. 38, No. 3,
(March 2007), pp. 918-922, ISSN 0039-2499

[41] Kim, K.H., Sekiguchi, K., Furuuchi, M. & Sakamoto, K. (2011). Seasonal variation of
carbonaceous and ionic components in ultrafine and fine particles in an urban area of
Japan. *Atmospheric Environment*, Vol. 45, No. 8, (March 2011), pp. 1581-1590, ISSN
1352-2310

[42] Kim, Y.J., Kim, K.W. & Oh, S.J. (2001). Seasonal characteristics of haze observed by
continuous visibility monitoring in the urban atmosphere of Kwangju, Korea. *Environmental Monitoring and Assessment*, Vol. 70, No. 1-2, (July 2001), pp. 35-46, ISSN
0167-6369

[43] Kittelson, B.D. (1998). Engines and nanoparticles: a review. *Journal of Aerosol Science*, Vol. 29, No. 5-6, (June 1998), pp. 575–588, ISSN 0021-8502

[44] Kittelson, D., Watts, W. & Johnson, J. (2006). On-road and laboratory evaluation of combustion aerosols – Part1: summary of diesel engine results. *Journal of Aerosol Science*, Vol. 37, No. 8, (August 2006), pp. 913–930, ISSN 0021-8502

[45] Kittelson, D.B., Watts, W.F. & Johnson, J.P. (2004). Nanoparticle emissions on Minnesota highways. *Atmospheric Environment*, Vol. 38, No. 1, (January 2004), pp. 9–19, ISSN 1352-2310

[46] Klems, J.P., Pennington, M.R., Zordan, C.A., McFadden, L. & Johnston, M.V. (2011). Apportionment of motor vehicle emissions from fast changes in number concentration and chemical composition of ultrafine particles near a roadway intersection. *Environmental Science and Technology*, Vol. 45, No. 13, (July 2011), pp. 5637-5643, ISSN 0013-936X

[47] Knol, A., de Hartog, J., Boogaard, H., Slottje, P., van der Sluijs, J., Lebret, E., Cassee, F., Wardekker, J.A., Ayres, J., Borm, P., Brunekreef, B., Donaldson, K., Forastiere, F., Holgate, S., Kreyling, W., Nemery, B., Pekkanen, J., Stone, V., Wichmann, H.E., Hoek, G., 2009. Expert elicitation on ultrafine particles: likelihood of health effects and causal pathways. *Particle and Fibre Toxicology*, Vol. 6, No. 19, (July 2009), 16 pp., ISSN 1743-8977

[48] Kudo, S., Sekiguchi, K., Kim, K.H. & Sakamoto, K. (2011). Spatial distributions of ultrafine particles and their behavior and chemical composition in relation to roadside sources. *Atmospheric Environment*, Vol. 45, No. 35, (November 2011), pp. 6403-6413, ISSN 1352-2310

[49] Kulmala, M., Pirjola, L., Makela & J. (2000). Stable sulphate clusters as a source of new atmospheric particles. *Nature*, Vol. 404, No. 6773, (March 2000), pp. 66–69, ISSN 0028-0836

[50] Kulmala, M., Vehkamäki, H., Petäjä, T., Dal Maso, M., Lauri, A., Kerminen, V.-M., Birmili, W. & McMurry, P.H. (2004). Formation and growth rates of ultrafine atmospheric particles: a review of observations. *Journal of Aerosol Science*, Vol. 35, No. 2, (March 2004), pp. 143-176, ISSN 0021-8502

[51] Kumar, P., Fennell, P. & Britter, R. (2008a). Effect of wind direction and speed on the dispersion of nucleation and accumulation mode particles in an urban street canyon. *The Science of The Total Environment*, Vol. 402, No. 1, (August 2008), pp. 82–94, ISSN 0048-9697

[52] Kumar, P., Fennell, P. & Britter, R. (2008b). Measurements of particles in the 5–1000 nm range close to road level in an urban street canyon. *Science of The Total Environment*, Vol. 390, No. 2-3, (February 2008), pp. 437-447, ISSN 0048-9697

[53] Kumar, P., Fennell, P., Hayhurst, A.N. & Britter, R.E. (2009). Street versus rooftop level concentrations of fine particles in a Cambridge street canyon. *Boundary-Layer Meteorology*, Vol. 131, No. 1, (April 2009), pp. 3-18, ISSN 0006-8314

[54] Kumar, P., Robins, A., Vardoulakis, S. & Britter, R. (2010). A review of the characteristics of nanoparticles in the urban atmosphere and the prospects for developing regulatory controls mode particles in an urban street canyon. *Atmospheric Environment*, Vol. 44, No. 1, (August 2008), pp. 5035-5052, ISSN 1352-2310

[55] Kumara, P., Robins, A., Vardoulakis, A., Paul Quincey, P. (2011). Technical challenges in tackling regulatory concerns for urban atmospheric nanoparticles. *Particuology*, Vol. 9, No. 6, (December 2011), pp. 566– 571, ISSN 1674-2001

[56] Maynard, A.D. & Aitken, R.J. (2007). Assessing exposure to airborne nanomaterials: current abilities and future requirements. *Nanotoxicology*, Vol. 1, No. 1, (March 2007), pp. 26-41, ISSN 1743-5390

[57] Monks, P.S., Granier, C., Fuzzi, S., Stohl, A., Williams, M.L, Akimoto, H., Amanni, M., Baklanov, A. & et al. (2009. Atmospheric composition change – global and regional air quality. *Atmospheric Environment*, Vol. 43, No. 33, (October 2009), pp. 5268–5350, ISSN 1352-2310

[58] Morawska, L., Ristovski, Z., Jayaratne, E.R., Keogh, D.U. & Ling, X. (2008). Ambient nano and ultrafine particles from motor vehicle emissions: characteristics, ambient processing and implications on human exposure. *Atmospheric Environment*, Vol. 42, No. 35, (November 2008), pp. 8113–8138, ISSN 1352-2310

[59] Naga, S., Guptaa, K. & Mukhopadhyay, U.K. (2005). Size distribution of atmospheric aerosols in Kolkata, India and the assessment of pulmonary deposition of particle mass. *Indoor and Built Environment*, Vol. 14, No. 5, (October 2005), pp. 381-389, ISSN 1420-326X

[60] Nel, A., Xia, T., Madler, L. & Li, N. (2006). Toxic potential of materials at the nanolevel. *Science*, Vol. 311, No. 5761, (February 2006), pp. 622–627, ISSN 0036-8075

[61] Ntziachristos, L., Ning, Z., Geller, M.D. & Sioutas, C. (2007). Particle concentration and characteristics near a major freeway with heavy duty diesel traffic. *Environmental Science and Technology*, Vol. 41, No. 7, (April 2007), pp. 2223–2230, ISSN 0013-936X

[62] O'Dowd, C. & Hoffmann, T. (2005). Coastal new particle formation: a review of the current state-of-the-art. *Environmental Chemistry*, Vol. 2, No. 4, pp. 245–255, ISSN 1448-2517

[63] O'Dowd, C., Aalto, P., Hameri, K., Kulmala, M. & Hoffmann, T. (2002). Aerosol formation: atmospheric particles from organic vapours. *Nature*, Vol. 416, No. 6880, (April 2002), pp. 497-498, ISSN 0028-0836

[64] O'Dowd, C., Facchini, M.C., Cavalli, F., Ceburnis, D., Mircea, M., Decesari, S., Fuzzi, S., Yoon, Y.J. & Putaud, J.-P. (2004). Biogenically driven organic contribution to marine aerosol. *Nature*, Vol. 431, No. 7009, (October 2004), pp. 676–680, ISSN 0028-0836

[65] Oberdörster, G., Oberdörster, E. & Oberdörster, J. (2005). Nanotoxicology: an emerging discipline evolving from studies of ultrafine particles. *Environmental Health Perspectives*, Vol. 113, No. 7, (July 2005), pp. 823–839, ISSN 0091-6765

[66] Oberdörster, G., Sharp, Z., Atudorei, V., Elder, A., Gelein, R., Kreyling, W. & Cox, C. (2004). Translocation of inhaled ultrafine particles to the brain. *Inhalation Toxicology*, Vol. 16, No. 6-7, (June 2004), pp. 437-445, ISSN 0895-8378

[67] Pekkanen, J., Peters, A., Hoek, G., Tiittanen, P., Brunekreef, B., De Hartog, J., Heinrich, J., Ibald-Mulli, A., Kreyling, W.G., Lanki, T., Timonen, K.L. & Vanninen, E. (2002). Particulate air pollution and risk of ST-segment depression during repeated submaximal exercise tests among subjects with coronary heart disease: The exposure and risk assessment for fine and ultrafine particles in ambient air (ULTRA) study. *Circulation*, Vol. 106, No. 8, (August 2002), pp. 933-938, ISSN 00097322

[68] Pekkanen, J., Timonen, K.L., Ruuskanen, J., Reponen, A. & Mirme, A. (1997). Effects of ultrafine and fine particles in urban air on peak expiratory flow among children with asthmatic symptoms. *Environmental Research*, Vol. 74, No. 1, pp. 24-33, ISSN 0013-9351

[69] Penttinen, P., Timonen, K.L., Tiittanen, P., Mirme, A., Ruuskanen, J. & Pekkanen, J. (2001a). Ultrafine particles in urban air and respiratory health among adult asthmatics. *European Respiratory Journal*, Vol. 17, No. 3, (March 2001), pp. 428-435, ISSN 0903-1936

[70] Penttinen, P., Timonen, K.L., Tiittanen, P., Mirme, A., Ruuskanen, J. & Pekkanen, J. (2001b). Number concentration and size of particles in urban air: Effects on spirometric lung function in adult asthmatic subjects. *Environmental Health Perspectives*, Vol. 109, No. 4, (April 2001), pp. 319-323, ISSN 0091-6765

[71] Peters, A., Wichmann, H.E., Tuch, T., Heinrich, J. & Heyder, J. (1997). Respiratory effects are associated with the number of ultrafine particles. *American Journal of Respiratory and Critical Care Medicine*, Vol. 155, No.4, (April 1997), pp. 1376-83, ISSN 1073-449X

[72] Pey, J., Querol, X., Alastuey, A., Rodríguez, S., Putaud, J.P. & Van Dingenen, R. (2009). Source apportionment of urban fine and ultra fine particle number concentration in a Western Mediterranean City. *Atmospheric Environment*, Vol. 43, No. 29, (September 2009), pp. 4407–4415, ISSN 1352-2310

[73] Raes, F. (1995). Entrainment of free tropospheric aerosols as a regulating mechanism for cloud condensation nuclei in the remote marine boundary layer. *Journal of Geophysical Research*, Vol. 100, No. D2, (February 1995), pp. 2893–2904, ISSN 0148-0227

[74] Ramanathan, V. & Feng, Y. (2009). Air pollution, greenhouse gases and climate change: Global and regional perspectives. *Atmospheric Environment*, Vol. 43, No. 1, (January 2009), pp. 37–50, ISSN 1352-2310

[75] Riipinen, S., Kulmala, M., Arnold, F., Dal Maso, M., Birmili, W., Saarnio, K., Teinilä, K., Kerminen, V., Laaksonen, A. & Lehtinen, K. (2007). Connections between atmospheric sulphuric acid and new particle formation during QUEST III-IV campaigns in Heidelberg and Hyytiälä. *Atmospheric Chemistry and Physics*, Vol. 7, No. 8, (April 2007) pp. 1899–1914, ISSN 1680-7316

[76] Ristovski, Z.D., Jayaratne, E.R., Lim, M., Ayoko, G.A. & Morawska, L. (2006.) Influence of diesel fuel sulphur on the nanoparticle emissions from city buses. *Environmental Science and Technology*, Vol. 40, No. 4, (February 2006), pp. 1314–1320, ISSN 0013-936X

[77] Ristovski, Z.D., Jayaratne, E.R., Morawska, L., Ayoko, G.A., Lim, M. (2005). Particle and carbon dioxide emissions from passenger vehicles operating on unleaded petrol and LPG fuel. *Science of The Total Environment*, Vol. 345, No. 1-3, (June 2005), pp.93–98, ISSN 0048-9697

[78] Rosenbohm, E., Vogt, R., Scheer, V., Nielsen, O., Drieseidler, A., Baumbach, G., Imhof, D., Baltensperger, U., Fuchs, J. & Jaeschke, W. (2005). Particulate size distributions and mass measured at a motorway during the BAB II campaign. *Atmospheric Environment*, Vol. 39, No. 31, (October 2005), pp. 5696–5709, ISSN 1352-2310

[79] Rückerl, R., Phipps, R.P., Schneider, A., Frampton, M., Cyrys, J., Oberdörster, G., Wichmann, H.E. & Peters, A. (2007). Ultrafine particles and platelet activation in patients with coronary heart disease--results from a prospective panel study. *Particle and Fibre Toxicology*, Volume 4, (January 2007), pp. 1, ISSN 17438-977

[80] Ruuskanen, J., Tuch, Th., Ten Brink, H., Peters, A., Khlystov, A., Mirme, A., Kos, G.P.A., Brunekreef, B., Wichmann, H.E., Buzorius, G., Vallius, M., Kreyling, W.G. & Pekkanen, J. Concentrations of ultrafine, fine and PM2.5 particles in three European cities. *Atmospheric Environment*, Vol. 35, No. 21, (July 2001), pp. 3729-3738, ISSN 1352-2310

[81] Seinfeld, J.H. & Pandis, S.N. (2006). *Atmospheric Chemistry and Physics: From Air Pollution to Climate Change* (2nd edition), John Wiley & Sons, ISBN 978-0-471-72018-8, Hoboken, New Jersey

[82] Shi, J. & Harrison, R.M. (1999). Investigation of ultrafine particle formation during diesel exhaust dilution. *Environmental Science and Technology*, Vol. 33, No. 21, (September 1999), pp. 3730–3736, ISSN 0013-936X

[83] Shi, J., Evans, D., Khan, A., Harrison, R., 2001. Sources and concentration of nanoparticles (<10 nm diameter) in the urban atmosphere. *Atmospheric Environment*, Vol. 35, No. 7, (July 2001), pp. 1193–1202, ISSN 1352-2310

[84] Sioutas, C., Delfino, R. J. & Singh, M. (2005). Exposure assessment for atmospheric ultrafine particles (UFPs) and implications in epidemiologic research. *Environmental Health Perspective*, Vol. 113, No. 8, (August 2005), pp. 947-955, ISSN 0091-6765

[85] Slezakova, K., Morais S. & Pereira M.C. (2012). Traffic–related air pollution: legislation versus health and environmental effects, In: *Environmental Health – Emerging Issues and Practice*, J. Oosthuizen (Ed.), pp. 103–124, Intech, ISBN 978-953-307-854-4, Rijeka, Croatia

[86] Slezakova, K., Morais S. & Pereira M.C. (2012). Air pollution: particulate matter, In: *Encyclopedia of Environmental Management*, S.E. Jorgensen (Ed.), in press, CRC Press, ISBN 9781-439-829-271, Boca Raton, Florida

[87] Stölzel, M., Breitner, S., Cyrys, J., Pitz, M., Wölke, G., Kreyling, W., Heinrich, J., Wichmann, H.E. & Peters, A. (2007). Daily mortality and particulate matter in different size classes in Erfurt, Germany. *Journal of Exposure Science and Environmental Epidemiology*, Vol. 17, No. 5, (August 2007), pp. 458-467, ISSN 1559-0631

[88] Strawa, A.W., Kirchstetter, T.W., Hallar, A.G., Ban-Weiss, G.A., McLaughlin, J.P., Harley, R.A. & Lunden, M.M. (2010). Optical and physical properties of primary on-road vehicle particle emissions and their implications for climate change. *Journal of Aerosol Science* Vol. 41, No. 1, (January 2010), pp. 36-50, ISSN 0021-8502

[89] Terzano, C., Di Stefano, F., Conti, V., Graziani, E. & Petroianni, A. (2010). Air pollution ultrafine particles: Toxicity beyond the lung. *European Review for Medical and Pharmacological Sciences*, Vol. 14, No. 10, (October 2010), pp. 809-821, ISSN 1128-3602

[90] Tranfield, E.M. & Walker D.C. (2012). Understanding of Human Illness and Death Following Exposure to Particulate Matter Air Pollution, In: *Environmental Health – Emerging Issues and Practice*, J. Oosthuizen (Ed.), pp. 81-102, Intech, ISBN 978-953-307-854-4, Rijeka, Croatia

[91] Tsai, Y.I. (2005). Atmospheric visibility trends in an urban area in Taiwan 1961-2003. *Atmospheric Environment*, Vol. 39, No. 30, (September 2005), pp. 5555-5567, ISSN 1352-2310

[92] Tunved, P., Hansson, H., Kerminen, V., Strom, J., Dal Maso, M., Lihavainen, H., Viisanen, Y., Aalto, P., Komppula, M. & Kulmala, M. (2006). High natural aerosol loading over boreal forests. *Science*, Vol. 312, No. 5771, (April 2006), pp. 261–263, ISSN 0036-8075

[93] United States Environmental Protection Agency (USEPA). (2006). *National Ambient Air Quality Standards for Particulate Matter; Final Rule*, Federal Register, Vol. 71, No. 200 (October 2006), pp. 61144, August, 2012, available from <http://www.gpo.gov/fdsys/pkg/FR-2006-10-17/html/06-8477.htm>

[94] United States Environmental Protection Agency (USEPA). (2009). *Assessment of the Impacts of Global Change on Regional U.S. Air Quality: A Synthesis of Climate Change Impacts on Ground-Level Ozone*, EPA 600-R-07-094F, Office of Research and Develop-

ment, National Centre for Environmental Assessment, Research Triangle Park, North Carolina

[95] United States Environmental Protection Agency (USEPA). (2012a). *Characteristics of Particles - Particle Size Categories*, June 2012, Available from: <http://www.epa.gov/ apti/bces/module3/category/category.htm>

[96] United States Environmental Protection Agency (USEPA). (2012b). *Our Nation's Air: Status and Trends through 2010*, EPA-454/R-12-001, Office of Air Quality Planning and Standards, Research Triangle Park, North Carolina

[97] Van Dingenen, R., Raes, F., Putaud, J.-P., Baltensperger, U., Charron, A., Facchini, M.-C., Decesari, S., Fuzzi, S., Gehrig, R., Hansson, H.-C. & et al. (2004). A European aerosol phenomenology - 1: physical characteristics of particulate matter at kerbside, urban, rural and background sites in Europe. *Atmospheric Environment*, Vol. 38, No. 16, (May 2004), pp. 2561–2577, ISSN 1352-2310

[98] von Klot, S., Wölke, G., Tuch, T., Heinrich, J., Dockery, D.W., Schwartz, J., Kreyling, W.G., Wichmann, H.E. & Peters, A. (2002). Increased asthma medication use in association with ambient fine and ultrafine particles. *European Respiratory Journal*, Vol. 20, No. 3, (September 2002), pp. 691-702, ISSN 0903-1936

[99] Wåhlin, P., Palmgren, F., Dingenen, R., & Raes, F. (2001). Pronounced decrease of ambient particle number emissions from diesel traffic in Denmark after reduction of the sulphur content in diesel fuel. *Atmospheric Environment*, Vol. 35, No. 21, (July 2001), pp. 3549–3552, ISSN 1352-2310

[100] Weber, R., Marti, J.J., McMurray, P., Eisele, F.L., Tanner, D.J. & Jefferson, A. (1996). Measured atmospheric new particle formation rates: implications for nucleation mechanisms. *Chemical Engineering Communications*, Vol. 151, No. 1, (January 1996), pp. 53–64, ISSN 0098-6445

[101] Weber, R., Marti, J.J., McMurray, P., Eisele, F.L., Tanner, D.J. & Jefferson, A. (1997). Measurement of new particle formation and ultrafine particle growth rates at a clean continental site. *Journal of Geophysical Research D: Atmospheres*, Vol. 102, No. 4, (February 1997), pp. 4375–4386, ISSN 0148-0227

[102] West, J.B. (2008). *Pulmonary Pathophysiology: the Essentials*, (7th edition), Lippincott Williams & Wilkins, ISBN 978-0-7817-6414-8, Baltimore, Philadelphia

[103] Westerdahl, D., Fruin, S., Sax, T., Fine, P. & Sioutas, C. (2005). Mobile platform measurements of ultrafine particles and associated pollutant concentrations on freeways and residential streets in Los Angeles. *Atmospheric Environment*, Vol. 39, No. 20, (June 2005), pp. 3597–3610, ISSN 1352-2310

[104] Wichmann and Peters, H.E., Spix, C., Tuch, T., Wolke, G., Peters, A., Heinrich, J., Kreyling, W.G & Heyder, J. (2000). Daily mortality and fine and ultrafine particles in Erfurt, Germany part I: role of particle number and particle mass. *Research report*

(Health Effects Institute), No. 98, (November 2000), pp.5-86; discussion 87, ISSN 1041-5505

[105] World Health Organization (WHO). 2000. *Particulate Matter, Chapter 7.3*; WHO Regional Publications, European Series: Copenhagen, Denmark; pp. 1–40, August 2012, <http://www.euro.who.int/__data/assets/pdf_file/0019/123085/AQG2ndEd_7_3Particulate-matter.pdf>

Pharmacoepidemiology and Pharmacosurveillance in Public Health

Epidemiology of Patients Diagnosed with Prescription and Non-Prescription Drug Overdose at the Riyadh Security Forces Hospital Between January 2007 and December 2011

Naser Al-Jaser, M. Cli. Epi and Niyi Awofeso

Additional information is available at the end of the chapter

1. Introduction

There is global concern concerning the higher rate of drug overdose morbidity and mortality, particularly from opioid medicines.[1] Drug overdose is one of the leading causes of death in many countries.[2] In the US, prescription drug mortality rate is higher than the death rate from illicit drugs, and drug overdose mortality currently exceeds mortality from motor vehicle accidents.[3] Moreover, there has been a tenfold increase in painkiller prescriptions in the US over the past 15 years.[4] In Saudi Arabia, there has been a significant increase in the use of prescription drugs compared with the previous decade, as the Ministry of Health stated in its 2009 annual report.[5] A number of studies have been conducted that investigate the epidemiology of drug overdose in Saudi Arabia. However, most of these studies were conducted in the late twentieth century.[6,7]

The purpose of this research is to investigate prescription and non-prescription overdose cases admitted to the emergency department of the Security Forces Hospital, Riyadh, from 2007 to 2011. The study sought to identify demographic characteristics of patients who were admitted to the emergency department with drug overdose, including age, gender, income and occupation.

The findings of this study have a number of implications for the Security Forces Hospital and drug overdoses in Saudi Arabia, particularly for elderly patients who take Warfarin continuously. Further, it appears that parents leave their medications unsecured and unprotected from children; thus, preventive and awareness programs are needed to address these issues.

2. Literature review

An Adverse Drug Event (ADE) is defined as an injury resulting from medical intervention related to a drug.[8] It is considered a major problem in medicine because it results in hospital admissions. ADEs include harm caused by the drug, such as adverse drug reactions and overdoses, and harm resulting from using the drug, such as dose reductions and discontinuation of drug therapies.[9] Previous studies have found that ADEs account for 3.9–6.2 per cent of hospital admissions. Further, drug overdoses account for a higher hospital admission rate of ADEs.[10,11]

Drug overdose can be defined as intentionally or unintentionally administering a higher dose of prescription or non-prescription drugs than recommended.[12] Drug overdose is considered a major health problem, particularly in developed countries. In the United States (US), the Centers for Disease Control and Prevention (CDC) recently reported that fatal overdoses from opiate painkillers currently exceed those from cocaine and heroin combined. [12] The rate of prescription drug use is increasing globally.[13] In Saudi Arabia, there has been a significant increase in prescription drug use since 2000 compared with the previous decades; however, there is a dearth of information relating to drug use and overdoses.[5]

In many Asian countries, drug overdose mortality is considered a major problem. For example, a study in northern Thailand which investigated the overdose mortality rate of injecting drug users between 1999 and 2002 found a death rate of 8.97 per 1,000 people among 861 drug users who were Human Immunodeficiency Virus (HIV)-negative.[14] A study in Xichang City, China, found a heroin overdose mortality rate of 4.7 per 100 people among 379 people who injected drugs during 2002 to 2003.[15] Further, in a review conducted in several central Asian countries, emergency medical services stated that there were 21 drug overdose deaths in Tajikistan and 57 in Kyrgyzstan in 2006.[1]

Many European countries also consider drug overdose a major concern, and it is considered one of the leading causes of death. The average mortality rate is 21 deaths per 1 million people aged 15–64.[16] Drug overdose in Europeans aged 15–39 accounted for 4 per cent of all deaths. Males were at a greater risk than females in all countries, with males accounting for 81 per cent of all drug-related deaths reported in European countries. The male to female ratio varied across countries, with the lowest rate in Poland (4:1) and the highest rate in Romania (31:1). The most common drugs used in almost all countries were opioids, which accounted for 90 per cent of drugs used in five countries and 80–90 per cent in 12 countries.[16]

Drug overdose is also considered a major public health threat in the US. There, the drug overdose mortality rate among adults increased from 4 per 100,000 people in 1999 to 8.8 per 100,000 in 2006. Moreover, deaths from drug overdose increased from 11,155 in 1999 to

22,448 in 2005, which can be attributed mainly to prescription drugs rather than illicit drugs. [3] Drug overdose is the second leading cause of death among all unintentional deaths in the US. The most common drugs that caused death by overdose were heroin, cocaine and pain-killers. The use of prescription medicines has increased, thus contributing to the death rate. [4] According to the CDC, from 2005 to 2007, prescription drugs such as benzodiazepine, anti-depressants and opioid medicines were found in 79 per cent (2,165 cases) of all substance overdoses.[17]

In Australia, there appears to be a lower risk of drug overdose than in other countries. For instance, the rate of death from opioids was 101.9 per 1 million people in 1999 and 31.3 deaths per 1 million in 2004.[18] Moreover, in 2005, the Illicit Drug Reporting System distributed a survey among intravenous drug users and found that 46 per cent had experienced an overdose.[18] It was also found that 357 deaths were caused by opioid overdose and 40 per cent of deaths occurred in New South Wales. Males accounted for 75 per cent of overdose deaths, and those aged 25–34 were most at risk, accounting for 40 per cent of deaths.[19] Recently released Australian prisoners are at significantly increased risks of illicit drug overdose and deaths.[20]

In Saudi Arabia, studies have noted an increase in drug overdoses in localised cohorts over the past several decades. However, there are no significant statistics for drug overdose morbidity and mortality in Saudi Arabia as a whole.[6,21] Several studies have been undertaken in Saudi Arabia to investigate the drug overdose in hospitals. Moazzam's and Aljahdali's studies found that paracetamol accounted for 24.1 per cent of 170 drug overdose cases and 30 per cent of 79 cases, respectively.[21,22] Ahmed's study found that mefenamic acid accounted for 20 per cent of 50 cases investigated.[6] The rate of death amongst drug overdose was investigated in some studies in Saudi Arabia. Ahmed stated that there was one death among 106 drug overdoses admitted between 1992 and 1994.[6] Elfawal investigated 249 deaths from substance overdose between 1990 and 1997, and found 20 per cent of cases related to medically prescribed drugs.[7] Aljahdali and Ahmed found females accounted for a higher percentage of drug overdose cases.[6,22] Moazzam and Elfawal found males were represented in a higher percentage of cases.[7,21]

Drug overdoses could result from non-prescription substances such as herbal medicines.[23] The problem with herbal remedies relates to limited control and regulation among stores that provide them.[24] Many people believe that herbal substances are harmless and that it is safe to administer excessive amounts because they come from natural sources.[25] Although the rate of usage has increased, fewer than half of patients consult their physicians before administrating herbal remedies.[26] Further, the accurate dosage of herbal medicines is variable, and there are no guidelines to determine correct dosage.[25]

Drug overdoses could result from administering illicit drugs such as heroin and hashish. [27,28] As Saudi Arabia is a strict Islamic country, and Islam prohibits the use of illicit drugs, overdose cases involving illicit drugs are rare.[22] However, according to a world drug report, Saudi Arabia is considered a major market of phenethylline (Captagon) in the Middle East. The Saudi government confiscated more than 10 million pills in one seizure in 2010. However, the prevalence of amphetamines in Saudi Arabia is low compared with other western countries: in 2006, the prevalence of amphetamines in Saudi Arabia was 0.4 per 100,000 people, whereas in Australia and the US, the prevalence was 2.7 and 1.5 per 100,000 people respectively. Further, the prevalence of opioids and cannabis was 0.06 and 0.3 per 100,000 respectively in Saudi Arabia, 0.4 and 10.6 per 100,000 respectively in Australia and 5.9 and 13.7 per 100,000 respectively in the US. Therefore, the prevalence of opioids and cannabis are markedly lower in Saudi Arabia than in Australia and the US.[13]

Suicide is one of the major motivations and outcomes of intentional drug overdose.[29] Suicide accounts for 2 per cent of all deaths in the world. In 2005, there were about 800,000 deaths from suicide, and about 56 million deaths globally.[30] Drugs cause 11 per cent of suicides in Australia.[30] A study found that suicide is a greater risk among people who had a history of drug overdoses compared with people who did not.[31] Another study found a positive correlation between suicide and drug overdose.[32] Moreover, research has found that committing suicide by administering drugs is common among adolescents.[33] One study found suicide was associated with both prescription and non-prescription drugs, with a strong association between opiates and suicide, and opioid users were 14 times more likely to attempt suicide compared with non-opioid users.[34]

The excessive availability of medicines in households is due to the relative affordability of drugs, which can be bought from a range of places including markets, internet pharmacies and cosmetic stores. For instance, patients can purchase prescription drugs from an internet pharmacy without a prescription.[35] One survey investigated how easy it was for adolescents to acquire prescription medications. The question asked was 'which is easiest for someone your age to buy: cigarettes, beer, marijuana or prescription drugs without prescription?' Nineteen per cent of respondents said it was easier to buy prescription drugs compared to 13 per cent in the previous year.[36]

Two main factors contribute to the excessive availability of medicines: physicians and patients. Physicians appear to prescribe more medicines than in the past. For example, there was a 300 per cent increase in the prescription of painkillers in the US in 1999.[35,37] According to the National Institute on Drug Abuse (NIDA), the number of potentially addictive drug prescriptions for pain rose to 200 million in 2011.[38] There is also an association between patient death and physicians who frequently prescribe painkillers. Dhalla published a study in Ontario in 2011 that investigated the opioid prescription rate in family physicians and their relation to opioid-related deaths. He found that 20 per cent of physicians have a prescription rate that is 55 times higher than the 20 per cent of physicians who prescribed the lowest. The top 20 per cent of physicians were responsible for 64 per cent of patient deaths caused by painkillers.[39] In addition, many people falsely reporting symptoms in order to obtain a prescription and this is defined as drug seeking behaviour. The most drugs associated with drug seeking behaviour are benzodiazepine and opioids.[40]

Alcoholism is considered a major risk factor for intentional overdoses. Several studies state that the risk of drug overdose from prescription medicines is higher among people who drink alcohol.[41-43] A study by Li in 2011 investigated trends of paracetamol overdose in US emergency departments from 1993 to 2007 using data from physicians' diagnoses codes and cause of injury codes. The author found those who drank alcohol were 5.48 times more likely to overdose compared to people who did not drink alcohol, and the p-values were statistically significant.[41]

A study published by Wazaify in 2005 examined OTC drugs and prescription drug overdoses for three months, as well as the potential risk factors. The study investigated 247 overdose cases, excluding alcohol intoxication and spiked drinks. He found alcohol was a major risk factor for overdoses of both OTC and prescription drugs, and that alcohol contributed more to OTC drug overdoses (32.2 per cent) than prescription drugs combined with OTC drugs (24.7 per cent).[42] Moreover, the prescription drug overdose death rate increased with alcohol consumption. West Virginia found 32.9 per cent of overdose deaths were associated with alcohol consumption.[43] Another study on paracetamol overdose found more than one-third of drug overdoses were associated with alcohol consumption at the time of overdose, and it was slightly higher in males (12 per cent) than females (11 per cent).[44] In addition, people who consumed alcohol could overdose on lower doses of paracetamol compared with those who did not consume alcohol.[45] Paulozzi conducted a study on methadone overdose and found that the concentration of methadone was lower when alcohol was involved.[28] Mixing drugs with alcohol is therefore considered a risk factor for drug overdose.[46]

Violence involving sex and family could also be associated to intentional drug overdose. [33,47] A study by Budnitz investigated the pattern of acetaminophen overdoses in the emergency department from two components of the National Electronic Injury Surveillance System. Of the 2,717 annual acetaminophen overdose cases, 69.8 per cent were related to self-directed violence. Further, females had a greater rate of self-directed violence (27.2 per 100,000) compared with males (14.4 per 100,000).[33] Violence and strife have also contributed to the increased rate of illicit drug use in the US.[47]

Drug overdoses can be associated with people who take drugs for recreational purposes. According to the Centers for Disease Control and Prevention (CDC), opioids are involved in more overdose deaths than heroin and cocaine combined, and they are often associated with recreational use.[4] Further, several studies found that recreational use contributed to many of the drug overdoses presenting to emergency departments. For example, a study found that 15.4 per cent of 500 overdose cases presented to emergency departments resulted from recreational use.[48] Further, a survey of 975 students found that 16 per cent abused medicine for recreational purposes.[49]

Buykx found that many people overdose on drugs after they experience interpersonal conflicts.[31] Britton's 2010 study investigated the risk factors of non-fatal overdoses over 12 months. The author recruited 2,966 participants and found that 23.5 per cent of all overdose cases had experienced sexual abuse. Moreover, victims of sexual abuse were 2.02 times more likely to overdose, and the result was statistically significant.[50] Other forms of physical abuse were also addressed in the study: 33.4 per cent of all overdose cases had experienced physical abuse, and they were 1.91 times more likely to overdose, which was statistically significant.[50]

The level of a medicine's purity could lead to a drug overdose, particularly for people using non-prescription medicines. Previous studies have found the fluctuation of heroin purity contributed to the overdose rate.[51] Moreover, in a survey of healthcare providers that asked about risk factors for opioid overdose, approximately 90 per cent mentioned the fluctuation of opioid purity.[52] Of 855 heroin users, 29 per cent split the tablets in half when the purity was unknown.[53] In addition, a study stated that many heroin users believed that purity fluctuation contributed to drug overdose.[54] Conversely, several studies on heroin (e.g. Toprak and Risser) found no association between drug overdose and purity.[55,56]

Other factors that contribute to intentional drug overdose include psychiatric illness, marital problems and family size.[6] Ahmed found that psychiatric illness was a greater risk among males than females, and it was a risk factor in 10 of the 50 cases he investigated. Further, five cases had experienced marital problems.[6] Family size could be a major factor in drug overdose. Large families are common in Saudi culture. A 2011 study by Bani found that 43 per cent of participants had six to eight family members.[57] A study by TNS Middle East of demographic characteristics in Saudi Arabia in 2006 found that 40 per cent of Saudi families are considered large, with six or more members.[58] Aljahdali found that large family size was a risk factor in drug overdoses: 59 per cent of the 79 cases in his study had more than five family members This could indicate that because large families have more children, parental supervision amongst the children is lowered, potentially increasing the chance of the unsupervised ingestion of drugs.[22]

A previous drug overdose might also be a risk factor for another drug overdose, as many studies have attested.[59],[60],[46] For example, Kinner's study in 2012 investigated the risk factors of non-fatal overdoses among illicit drug users, recruiting 2,515 illicit drug users in Vancouver, Canada. The author found an association between drug overdoses and previous drug experiences; people with previous overdoses were four times more likely to overdose compared with people who had no previous experience.[59] This finding is similar to that of a study by Hall in 2008, which investigated the pattern of unintentional drug overdose caused by prescription drugs, recruiting 295 participants. The author found that people who had experienced a previous overdose had a 30.2 per cent chance of overdose compared with 14.4 per cent of people who had not.[60] In addition, a New York study that investigated the risk factors of heroin users found that participants who had overdosed were 28 times more likely to overdose than those who had not experienced a previous overdose.[46] In contrast, some previous studies found no associations between drug overdose and previous overdose experience.[59]

Doctor shopping is considered the most common method of obtaining prescription drugs for legal and illegal use.[61-64] It is defined as patients visiting several doctors to obtain prescription medicines without medical need, and it is considered one of the major mechanisms of diversion.[35] Several studies have found that doctor shopping contributes to drug overdose. For example, the author Hall found that doctor shopping contributed to 21.4 per cent of 259 overdose cases.[65] Further, it found that 19 per cent of participants who overdosed acquired their medicines through doctor shopping.[49] Moreover, doctor shopping is attributed to a higher rate of drug overdose death.[65,66] Several studies have stated that controlling doctor shopping would assist in preventing drug overdoses.[35,67]

The consumption of prescription drugs, especially opioids, has increased due to their euphoric and energising effects.[4] For example, methamphetamine and alprazolam users tend to redose every three-to-eight hours to maintain the euphoric effect.[46] Further, drug users tend to abuse cocaine to feel euphoric and increase a feeling of sexual desirability.[68] Some medicines do not enhance euphoria until taken in higher doses. For example, drug users take higher doses of benzodiazepine to experience the euphoria effect. [24] Many fatal overdoses occur when larger doses of medicines have been taken to achieve the euphoric effect.[37]

Long-term therapy could be related to overdoses, especially in patients suffering from chronic pain. Further, such patients have easy access to painkillers in the home, which increases the chance of a fatal overdose.[69] Previously, long-term therapy was restricted to cancer patients; however, currently, it is commonly used for chronic pain in non-cancer patients. Unfortunately, the latter have been associated with higher overdose rates.[70] One of the reasons for drug overdose in chronic patients is inadequate pain management.[69,70] The critical issue with chronic pain is pain management, and inadequate pain management could lead to increased doses of painkillers and consequently, an increased rate of drug overdoses.[71]

Calculating the dose is an important factor, and miscalculated doses could lead to unintentional overdoses.[72] Many parents have difficulty measuring and calculating the appropriate dose of paracetamol for their children.[73] One survey asked 100 caregivers if they were able to determine the appropriate dose for their children; only 30 per cent were able to do so.[73] Hixson conducted a study in 2010 to compare the ability of parents to calculate the appropriate dose of acetaminophen using product information leaflets or the Parental Analgesia Slide. Participants were divided into two groups, and a questionnaire was distributed to each group. The author found that caregivers using the Parental Analgesia Slide had fewer dosing errors than caregivers using product information leaflets, but the difference was not statistically significant.[74] Limited literacy and numeracy skills are also associated with poor clinical outcomes and overdoses. Many people with limited numeracy skills are confused with dosing instructions and warning labels. Moreover, people could be confused with the information on the labels of prescription medicines.[75]

Mental states could be a major risk factor of drug overdose, as patients with mental disorders and drug addictions are more vulnerable.[76] For example, Hasin's study found that 15–20 per cent of patients with mental disorders overdosed on drugs at least once in their lives, and patients with depressive disorders were 3.7 times more likely to overdose.[76] Fischer's study found that people with mental problems were 1.51 times more likely to overdose than people without mental problems, but this result was not statistically significant.[77]

Children are considered at greater risk of drug overdose for several reasons. Inappropriate storage and disposal of medicines can contribute to this risk.[78] For example, according to the CDC and Prevention, one of the main causes of drug overdose reported to emergency departments is the unsupervised ingestion of OTC and prescription medicines. Further, the CDC stated that of the 72,000 overdose cases presented to emergency departments in 2004, more than 26,000 were caused by OTC drugs.[79] Additionally, Li's study found that children under the age of five accounted for a higher percentage of drug overdose cases in emergency departments,[41] while another study which investigated 3,034 overdose cases among children found 97 per cent of the cases resulted from the unsupervised ingestion of drugs.[80]

Older age is associated with a higher drug overdose rate for several reasons. First, elderly people aged 65 years and over tend to have more medical problems; thus, they may take many medicines that might interact with each other and cause an overdose.[79] Second, many elderly people live independently and might find it difficult to calculate the correct dose. In addition, they may not recognise the symptoms of drug overdose when it occurs. [81] Suicide attempts are common among elderly people by taking an excessive amount of a drug. Several factors contribute to suicide attempts, such as old age, failing physical and mental health, reduced income and social support.[82]

Maintaining a dose is an important factor in preventing intentional overdoses among chronic patients.[83,84] When medicines such as Warfarin have a narrow therapeutic index, it is critical to adjust the appropriate dose.[83] Physicians prefer not to dispense Warfarin because of the uncertainty of patient compliance with monitoring, dietary implications and the fear of haemorrhagic complications.[85] The initial dose is challengeable, which could result in bleeding, and many patients might overdose at the beginning because they might have Warfarin sensitivity or a poor metabolism, thus requiring reduced dose. The maintenance of the dose depends on several factors, such as weight, diet, disease state and concomitant use of other medications, as well as genetic factors.[84] Genetic variability is considered a major factor in determining Warfarin overdose. There are two genes which are cytochrome P450, family 2, subfamily C, polypeptide 9 (CYP2C9), and vitamin K epoxide reductase complex, subunit 1 (VKORC1) contributing significantly to the variability among patients in dose requirements for Warfarin.[84],[86]

Misunderstanding and misreading the abbreviation of prescriptions can lead to medication errors and overdoses. One report demonstrated that a woman had a severe digoxin overdose because her nurse misread the pharmacist's instructions. The pharmacist had used the abbreviation (=), which was unclear because the pen had trailed ink.[87] Maged conducted a study in Saudi Arabia in 2010 to investigate medication errors in prescription medicines. Of the 529 dosing errors, the author found that 46 per cent caused overdoses. The two main errors were the route and frequency of the medicines.[88] Further, many parents have difficulty understanding the instructions to administer appropriate doses for their children. A study in 2008 examined caregivers' understandings of the age indication of OTC drugs and cough medications. Of the 182 participants whose misunderstood dose instruction, the author found that more than 80 per cent had given medicine to their infants when they should have consulted a physician first.[75]

Many people believe that using excessive amounts of OTC medicines is safe and effective. Some people believe that if a medicine is OTC, it is safe to consume in large quantities.[33], [44] For example, paracetamol is considered a safe medication. However, it has a narrow therapeutic index, so the dangerous dose is close to the recommended dose, and an excessive dose could lead to liver toxicity.[33] Simkin's study found that 20 per cent of the 60 participants did not know the dose that could cause death, and 15 per cent believed that 100 tablets or more would cause death.[44] Advertising and media could contribute to the excessive amounts of OTC drugs administered; for example, advertisements could suggest that the consumption of large amounts is effective before seeing a doctor.[89] Wazaify claims that there is aggressive marketing and advertising for OTC medicines.[42]

There is a higher risk of drug-related deaths among recently released prisoners,[20,90] who are associated with overdoses in the first few weeks after release.[90,91] Many studies state that the leading cause of death for recently released prisoners is accidental drug overdose. [92] For example, a study found that recently released prisoners have an overdose rate that is 12 times higher than the general population.[91] In addition, another study found that the overdose mortality rate is three-to-eight times higher in the first two weeks after release compared to the subsequent 10 weeks.[20] The reasons for higher overdose rates are not understood; however, previous studies have suggested that possible reasons include poor housing, unemployment, psychosocial problems and barriers to health care.[93-95]

Another major factor related to the increase in drug overdose rates is the lack of education, which includes the education of healthcare providers, miscalculation of doses, and limited literacy and numeracy.[35,45,67] Manchikant states that many healthcare providers, such as physicians and pharmacists, do not have adequate education regarding drug misuse.[35] In 2012, Taylor investigated the pattern of acetaminophen overdose in the military and found that a lack of education was a risk factor.[45] The CDC stated that the majority of healthcare providers have the minimum education background regarding prescription drug misuse, and they could prescribe addictive medicines without being aware of the risks involved.[67] Wallace demonstrated that physicians have limited knowledge in detecting, investigating and managing acetaminophen overdoses. Further, Wallace's study proved that the management of overdoses improved when physicians had more knowledge. A management flowchart for paracetamol poisoning was introduced to help physicians treat overdose cases.[96]

Income could be a major factor in drug overdose. People with low incomes could have lower education and numeracy levels compared to those with higher incomes. This is supported by Lokker's study of parental misinterpretations of OTC medication labels, which found that 42 per cent of parents who misinterpreted the labels had an income of less than $20,000 per annum.[75] Further, people with low incomes had more motivation to misuse prescription medicines compared to those with higher incomes.[97] In addition, low-income people were six times more likely to overdose on prescription painkillers, and a US study found that low-income people accounted for 45 per cent of prescription overdose deaths.[37] The CDC also noted that low-income people are at a greater risk of drug overdose.[67]

In contrast, Yu's study in 2005 investigated drug misuse admissions to the emergency department in a large metropolitan teaching hospital in Taipei, Taiwan. The author found that those on high-incomes were more likely to misuse drugs than low and medium income people, and the result was statistically significant.[98] Another study by Hall, which examined the pattern of unintentional drug overdoses, categorised participants' incomes into four quartiles. He found that the higher-quartile income had a greater risk of drug overdose (24.7 per 100,000 people) than the other quartiles. Further, doctor shopping is related to the higher quartile; 58 per cent of doctor shoppers were represented by the higher-quartile income. [60] Paulozzi's study also categorised income into four quartiles and found that the higher-quartile income was at a greater risk of death from methadone overdose (29.9 per cent) and other opioid analgesics (33.1 per cent).[28]

Adverse Drug Reaction (ADR) consider as the fifth leading cause of death and illness in the developed world with direct medical costs estimated to be US$30–130 billion annually in the US and claiming 100,000-218,000 lives annually.[99] Despite this, health-related associations estimate that 95 per cent of all ADRs in Canada and the US are not reported.[100] Many drugs have caused adverse drug reactions after there have been proved, and this were attributed to the drug safety issue. For example in Canada, 3–4 per cent of drugs approved will eventually be withdrawn from the market because of safety issues, Faster approval of new drugs has the potential to produce more safety problems once drugs are on the market. Many agencies have launched post marketing surveillance and pharmacosurveillance systems, and these are aimed to generate safety signals for marketed drugs.[101]

Identifying patterns of drug overdose will help to implement evidence-based policies. In a study in the UK on the effects of the withdrawal of Distalgesic (a prescription-only analgesic compound) from the market, the author found an 84 per cent reduction in intentional drug overdoses presenting to emergency departments in hospitals compared with the three years before the drug was withdrawn. Further, there was a marked reduction in tablet sales after the medicine was withdrawn, from 40 million in 2005 to 500,000 in 2006. Thus, identifying drugs that are commonly involved in overdoses will help in reducing the overdose rate.[102]

3. Methodology

An emergency department visit for drug overdose was the primary outcome measure, including unintentional and intentional overdoses. Drug overdoses are identified by physicians in the emergency department using the terms overdose, poisoning and drug relayed problem. Secondary measures include the patient's age, gender, interior personal occupation, Length of Stay (LOS) in the emergency department, patient type, drug level, previous admission, previous overdose and measurement outcome.

In this research, participants are categorised into three groups. First, interior personnel are identified as people who work in the Ministry of Interior. The second group is interior personnel relatives, where each employee has the right to have his family treated in the hospital. The third group is called exceptional people; many people do not belong to the Ministry of Interior, but they seek treatment in the hospital because they have acquired an exceptional letter, as they require special health intervention.

Overdose cases obtained in the study are divided according to prescription and non- prescription drugs in order to test the hypothesis of the study. Moreover, the number of medicines involved in the cases is addressed and the drugs are categorised into three groups: single, double and triple. In addition, drug level is addressed in the study and it is standardised to moderate or severe according to the level of drug in the body. The LOS of patients was determined by calculating the period between the time of admission and the time of discharge from the emergency department, or the time when admitted to the inpatient management is included in the study and all cases are divided into two categories: discharged from the emergency department and admitted to the inpatient department.

Descriptive statistics such as frequencies and cross-tabulations were obtained to describe the various motives reported by the sample. All drugs involved in overdoses were obtained, as well as their frequency, to identify the medicine that accounted for the highest percentage. Further, the medicines used in overdoses were tabulated according to their medical indication of use and then each medicine was categorised according to their medical indication group. Fisher and chi-square tests were conducted to test the differences between categorical variables. As the chi-square prefers two-by-two tables and each cell must have at least five cells, the patients' type needed to be re-categorised into two groups: interior and non-interior. Although the patients' type was allocated to two groups, one of the cells had less than five, so a Fisher exact test was used.

The data was obtained from medical records, which raises the issue of confidentiality. However, the anonymity of participants will be protected, and only de-identified data was accessed. A letter was obtained from the hospital to ensure the anonymity of the research. The data was obtained only from files that were considered essential for the research. No patient was contacted as part of this study. Each participant will have a unique three-digit code. The data collection complies with the National Health and Medical Research Council's National Statement on Ethical Conduct in Human Research. Further, the study has been approved by the Security Forces Hospital's Research Committee. In addition, the UWA's Human Research Ethics Committee has approved this study.

4. Results

4.1. Demographic characteristics

One hundred and forty drug overdose cases were admitted to the emergency department of the Riyadh Security Forces Hospital between 1 January 2007 and 31 December 2011. Table 1 describes the demographic characteristics of patients associated with drug overdose, and the findings are discussed below. Females accounted for 57.90 per cent of cases and males accounted for 42.10 per cent. In this study, there is a variety in age distribution, with patients aged between 11 months and 86 years. The patients' ages were divided into seven groups:

(0.01–1.12), (2.00–9.12), (10.00–19.12), (20.00–29.12), (30.00–44.12), (45.00–59.12) and (over 60 years). This study demonstrates that groups (2.00–9.12 years) and (over 60 years) accounted for the highest percentage of drug overdose cases (22.9 per cent).

Characteristics	Number	Per cent
Gender:		
Male	59	42.1
Female	81	57.9
Age groups:		
0.01–1.12 years	8	5.7
2.00–9.12 years	32	22.9
10.00–19.12 years	9	6.4
20.00–29.12 years	25	17.9
30.00–44.12 years	19	13.6
45.00–59.12 years	15	10.7
Over 60 years	32	22.9
Type:		
Interior Personnel	30	21.4
Relatives	105	75.0
Exceptional people	5	3.60
Income groups:		
Less than 22,000 USD	37	27.4
22,001–45,000USD	69	51.1
45,001–67,001USD	18	13.3
More than 67,001 USD	11	8.1

Table 1. Socio-demographic characteristics of drug overdose cases.

The interior personnel relatives group accounted for the highest percentage of cases (n=105, 75 per cent), and interior personnel and exceptional people accounted for 21.4 and 3.60 per cent respectively. Income was divided into four groups that were represented by United State Dollar (USD) per annum: (less than 22,000 USD), (22,001–45,000USD), 3 (45,001–

67,001USD) and (more than 67,001 USD). The study showed that (22,001–45,000USD) group represents the highest percentage of participants.

According to Table 2, 96.4 per cent of all drug overdose cases reported to the emergency department between January 2007 and December 2011 were caused by prescription medicines. Previous overdoses were addressed in the study, and only eight patients were found to have previous overdose experiences. Further, the study found that 53.6 per cent of cases were associated with previous admission, and patients with one previous admission represented 20 per cent of all participants who had been admitted previously. In the study, some patients used more than one drug to overdose. It found that 91.4 per cent of patients were taking one drug, while double and triple drugs accounted for 7.9 per cent and 0.7 per cent respectively. In addition, 67.5 per cent of the cases were found to have moderate drug levels, while severe drug levels accounted for 26.4 per cent of cases.

LOS groups were categorised into the following: (less than five hours), (5.01–10.01 hours), (10.01–15.00 hours), (15.01–20.00 hours), (20.01–35.00 hours) and (over 40 hours). It found that 50.0 per cent of all cases reported to the emergency department stayed for less than five hours, and these cases were either discharged or transferred to the inpatient admission department. The study found that 106 drug overdose cases were referred to the inpatient admission department.

Interior relatives accounted for 75 per cent of all overdose cases in the study. It found that 28.6 per cent of the cases were aged 2–9.12 years. Further, 54 per cent of the participants' income was between (22,001–45,000USD) per annum. Eight cases were associated with previous overdose cases, and seven of them were relatives. Moreover, 49.5 per cent of cases stayed in the emergency department for less than five hours. Further, there were 34 discharged cases in the study, 28 of which were relative cases.

The outcome of a drug overdose is statistically different between patients' type (one-sided p-value = 0.007). It found that the inpatient admission department accounted for 93.3 per cent for all interior personnel cases, while non-interior people who were relatives and exceptional people accounted for 78 per cent of the cases, and the difference of outcome management among patient type is significant. By using the Fisher exact test, previous admission is statistically relevant to patient type (one-sided p-value = 0.033). It found that 70 and 50.1 per cent of interior and non interior cases were associated with previous admission; thus, the difference is significant. The difference between drug level and outcome management was tested using a chi-square test, and a significant difference was found. It found that 72.6 per cent of moderate-level cases were admitted to the inpatient department and 91.9 per cent of severe-level cases were admitted to the inpatient department. The management outcome from admission is statistically relevant to the level of drug (one-sided p-value = 0.008). The difference between gender and patients' type was tested using the Fisher exact test; thus, gender is statistically relevant to patients' type (one-sided p-value = 0.000).

Characteristics	Number	Per cent
Previous overdose:		
Yes	8	5.7
No	132	94.3
Previous admission:		
Yes	75	53.6
No	65	46.4
Number of previous admissions:		
0	65	46.4
1	28	20.0
2	21	15.0
3	8	5.7
4	6	4.3
5	4	2.9
7 and more	8	5.6
Drug kind:		
Prescription	135	96.4
Non-prescription	5	3.6
Drug combination		
Single drug	128	91.4
Double drugs	11	7.9
Triple drugs	1	0.7
Drug level:		
Moderate	95	67.9
Severe	37	26.4
LOS groups:		
Less than five hours	70	50.0
5.01–10.01 hours	24	17.1
10.01–15.00 hours	12	8.6
15.01–20.00 hours	13	9.3
20.01–35.00 hours	10	7.1
Over 40 hours	11	7.9
Outcome management:		
Discharge	34	24.3
Inpatient admission	106	75.7

Table 2. Characteristics of drug overdose cases

4.2. Drug overdose percentages and rates

The means of LOS age and income per annum of patients in the emergency department are addressed, and it was found that the average LOS was around 11 hours, average age was 33 years and four months, and average income was around 35,951 USD.

The number of drug overdose cases was calculated for each year of the study. The annual number of emergency admissions was requested from the medical records department to identify the rate of drug overdose cases among all emergency cases. All results are shown in Table 3. According to the results, the rate of drug overdose reduced between 2007 and 2011.

Year	Number of cases	Number of emergency cases	Rate
2007	33	9576	3.45 per 1,000
2008	30	9131	3.26 per 1,000
2009	26	8707	2.99 per 1,000
2010	26	8209	3.17 per 1,000
2011	25	7883	3.17 per 1,000

Table 3. Number and rate of drug overdose for each year in the study

Most patients overdosed on one drug. Fifty-eight prescription and non-prescription medicines were included in the study. These medicines were categorised in terms of medical indication purpose. Seven drug categories were found in the study, and each one involved more than seven cases. Further, anti-coagulants and analgesics accounted for 35.3 per cent of drug overdose cases. These categories were investigated in terms of age groups. The findings show that 55 per cent of anti-coagulant overdose cases occurred in patients aged over 60 years, while 41 per cent of analgesic overdose cases occurred in patients aged 20–30 years. According to the findings, Warfarin accounted for the highest percentage of drug overdoses. Warfarin accounted for 85 per cent of overdoses in patients aged over 50 years, while two cases occurred in children and middle-aged people respectively. Further, people in lower and middle-income groups accounted for 85.7 per cent of anti-coagulant cases.

The results show that four patients from age (20.00–29.12 years), had a previous overdose, and this age group represented 50 per cent of patients associated with previous overdoses. Moreover, two patients overdosed on OTC medicines twice, and one patient overdosed twice on Warfarin. Two deaths occurred from drug overdoses: one death was a patient who overdosed on paracetamol twice, and the other was attributed to amphetamine. In addition, there were 18 overdose cases aged from 15 to 25 years. It found that analgesics and antipsychotics accounted for 38.8 and 22.2 per cent of the cases respectively. Cholesterol-lowering and diabetic medicines were involved in two cases and antihistamine and antiepileptic drugs were involved in one case each.

As the hospital belongs to the Ministry of Interior, it is important to identify the occupations that are more involved in drug overdoses. There were 30 interior personnel cases, and eleven positions represented all interior personnel drug overdose cases. The system of occupation in the Ministry of Interior has two major categories: officer and non-officer. Non-officer personnel presented at a higher rate in drug overdoses than non-officer personnel. In this study, five of 30 cases belong to officers and the rest belong to non-officers.

Position name	Frequency
Soldier	7
First soldier	5
Captain	4
First Sargent	3
Sargent	2
Staff-Sargent	2
Unknown	2
Colonel	1
Corporal	1
Chief-Sargent	1
Porter	1
Senior-Sargent	1

Table 4. Occupations of interior personnel cases and their frequency

5. Discussion

We found that females accounted for a higher percentage of drug overdose cases than males, which is similar to findings in previous studies.[6,22,103,104] In contrast, Alfawal's study found that males accounted for 88 per cent of the cases.[7] Further, it found that (2.00–9.12 years) and (over 60 years) patients accounted for the highest percentage, at 22.9 per cent of cases. Previous studies associated the elderly with a higher percentage of drug overdoses, and this study had a similar result.[79,82] Further, the CDC found that the highest risk group of drug overdose among children was amongst those aged two years.[80] This research reached the same conclusion. Thus, most cases might have occurred unintentionally because previous studies demonstrated that children and the elderly are at a higher risk of unintentional overdose.[80]

The finding stated that 75.7 per cent of cases were referred to the inpatients admission department. According to the medical records department supervisor, this high percentage is not because most cases were severe; rather, many cases that were presented and discharged from the emergency department were missing and did not register to the medical files. There are two possible reasons for missing drug overdose cases. First, there is a higher load on emergency physicians; so many diagnostic forms are not fully completed. Second, many cases present to the emergency department have not been registered in the patients' medical records, so some overdose cases may have been missed and not caught by the ICD-9-CM. This explains why there were only 140 drug overdose cases in the five-year period. A study conducted in the National Guard Hospital in Riyadh, which is considered larger than the

Security Force Hospital, found nine drug overdose cases per month,[105] compared to this study, which found around three cases per month. This is further evidence that there might be missing cases.

Fifty-eight medicines were involved in the drug overdose cases, and the most common drug was Warfarin, which caused 29 overdose cases. This finding differs from previous studies conducted in Saudi Arabia, which found that OTC medicines accounted for a large percentage of drug overdoses. Moazzam's and Aljahdali's studies found that paracetamol accounted for 24.1 per cent of 170 drug overdose cases and 30 per cent of 79 cases, respectively. [21,22]Ahmed's study found that mefenamic acid accounted for 20 per cent of 50 cases investigated.[6] Moreover, Malik's study found that the most common drugs used were analgesics and non-steroid anti- inflammatory drugs.[104] AbuMadini's study found that 80 per cent of cases were caused by paracetamol,[103] which was the second most common medicine in this study (12 cases).

According to the findings, children aged 2–9 years accounted for 22.4 per cent of drug overdose cases. This might indicate that many parents leave medicines unprotected from children, so children might administer excessive amounts of drugs accidentally. Education and awareness campaigns should be conducted to educate people about the risk of leaving medicines unprotected, as well as how to store their medicines correctly.[1,75,106, 107] Further, leaving medicines unsecured from children can contribute to an increase in the rate of drug overdose.[78,108,109] According to the American Association of Poison Control Centers, in 2009, prescription and OTC drugs caused more than 30 per cent of children's death in the US.[110]

Many policy and prevention measures can be implemented to protect children from drug overdoses, such as child-resistant packaging (CRP), product reformulations and heightened parental awareness. CRP reduced the drug overdose mortality rate of children by 45 per cent between 1974 and 1992.[22,80] Medication packaging will not protect children from overdose, and it becomes ineffective if the medication is not re-secured correctly.[109] Further, packaging has not proved to be effective, as young children have the dexterity to open these containers.[111] Some prevention programs have been conducted to educate parents about storing medicine in safe places. The Preventing Overdoses and Treatment Exposures Task Force (PROTECT) launched a program called 'Up and Away', which aims to educate parents about effectively storing medicines, and it emphasises the need to return medicines to a safe storage location immediately after every use to prevent children from reaching them.[109]

Other strategies might be helpful in preventing drug overdoses in children. For example, the use of adaptors on bottles of liquid medication so that the medication can be accessed only with a needleless syringe; parents should not allow children to drink medicine directly from the bottle; and using unit dose packaging might reduce the amount of accidental drug ingestion. These strategies are highly recommended for common medicines such as OTC drugs.[80]

As children account for a higher percentage of drug overdose cases, parents' misunderstanding and miscalculation of doses can contribute to a higher percentage of overdoses. Contributing factors include limited literacy and numeracy, particularly in age indication. This problem is emphasised in terms of OTC medicines, as no instructions are provided directly by healthcare providers.[28,112] Applying simple language instructions and warning labels in the leaflets of medicines might be helpful in terms of calculating correct doses.[75] Further, healthcare providers should request that parents with low literacy levels use one product for all children in the family, which might help to prevent dose miscalculation.[73]

Another major factor contributing to drug overdoses in children is the availability of unused drugs in homes.[113] The solution for this problem is medication disposal. Campaigns for the disposal of medications have been used in many countries, which would help to reduce accidental drug overdoses in children, intentional drug abuse and the accumulation of drugs by elderly people, as well as protect the physical environment and eliminate waste in the healthcare system.[113,114] The government of Ireland launched a campaign called Dispose of Unused Medicines Properly (DUMP), which encouraged the public to return unused or expired medicines to community pharmacies. The project was launched in 2005, and 9,608 items were returned in the first year and 2,951 kilograms were returned in 2006. The most common medicine group returned was the nervous system class, which accounted for 26.3 per cent.[115]

A study conducted in Saudi Arabia in 2003 identified the issue of unused and expired medicines in Saudi dwellings. The study recruited 1,641 households in 22 cities. The study found that more than 80 per cent of Saudi families had more than five medicines, with an average of more than two medicines that were expired or unused. The most common drugs found in the participants' houses were respiratory drugs (16.8 per cent), followed by central nervous system (CNS) agents (16.4 per cent) and antibiotics (14.3 per cent). Of the 2,050 CNS medications, OTC analgesics (including non-steroidal anti-inflammatory agents) constituted 49.9 per cent of the total (n = 1,023). Further, 51 per cent of all medicines found were not currently used and, of these, 40 per cent were expired. So medication wastage can provide greater opportunity to access prescription drugs in Saudi Arabia. The study recommended disposal medication campaigns to reduce the danger of available unused and expired medicines.[116]

According to the results a large number of medicines were involved in drug overdose, and thus might indicated that many patients have excessive amount of medicines in there dwelling. One reason might contribute to the excessive amount of medicines is drug seeking behaviour. Warfarin accounted for the highest percentage of drug overdoses. Eighty-five per cent of all Warfarin overdoses occurred in patients aged over 50 years, while two cases occurred in children and the middle-aged, respectively. This might indicate that the overdoses occurred unintentionally. One of major reasons for Warfarin overdoses is that it has a narrow therapeutic index; thus, administrating a larger dose would easily lead to overdoses. [117] Further, Warfarin is associated with complex pharmacology and inherent risk of outcome. As it is used continuously, maintaining the dose is critical to ensure safe and effective therapy.[117]

According to the results, females accounted for a higher percentage of drug overdoses. Several factors might contribute to this. First, family conflict was stated as a higher-risk factor of drug overdoses in women. Aljahdali's study found that 80 per cent of the 79 overdose cases investigated were female, and 60 per cent had family conflicts.[22] Further, a study was conducted in the King Fahd Hospital of the University (KFHU) to investigate cases of deliberate self-harm presented to the emergency department of the hospital. The study recruited 362 cases, and the female to male ratio was 1.8:1. The study found that 71 per cent of cases were drug overdoses, of which 50.3 per cent were caused by family problems.[103] Moreover, a study was conducted in Saudi Arabia in KFHU to investigate non-fatal, deliberate self-harm cases. There were 55 cases investigated over nine months, and 80 per cent of them were female. The most common method used was self-poisoning (drug and chemical). The study found that family conflict was the main factor, contributing to 50.9 per cent of cases.[118]

The rate of drug overdose for each year of the study period was reduced from 3.45 to 3.17 per 1,000. However, the number of emergency admissions also reduced annually. This result contrasts with previous studies. For example, Moazzam found an increased rate of drug poisoning in the alQassim region in Saudi Arabia, from 6.6 per 100,000 in 1999 to 10.7 per 100,000.[21] Further, Malik found that the number of drug overdose cases presented in Asir Center Hospital increased from two cases in 1989 to 22 cases in 1993.[104] This indicates that there were perhaps more preventive and awareness programs in Saudi Arabia in the previous years.

There are several pharmacyosurveillance implications; one of them is collecting data regarding motivations and causes of drug overdose. According to the finding most of the cases occurred in elderly and children, so targeting these groups of people would help in reducing the rate of drug overdose cases.[119] Further, another implication would be the use of Electronic prescription. It is defined as a tool for prescribers to electronically prepare and send an accurate, error-free and understandable prescription directly to a pharmacy. Previous study found that electronic prescription system reduced medical errors by 55 per cent - from 10.7 to 4.9 per 1000 patient-days.[120] According to the results the rate of drug overdose cases in the emergency department decreased between 2007 and 2011, and this was attributed for using electronic prescription system in the hospital.

Drug related problems account for large amount of money in hospital cost. For example, in US a probability model in 2002 estimated that morbidity and mortality associated with DRPs account for $76.6 billion in hospital cost. Further, a study conducted in Saudi Arabia in 2008 found that the estimate cost of one day admission for drug related problem is 666$. So Implementing preventable measures such as pharmacosurveillance system would be a cost effective.[105]

Some policies might be implemented to reduce the risk of drug overdose cases. As Warfarin accounted for the highest percentage of drug overdoses, particularly in elderly people, further dose instruction should be given to elderly patients to ensure they have understood the instructions correctly.[85] Further, patients acquired Warfarin from hospital; thus, if the quantity of medicine dispensed is reduced, drug overdose cases might be prevented. In addition, children accounted for the highest percentage of drug overdose cases, so policymakers should implement awareness courses to educate parents to secure and protect medicines from children.[80] There was a wide range of medicines involved in drug overdose cases, so further dose instruction is needed. Moreover, patients must be educated regarding the dangers of overdosing.

6. Conclusion

Despite religious, cultural and legal deterrents, occasional cases of drug overdoses occur in the Saudi population.

The main limitations of this study mainly in relate to the quality of data available in patients' medical records, as many files might not be fully documented, and some variables related to research are not found in the medical records (e.g. education level). Moreover, as the income level is identified based on the household occupation, a number of files did not document the household occupation; thus, some patients' incomes were not available. The sample size is considered small, as there are few statistically significant associations between variables. Thus, the findings relating to associations between variables might not represent the actual validity of the associations between the independent and outcome variables. In addition, the data in this study was collected from a single institution, and the patients of drug overdoses have special characteristics that might not be similar to the general Saudi population. For example, all people treated in the hospital obtain medicines from the pharmacy without any charge. Further, One of the limitations of this study is that it does not state the reasons for drug overdoses, and it does not identify if overdoses occurred intentionally or accidentally.

Some significant findings were made, such as Warfarin causing 29 overdose cases, and patients aged over 50 accounting for 85 per cent of all Warfarin cases. This finding signifies a problem with Warfarin in elderly patients, and further research is needed to identify the major cause of this high percentage and to assist in implementing preventive measures to protect the elderly from the risk of overdosing. Further, children accounted for a high percentage of drug overdoses, and the study stated that 66.6 of anti-hypertensive overdoses were children. Thus, further research should be conducted to identify the reasons why children overdose so they can be protected from drug overdoses.

These findings could help the hospital to implement preventive strategies and policies. As many cases occur accidentally, education and awareness programs are required regarding dose instructions and the storage and disposal of medicines. Further, many patients keep excessive amounts of medicines in their dwellings, so reducing the amount of medicines provided to chronic patients would help to reduce drug overdose cases. Education of physicians on drug-seeking behaviour of patients is important. Further, special courses in dose instructions could be implemented for elderly patients, as well as programs that target parents regarding dose calculations for their children and the safe storage of medicines. In addition, clinical guidelines for overdose management need to be standardised, and the surveillance and recording of overdose information should be improved. Lastly, improved education is required for the public and for health workers in order to prevent drug interactions that might precipitate overdoses.

Author details

Naser Al-Jaser, M. Cli. Epi and Niyi Awofeso

School of Population Health, University of Western Australia, Australia

References

[1] Coffin P. Overdose: A Major Cause of Preventable Death in Central and Eastern Europe in Central Asia:Vilnius; 2008 [cited 17/5/2012]. Available from: http://www.harm-reduction.org/images/stories/library/od_report_2008_en.pdf

[2] Warner M, Chen LH, Makuc DM. Increase in fatal poisonings involving opioid analgesics in the United States, 1999-2006. NCHS data brief. 2009 (22):1.

[3] CDC. Prescription Drug Overdose: State Health Agencies Respond. 2008. Available from: http://www.cdc.gov/HomeandRecreationalSafety/pubs/RXReport_web-a.pdf

[4] CDC. Unintentional Drug Poisoning in the United States.; 2006 [cited 11/5/2012]. Available from: http://www.cdc.gov/HomeandRecreationalSafety/pdf/poison-issue-brief.pdf

[5] statistics dgo. Health statistics year book, new outpatient and inpatients in Mental Health Departments. Riyadh: MOH; 2009. Available from: http://www.moh.gov.sa/en/Ministry/Statistics/book/flash/1430/MOH_Report_1430.html

[6] Ahmed M. Drug-associated admissions to a district hospital in Saudi Arabia. Journal of clinical pharmacy and therapeutics. 1997;22(1):61-66.

[7] Elfawal M. Trends in fatal substance overdose in eastern Saudi Arabia. Journal of Clinical Forensic Medicine. 1999;6(1):30-34.

[8] Jha AK, Kuperman GJ, Teich JM, Leape L, Shea B, Rittenberg E, et al. Identifying adverse drug events development of a computer-based monitor and comparison with chart review and stimulated voluntary report. Journal of the American Medical Informatics Association. 1998;5(3):305-314.

[9] Lazarou J, Pomeranz BH, Corey PN. Incidence of adverse drug reactions in hospitalized patients. JAMA: the journal of the American Medical Association. 1998;279(15): 1200-1205.

[10] Moore TJ, Cohen MR, Furberg CD. Serious adverse drug events reported to the Food and Drug Administration, 1998-2005. Archives of internal medicine. 2007;167(16): 1752.

[11] Budnitz DS, Pollock DA, Mendelsohn AB, Weidenbach KN, McDonald AK, Annest JL. Emergency department visits for outpatient adverse drug events: demonstration for a national surveillance system. Annals of emergency medicine. 2005;45(2): 197-206.

[12] CDC. Overdoses of Prescription Opioid Pain Relievers --- United States, 1999--2008. Prevention CfDC; 2011. Available from: http://www.cdc.gov/mmwr/preview/ mmwrhtml/mm6043a4.htm

[13] Santiago L, Altamirano P, Torreblanco M, Ruiz S. WORLD DRUG REPORT 2011. Vinne: (UNODC) UNOoDaC; 2011. Available from: http://www.unodc.org/docu- ments/data-and-analysis/WDR2011/World_Drug_Report_2011_ebook.pdf

[14] Quan VM, Vongchak T, Jittiwutikarn J, Kawichai S, Srirak N, Wiboonnatakul K, et al. Predictors of mortality among injecting and non-injecting HIV-negative drug users in northern Thailand. Addiction. 2007;102(3):441-446.

[15] Zhang L, Ruan Y, Jiang Z, Yang Z, Liu S, Zhou F, et al. An 1-year prospective cohort study on mortality of injecting drug users]. Zhonghua liu xing bing xue za zhi= Zhonghua liuxingbingxue zazhi. 2005;26(3):190.

[16] EMCDDA. THE STATE OF THE DRUGS PROBLEM IN EUROPE. Portugal: [cited 1/6/2012]. Available from: http://www.emcdda.europa.eu/publications/annual-re- port/2011

[17] CDC. Suicides Due to Alcohol and/or Drug Overdose. NVDRS; 2011 [cited 15/5/2012]. Available from: http://www.cdc.gov/ViolencePrevention/pdf/ NVDRS_Data_Brief-a.pdf

[18] Health AIo, Welfare. Statistics on Drug Use in Australia 2006. 2007 [cited 7/5/2012]. Report No.: 9781740246606. Available from: http://www.aihw.gov.au/publication-de- tail/?id=6442467962

[19] Degenhardt L, Roxburgh A. Accidental drug-induced deaths due to opioids in Aus- tralia. 2005 [cited 20/5/2012]. Available from: http://ndarc.med.unsw.edu.au/ resource/accidental-drug-induced-deaths-australia-1997-2001

[20] Merrall ELC, Kariminia A, Binswanger IA, Hobbs MS, Farrell M, Marsden J, et al. Meta-analysis of drug-related deaths soon after release from prison.Addiction. 2010;105(9):1545-1554.

[21] Moazzam M, Al-Saigul A, Naguib M, Al Alfi M. Pattern of acute poisoning in Al- Qassim region: a surveillance report from Saudi Arabia, 1999-2003. Eastern Mediter- ranean Health Journal. 2009;15(4):1005-1010.

[22] Al Jahdali, Antipsychotics SG. Pattern and risk factors for intentional drug overdose in Saudi Arabia. Canadian journal of psychiatry. 2004;49:331-334.

[23] WHO, Zhang X. WHO guidelines on safety monitoring of herbal medicines in pharmacovigilance systems. 2004 [cited 10/7/2012]. Report No.: 9241592214. Available from: http://apps.who.int/medicinedocs/documents/s7148e/s7148e.pdf

[24] Lessenger JE, Feinberg SD. Abuse of prescription and over-the-counter medications. The Journal of the American Board of Family Medicine. 2008;21(1):45-54.

[25] Saad B, Azaizeh H, Abu-Hijleh G, Said O. Safety of traditional Arab herbal medicine. Evidence Based Complementary and Alternative Medicine. 2006;3(4):433-440.

[26] Alkharfy K. Community pharmacists' knowledge, attitudes and practices towards herbal remedies in Riyadh, Saudi Arabia. East Mediterr Health J. 2010;16(9):988-993.

[27] Jane B, Trevor S, Andrew T, Bilal W, Alex W, Sunny M. The context of illicit drug overdose deaths in British Columbia, 2006. Harm Reduction Journal. 2009;6.

[28] Paulozzi LJ, Logan JE, Hall AJ, McKinstry E, Kaplan JA, Crosby AE. A comparison of drug overdose deaths involving methadone and other opioid analgesics in West Virginia. Addiction. 2009;104(9):1541-1548.

[29] De Leo D, Evans R. International suicide rates: recent trends and implications for Australia. 2006 [cited 25/5/2012]. Available from: http://www.health.gov.au/internet/main/publishing.nsf/content/1D2B4E895BCD429ECA2572290027094D/$File/intsui.pdf

[30] Suicides, Australia, 1994 to 2004. Canberra,; 2006 [cited 12/4/2012]. Available from: http://www.ausstats.abs.gov.au/ausstats/subscriber.nsf/0/FF573FA817DC3C84CA25713000705C19/$File/33090_1994 to 2004.pdf

[31] Buykx P, Ritter A, Loxley W, Dietze P. Patients Who Attend the Emergency Department Following Medication Overdose: Self-reported Mental Health History and Intended Outcomes of Overdose. International Journal of Mental Health and Addiction. 2011:1-11.

[32] Bohnert ASB, Roeder KM, Ilgen MA. Suicide attempts and overdoses among adults entering addictions treatment: Comparing correlates in a US national study. Drug and alcohol dependence. 2011;119(1-2):106-12.

[33] Budnitz DS, Lovegrove MC, Crosby AE. Emergency department visits for overdoses of acetaminophen-containing products. American Journal of Preventive Medicine. 2011;40(6):585-592.

[34] Darke S, Ross J. The relationship between suicide and heroin overdose among methadone maintenance patients in Sydney, Australia. Addiction. 2001;96(10):1443-1453.

[35] Manchikanti L. Prescription drug abuse: what is being done to address this new drug epidemic? Testimony before the Subcommittee on Criminal Justice, Drug Policy and Human Resources. Pain Physician. 2006;9(4):287.

[36] Leary E, Poisson M. prescription and over the counter drug abuse, Orange County Comprehensive Report. Santa Ana, california; 2010 [cited 2/5/2012]. Available from: http://www.duila.org/Assets/StreetTrends/Prescription and OTC Drug Abuse/ prescription-over-the-counter-drug-abuse-report.pdf

[37] CDC. Policy Impact: Prescription Painkiller Overdoses. 2011 [cited 9/5/2012]. Available from: http://www.cdc.gov/HomeandRecreationalSafety/pdf/PolicyImpact-PrescriptionPainkillerOD.pdf

[38] Devi S. USA homes in on prescription drug abuse. The Lancet. 2011;378(9790): 473-474.

[39] Dhalla IA, Mamdani MM, Gomes T, Juurlink DN. Clustering of opioid prescribing and opioid-related mortality among family physicians in Ontario. Canadian Family Physician. 2011;57(3):e92-e96.

[40] White J, Taverner D. Drug-seeking behaviour. Australian prescriber 1997 (20):68-70.

[41] Li C, Martin BC. Trends in emergency department visits attributable to acetaminophen overdoses in the United States: 1993,Äì2007. Pharmacoepidemiology and drug safety. 2011;20(8):810-818.

[42] Wazaify M, Kennedy S, Hughes CM, McElnay JC. Prevalence of over-the-counter drug-related overdoses at Accident and Emergency departments in Northern Ireland--a retrospective evaluation. Journal of clinical pharmacy and therapeutics. 2005;30(1):39-44.

[43] Toblin RL, Paulozzi LJ, Logan JE, Hall AJ, Kaplan JA. Mental illness and psychotropic drug use among prescription drug overdose deaths: a medical examiner chart review. The Journal of clinical psychiatry. 2010;71(4):491-496.

[44] Simkin S, Hawton K, Kapur N, Gunnell D. What can be done to reduce mortality from paracetamol overdoses? A patient interview study. QJM. 2012;105(1):41-51.

[45] Taylor LG, Xie S, Meyer TE, Coster TS. Acetaminophen overdose in the Military Health System. Pharmacoepidemiology and drug safety. 2012.

[46] Curtis M, Guterman L. Overdose Prevention and Response. 2009 [cited 6/5/2012]. Available from: http://harm.live.radicaldesigns.org/downloads/Overdose Prevention and Response Guide.pdf

[47] Shah N. Unintentional Illicit and Prescription Drug Overdose Death Trends, 2008. New Mexico Journal NME; 2009 [cited 7/5/2012]. Available from: http:// nmhealth.org/erd/pdf/ER prescription drug overdose 112009.pdf

[48] Craig DGN, Bates CM, Davidson JS, Martin KG, Hayes PC, Simpson KJ. Overdose pattern and outcome in paracetamol-induced acute severe hepatotoxicity. British journal of clinical pharmacology. 2011;71(2):273-282.

[49] Buykx P, Loxley W, Dietze P, Ritter A. Medications used in overdose and how they are acquired- an investigation of cases attending an inner Melbourne emergency department. Australian and New Zealand journal of public health. 2010;34(4):401-404.

[50] Britton PC, Wines JD, Conner KR. Non-fatal overdose in the 12 months following treatment for substance use disorders. Drug and alcohol dependence. 2010;107(1): 51-55.

[51] Darke S, Duflou J, Torok M. A reduction in blood morphine concentrations amongst heroin overdose fatalities associated with a sustained reduction in street heroin purity. Forensic science international. 2010;198(1-3):118-120.

[52] Mayet S, Manning V, Williams A, Loaring J, Strang J. Impact of training for healthcare professionals on how to manage an opioid overdose with naloxone: Effective, but dissemination is challenging. International Journal of Drug Policy. 2011;22(1): 9-15.

[53] HORYNIAK D, HIGGS P, LEWIS J, WINTER R, DIETZE P, AITKEN C. An evaluation of a heroin overdose prevention and education campaign. Drug and alcohol review. 2010;29(1):5-11.

[54] Maher L, Ho HT. Overdose beliefs and management practices among ethnic Vietnamese heroin users in Sydney, Australia. Harm Reduction Journal. 2009;6(1):6.

[55] Toprak S, Cetin I. Heroin Overdose Deaths and Heroin Purity Between 1990 and 2000 in Istanbul, Turkey*. Journal of forensic sciences. 2009;54(5):1185-1188.

[56] Risser D, Uhl A, Oberndorfer F, Stichenwirth M, Hirz R, Sebald D. Is there a relationship between street heroin purity and drug-related emergencies and/or drug-related deaths? An analysis from Vienna, Austria. Journal of forensic sciences. 2007;52(5): 1171-1176.

[57] Bani I. Prevalence and related risk factors of Essential Hypertension in Jazan region, Saudi Arabia. Sudanese Journal of Public Health 2011;6(2):45-50.

[58] East TM. Saudi Arabia's demographics - the winds of change. [cited 16/5/2012]. Available from: http://www.ameinfo.com/96723.html

[59] Kinner SA, Milloy M, Wood E, Qi J, Zhang R, Kerr T. Incidence and risk factors for non-fatal overdose among a cohort of recently incarcerated illicit drug users. Addictive Behaviors. 2012.

[60] Hall AJ, Logan JE, Toblin RL, Kaplan JA, Kraner JC, Bixler D, et al. Patterns of abuse among unintentional pharmaceutical overdose fatalities. JAMA: the journal of the American Medical Association. 2008;300(22):2613-2620.

[61] Trescot AM, Boswell MV, Atluri SL, Hansen HC, Deer TR, Abdi S, et al. Opioid guidelines in the management of chronic non-cancer pain. Pain Physician. 2006;9(1): 1.

[62] Reporting KASPE. A Comprehensive Report on Kentucky Prescription Monitoring Program Prepared by the Cabinet for Health and Family Services Office of the Inspector General. 2006 [cited 22/5/2012]. Available from: http://chfs.ky.gov/nr/rdonlyres/7057e43d-e1fd-4552-a902-2793f9b226fc/0/kaspersummaryreportversion2.pdf

[63] Manchikanti L, Damron K, Pampati V, McManus C. Prospective evaluation of patients with increasing opiate needs: prescription opiate abuse and illicit drug use. Pain Physician. 2004;7(3):339.

[64] Manchikanti L, Fellows B, Damron K, Pampati V, McManus C. Prevalence of illicit drug use among individuals with chronic pain in the Commonwealth of Kentucky: an evaluation of patterns and trends. The Journal of the Kentucky Medical Association. 2005;103(2):55.

[65] Hall AJ, Logan JE, Toblin RL, Kaplan JA, Kraner JC, Bixler D, et al. Patterns of abuse among unintentional pharmaceutical overdose fatalities. JAMA: the journal of the American Medical Association. 2008;300(22):2613.

[66] Hempstead K. Manner of death and circumstances in fatal poisonings: evidence from New Jersey. Injury Prevention. 2006;12(suppl 2):ii44-ii48.

[67] Strategies P. CDC Grand Rounds: Prescription Drug Overdoses – a U.S. Epidemic. [cited 13/5/2012]. Available from: http://www.cdc.gov/mmwr/preview/mmwrhtml/mm6101a3.htm

[68] Meehan TJ, Bryant SM, Aks SE. Drugs of Abuse: The Highs and Lows of Altered Mental States in the Emergency Department. Emergency medicine clinics of North America. 2010;28(3):663-682.

[69] Von Korff M, Kolodny A, Deyo RA, Chou R. Long-term opioid therapy reconsidered. Annals of internal medicine. 2011;155(5):325-328.

[70] Reidenberg M, Willis O. Prosecution of physicians for prescribing opioids to patients. Clinical Pharmacology & Therapeutics. 2007;81(6):903-906.

[71] Baehren DF, Marco CA, Droz DE, Sinha S, Callan EM, Akpunonu P. A statewide prescription monitoring program affects emergency department prescribing behaviors. Annals of emergency medicine. 2010;56(1):19-23. e3.

[72] Miles FK, Kamath R, Dorney SFA, Gaskin KJ, O'Loughlin EV. Accidental paracetamol overdosing and fulminant hepatic failure in children. Medical Journal of Australia. 1999;171:472-475.

[73] Buck M. Preventing Acetaminophen Overdosage. The Annals of Pharmacotherapy. 2000;34(32-4).

[74] HIXSON R, Franke U, Mittal R, Hamilton M. Parental calculation of pediatric paracetamol dose: a randomized trial comparing the Parental Analgesia Slide with product information leaflets. Pediatric Anesthesia. 2010;20(7):612-619.

[75] Lokker N, Sanders L, Perrin EM, Kumar D, Finkle J, Franco V, et al. Parental misinterpretations of over-the-counter pediatric cough and cold medication labels. Pediatrics. 2009;123(6):1464-1471.

[76] Hasin DS, Goodwin RD, Stinson FS, Grant BF. Epidemiology of major depressive disorder: results from the National Epidemiologic Survey on Alcoholism and Related Conditions. Archives of General Psychiatry. 2005;62(10):1097.

[77] Fischer B, Brissette S, Brochu S, Bruneau J, El-Guebaly N, Rehm J, et al. Determinants of overdose incidents among illicit opioid users in 5 Canadian cities. Canadian Medical Association Journal. 2004;171(3):235-239.

[78] Ozanne-Smith J, Centre MUAR, NPHPG. Pharmaceutical Poisoning to 0-19 Year Olds: National Public Health Partnership Public Health Planning and Practice Framework Trial. 2002 [cited 23/5/2012]. Report No.: 9780732614928. Available from: http://www.monash.edu.au/miri/research/reports/muarc193.pdf

[79] ACPM. Over The Counter Medications: Use In General and Special Population, Therapeutic Errors, Misuse, Storage and Disposal. Washington; 2011 [cited 28/4/2012]. Available from: http://www.acpm.org/resource/resmgr/timetools-files/otcmedstimetool.pdf

[80] Schillie SF, Shehab N, Thomas KE, Budnitz DS. Medication overdoses leading to emergency department visits among children. American Journal of Preventive Medicine. 2009;37(3):181-187.

[81] Conca AJ, Worthen DR. Nonprescription Drug Abuse. Journal of Pharmacy Practice. 2012 February 1, 2012;25(1):13-21.

[82] Gavrielatos G, Komitopoulos N, Kanellos P, Varsamis E, Kogeorgos J. Suicidal attempts by prescription drug overdose in the elderly: a study of 44 cases. Neuropsychiatric disease and treatment. 2006;2(3):359.

[83] Yin T, Miyata T. Warfarin dose and the pharmacogenomics of CYP2C9 and VKORC1--Rationale and perspectives. Thrombosis research. 2007;120(1):1-10.

[84] Klein T, Altman R, Eriksson N, Gage B, Kimmel S, Lee M, et al. Estimation of the warfarin dose with clinical and pharmacogenetic data. The New England journal of medicine. 2009;360(8):753.

[85] Nasser S, Mullan J, Bajorek B. Challenges of Older Patients' Knowledge About Warfarin Therapy. Journal of Primary Care & Community Health. 2012;3(1):65-74.

[86] AMA. Personalized health care report 2008: warfarin and genetic testing. 2008 [cited 15/7/2012]. Available from: http://www.ama-assn.org/ama1/pub/upload/mm/464/warfarin-brochure.pdf

[87] A misread abbreviation that led to a digoxin overdose. Prescriber. 2007;18(12):57-59.

[88] Majed AJ, Menyfah A, Mostafa A. Medication prescribing errors in a pediatric inpatient tertiary care setting in Saudi Arabia. BMC Research Notes. 2011;4(294):1-6.

[89]   Awofisayo S, Uwanta E. Colorimetric Detection and Measurement of Paracetamol Exposure in Patients Prior Dispensing at a Pharmaceutical Care Centre. Int J Cur Biomed Phar Res. 2012;2(1):249-251.

[90]   Bird SM, Hutchinson SJ. Male drugs-related deaths in the fortnight after release from prison: Scotland, 1996-99. Addiction. 2003;98(2):185-190.

[91]   Binswanger IA, Stern MF, Deyo RA, Heagerty PJ, Cheadle A, Elmore JG, et al. Release from prison--a high risk of death for former inmates. New England Journal of Medicine. 2007;356(2):157-165.

[92]   Binswanger IA, Blatchford PJ, Lindsay RG, Stern MF. Risk factors for all-cause, overdose and early deaths after release from prison in Washington state. Drug and alcohol dependence. 2011;117(1):1-6.

[93]   Iguchi MY, Bell J, Ramchand RN, Fain T. How criminal system racial disparities may translate into health disparities. Journal of health care for the poor and underserved. 2005;16(4 Suppl B):48-56.

[94]   Iguchi MY, London JA, Forge NG, Hickman L, Fain T, Riehman K. Elements of wellbeing affected by criminalizing the drug user. Public Health Reports. 2002;117(Suppl 1):S146.

[95]   Fontana L, Beckerman A. Recently released with HIV/AIDS: primary care treatment needs and experiences. Journal of health care for the poor and underserved. 2007;18(3):699.

[96]   Wallace C, Dargan P, Jones A. Paracetamol overdose: an evidence based flowchart to guide management. Emergency medicine journal: EMJ. 2002;19(3):202.

[97]   Rigg KK, Ibañez GE. Motivations for non-medical prescription drug use: A mixed methods analysis. Journal of substance abuse treatment. 2010;39(3):236-247.

[98]   Yu MC, Tang LH, Chang KS, Narayan K, Chen KT. Risk factors associated with emergency room drug abuse admissions in urban Taiwan, 1998-1999. Journal of Addictions Nursing. 2005;16(4):195-198.

[99]   Ernst FR, Grizzle AJ. Drug-related morbidity and mortality: updating the cost-of-illness model. JAPHA-WASHINGTON-. 2001;41(2):192-199.

[100] Mittmann N, Knowles SR, Gomez M, Fish JS, Cartotto R, Shear NH. Evaluation of the extent of under-reporting of serious adverse drug reactions: the case of toxic epidermal necrolysis. Drug safety. 2004;27(7):477-487.

[101] Lexchin J. Drug safety and Health Canada. The International Journal of Risk and Safety in Medicine. 2010;22(1):41-53.

[102] Corcoran P, Reulbach U, Keeley H, Perry I, Hawton K, Arensman E. Use of analgesics in intentional drug overdose presentations to hospital before and after the withdrawal of distalgesic from the Irish market. BMC clinical pharmacology. 2010;10(1):6.

[103]　AbuMadini M, Abdel Rahim S. Deliberate self-harm in a Saudi university hospital: A case series over six years (1994-2000). Arab Journal of Psychiatry. 2001;12(2):22-35.

[104]　Malik G, Bilal A, Mekki T, Al-Kinany H. Drug overdose in the Asir region of Saudi Arabia. Annals of Saudi Medicine. 1996;16(1):33.

[105]　Al-Olah YH, Al Thiab KM. Admissions through the emergency department due to drug-related problems. Ann Saudi Med. 2008;28(6):426-9.

[106]　Johnson EM, Porucznik CA, Anderson JW, Rolfs RT. State-Level Strategies for Reducing Prescription Drug Overdose Deaths: Utah's Prescription Safety Program. Pain Medicine. 2011;12:S66-S72.

[107]　Alliance DP. Preventing Overdose, Saving Lives: Strategies for Combating a National Crisis. 2009 [cited 17/5/2012]. Available from: http://www.drugpolicy.org/docUploads/OverdoseReportMarch2009.pdf

[108]　Medical JWGotNPFS, Committee SA, Staff NPF, Scotland SES, Executive SS, Medical S, et al. Prevention and Treatment of Substance Misuse: Delivering the Right Medicine: A Strategy for Pharmaceutical Care in Scotland: A Report of a Joint Working Group of the National Pharmaceutical Forum/Scottish Medical and Scientific Advisory Committee. 2005 [cited 23/5/2012]. Report No.: 9780755946938. Available from: http://www.scotland.gov.uk/Resource/Doc/57346/0017002.pdf

[109]　Budnitz DS, Salis S. Preventing medication overdoses in young children: an opportunity for harm elimination. Pediatrics. 2011;127(6):e1597-e1599.

[110]　Tucker C. Drug Takebacks Aim to Prevent Abuse, Protect Environment. Nations Health. 2011;41(2):1-3.

[111]　Maklad AI, Emara AM, El-Maddah EI, El-Refai MAAM. PEDIATRIC POISONING IN EGYPT. Journal of Applied Pharmaceutical Science. 2012;2(02):01-06.

[112]　Shah NG, Lathrop SL, Reichard RR, Landen MG. Unintentional drug overdose death trends in New Mexico, USA, 1990-2005: combinations of heroin, cocaine, prescription opioids and alcohol. Addiction. 2008;103(1):126-136.

[113]　Smolen A. Role of the Pharmacist in Proper Medication Disposal. US Pharm. 2011;36(7):52-55.

[114]　DHW. Prescription Drug Overdoses in Nova Scotia Working Group recommendations submitted to the Minister of Health and Wellness, the honourable Maureen MacDonald. [Nova Scotia Department of Health and Wellness]: Wellness DoHa; 2011 [cited 27/5/2012]. Available from: http://www.gov.ns.ca/DHW/Working-Group-Recommendations-Prescription-Drug-Overdoses.pdf

[115]　HENMAN MC. The DUMP campaign. 2009 [cited 19/5/2012]. Available from: http://www.tara.tcd.ie/bitstream/2262/56870/1/IPJUN09DUMPCAMPAIGN.PDF

[116] Abou-Auda HS. An economic assessment of the extent of medication use and wastage among families in Saudi Arabia and Arabian Gulf countries. Clinical therapeutics. 2003;25(4):1276-1292.

[117] Grice G, Milligan P, Eby C, Gage B. Pharmacogenetic dose refinement prevents warfarin overdose in a patient who is highly warfarin-sensitive. Journal of Thrombosis
and Haemostasis. 2008;6(1).207-209.

[118] Osman A, Ibrahim I. Deliberate Non-Fatal Self Harm in Patients Attending a General
Hospital in Saudi Arabia. Arab J. Psychiatr.1997;8(1):31-41.

[119] Dart RC. Monitoring risk: post marketing surveillance and signal detection. Drug
and alcohol dependence. 2009;105:S26-S32.

[120] Puspitasari IM, Soegijoko S. e-Prescription: An e-Health System for Preventing Adverse Drug Events in Community Healthcare. [cited 15/7/2012] Available from:
http://www.ijljecp.or.id/files/IJCP_2012_1_1_5-11.pdf

Research, Ethics, Social and Teaching Issues in Public Health

Chapter 8

The Role of Ethics in Public Health Clinical Research

C. N. Fokunang, E. A. Tembe-Fokunang, P. Awah,
M. Djuidje Ngounoue, P. C. Chi, J. Ateudjieu,
R. Langsi, Lazare Kaptue and O. M. T. Abena

Additional information is available at the end of the chapter

1. Introduction

The public health ethics look at the moral basis of the health of human as a guiding support put in place to maximize welfare, and therefore health as a component of welfare [1,2]. This view frames the core moral challenge of public health as balancing individual liberties with the advancement of good health outcomes.

An alternative view of public health ethics characterizes the fundamental problematic of public health ethics differently: what lies at the moral foundation of public health is social justice [2]. While balancing individuals' liberties with promoting social goods is one area of concern, it is embedded within a broader commitment to secure a sufficient level of health for all and to narrow unjust inequalities [2, 3]. Another important area of concern is the balancing of this commitment with the injunction to maximize good aggregate or collective health outcomes. Public health ethics has therefore a strong moral connection to broader questions of social justice, poverty, and systematic disadvantage [3,4].

1.1. Historical ethical perspective

Although there have been some manifested concerns about the vulnerability of human subjects implicated in clinical research for over a century, it was the scandals and tragedies of the Nazi doctors during the second World War that gave birth to the discipline of bioethics [4, 5]. Other recent concerns in bioethics are attempting to extend ethical debate beyond the one-to-one physician-patient relationship, to enter the domain of public health where focused is geared towards the health of the entire populations. In the Africa setting, these extended concerns are being driven in part by the persisting iniquities and disparities in the health status of the low income resource countries and the rich countries, the differences in access to health services, the differences in the effort put into solving health problems, whereby the larger health burdens of the South receive scarce research attention, and the fewer problems of the North receive most of the attention in what has been termed the 10/90 gap [6, 35]. More attempts made to redress these inequalities have led to greater research investment and North-South research collaboration with the aim of solving the major health problems affecting the population in the poor countries of the South [7, 35].

1.2. The Ethical fundamental principles

Four fundamental principles of ethics have been universally recognized namely; autonomy, beneficence, non-maleficence and justice. These principles universally deals with the respect for all other humans as moral equals, making sure that all our actions are intended to achieve results with less harm, and treating others with fairness and equity [8, 48].

1.2.1. Beneficence and non maleficence

The principle of beneficence and non-maleficence are best considered together as they are like mirror images of each other. Literally beneficence means doing good and non-maleficence means avoiding evil or harm [9, 38, 42].

1.2.2. The harm principle

It is likely that no classic philosophical work is cited more often in the public health ethics literature than John Stuart Mill's essay "On Liberty" [10]. In that essay, Mill defends what has come to be called the harm principle, in which the only justification for interfering with the liberty of an individual, against her will, is to prevent harm to others. The harm principle is relied upon to justify various infectious disease control interventions including quarantine, isolation, and compulsory treatment. In liberal democracies, the harm principle is often viewed as the most compelling justification for public health policies that interfere with individual liberty [10, 19]. For example, a prominent view in the United States is that it was not until the public became persuaded of the harmful effects of "second hand smoke" that the first signif-icant intrusion into smoking practices—the banning of smoking in public places—became politically possible. Perhaps because of the principle's broad persuasiveness, it is not uncom-mon to see appeals made about harm to others in less than obvious contexts [11]. Defenders of compulsory motorcycle helmet laws, for example, argued that the serious head injuries sustained by unprotected cyclists diverted emergency room personnel and resources, thus harming other patients[12, 32]. The harm principle has been interpreted to include credible threat of significant economic harm to others as well as physical harm. Regarding smoking policy, various restrictions on the behavior of smokers have been justified by appeal to the financial burden on the health care system of caring for smoking-related illnesses [13].

As with all such principles, questions remain about its specification. How significant must the threat of harm be, with regard to both its likelihood and magnitude of effect? Are physical harms to the health of others to be weighted more than economic harms or other setbacks to interests? Whether interpreted narrowly or broadly, there are limits to the public health cases that can plausibly be placed in the harm principle box [14, 15]. Moreover, in the context of commitments to social justice and general welfare, and the other justifications described above, too exclusive a focus on the harm principle can undermine otherwise justifiable government mandates and regulation. It is undeniable that individuals have much broader and more multi-dimensional interests than narrowly self-directed physical ones, and in that sense, it is not unreasonable to have a fairly expansive understanding of "harm" in a public health context [16-18]. The summary of the fundamental ethical principles and their applications in public health and biomedical research illustrated by Chilengi [17], is shown in table 1.

PRINCIPLES	DESCRIPTION	APPLICATION
AUTONOMY	Human beings are born as autonomous agents. This autonomy gives them the rights to self determination that must be respected. Autonomy demands that the wishes of all persons must be respected and we do so by asking their opinion or willingness to get involved or not	Informed Consent
NON-MALEFICENCE	*Primun non nocere*, Latin translation for first, do no harm. Research must primarily and actively seek not to do harm regardless of the extent of potential good that may arise from the research.	Evaluate foreseeable risks and minimize harm
BENEFICENCE	While minimizing harm research must be of benefit to individuals and society at large. Beneficence is a group of norms for providing benefits and balancing benefits against risks and costs	Maximize benefits
JUSTICE	A group of norms for distributing benefits risks and costs fairly. The benefits of research must equitably be shared by those who bore the cost and risk of the research.	Fair subject selection and fair distribution of benefits.

Table 1. Summary of fundamental ethical principles and their applications in public health and biomedical research [17].

2. Some challenges related to public health research ethics

There is no standardized method of organizing either the ethics of clinical practice, or the public health and biomedical research. Although these distinctive concerns are often dealt with under the broader term of bioethics, sometimes bioethics is presented as the equivalent of medical ethics. Whichever approach is preferred, a key question remains: what distinguishes public health ethics from medical ethics? The answer lies in the distinctive nature of public health [23,51].

Public health has four characteristics that provide much of the subject matter for public health ethics as follows: (1) its promotion involves a particular focus on prevention; (2) it is a public or collective good; (3) it involves an intrinsic outcome-orientation and (4) its promotion often entails government action; [11, 24-26].

First, in public health the main point of concern is the population, not individuals. Public health is, by its very nature, a public, communal good, where the benefits to one person cannot readily be individuated from those to another, though its burdens and benefits often appear to fall unevenly on different sub-groups of the population [25]. This raises a particular set of challenges the public health ethics has to address. Whose health are we concerned about, and then what sacrifices is it acceptable to ask of individuals in order to achieve it? Is there a difference between public health and population health? And why is public health a good worth promoting? [26]. Any answer to these questions has to take into account the fact that public health measures are often based on the prospect of benefit to individuals, not immediately securable benefits [23, 27].

Second, promoting public health involves a high degree of commitment to the prevention of disease and injury. However, although much of the discussion surrounding public health focuses primarily on this preventive aspect, public health agencies and services also involve diagnosing and treating illnesses, with all the attendant clinical services that those activities require [28, 29].

Achieving good public health results frequently requires government action: many public health measures are coercive or are otherwise backed by the force of law. Public health is focused on regulation and public policy, and relies less often on individual actions and services. In this as in all other areas of official state action, we therefore have to address tensions among justice, security, and the scope of legal restrictions and regulations [19, 30].

2.1. The rationale of public health programs and policies

Public health draws its fundamental legitimacy from the essential and direct role that health plays in human flourishing, whether that role is understood ultimately in terms of maximizing health or promoting health in the context of advancing social justice [31, 38]. This general justification is sometimes too broad, however, to provide sufficient moral warrant for specific public health policies and institutions, especially when, as is so often the case, these policies and institutions are implemented by the state and affect the liberty or privacy of corporate or individual persons (Beauchamp, 2010). This section puts forward six justifications or reasons that can be put forward to defend a particular public health institution or policy [32].

Two observations are worth making at the outset. First, public health policies are rarely defended by only one reason. Usually a mixed set of justifications can be provided. For example, tax policies intended to decrease cigarette consumption can be defended both by appeal to paternalism and by appeal to reducing the harms of second hand smoke to children in the home and in automobiles[20, 33]. Second, the impact of public health policies is often not uniform across all the individuals affected by the policy, and thus different justifications are sometimes put forward specific to these different people. This complexity is unavoidable, since it results from the nature of public health: The focus of public health is population health, but populations are rarely internally uniform with regard to all features that are morally relevant to any particular policy [28, 34-35]. Some people may stand to benefit from the policy while others may not. Moreover, in line with concerns about democratic legitimacy and state over-reaching, some members of the population may support the aims of the policy while others may object [36].

The first four of the justifications for public health policies- overall benefit, collective efficiency/ action, and fairness- speak specifically to the context in which some members of the affected population are not directly benefited by the policy or object to it [37]. The next two justifications appeal to the significance of harm, both to others and to oneself. They apply more specifically to traditional concerns about balancing respect for liberty with advancing health and are more prevalent in the public health ethics literature than the previous four. In the fifth justification, the argument is from a relatively uncontroversial Millian harm principle, and in the sixth justification, from somewhat more tendentious paternalistic principles [12, 38].

2.2. Some benefits of public health

It is difficult to estimate direct benefits of the majority of public health interventions since some of these interventions target many health problems and many interventions can contribute to reduce the burden of one health problem. Furtherer, it is known that some of health determinants like those associated to environment change naturally. At individual level, it is even more complicated as the efficacy of public health intervention is the absence of a particular health event that is difficult to justify by the intervention [39, 40].

Generally, we all benefit from having public health interventions, and from having trusted regulatory agencies such as the Centers for Disease Control and Prevention (CDC) or the Food and Drug Administration (FDA) make decisions about such interventions and their reach [16, 41]. All things considered, having public health regulation is better than not having it. Having public health decisions made on the basis of overall statistics and demographic trends is ultimately better for each one of us, even if particular interventions may not directly benefit some of us. Thus, the task of public health ethics is not necessarily to justify each particular intervention directly [16, 41]. Rather, public health interventions in general, as long as they stay within certain pre-established parameters, can be justified in the same way a market economy, the institution of private property, or other similarly broad and useful conventions that involve some coercive action but also enable individuals to access greater benefits can be justified: when properly regulated and managed, its existence is by and large better than its absence for everyone [43].

2.3. The public health policy action strategies

A related justification views health as a public good the pursuit of which is not possible without ground rules for coordinated action and near-universal participation. The public health is viewed as having the structure of a coordination or collective efficiency problem. For example, if one person (or a sufficient critical mass of such persons) decides not to abide by a public health regulation because the regulation does not directly benefit he or she otherwise objects, the ramifications will likely be felt by others in her environment and beyond (Daniels, 2008). Everybody has to participate because, failing their involvement, neither they nor anyone else can reap the benefit of a healthy society (Crawford, 2008).

The collective efficiency class of arguments relies on claims about the sheer number and technical complexity of the decisions that need to be made to protect health in the environment and in the market place, as well as the indivisible character of responses to some health threats [15, 21, 46].

2.4. Public health community engagement

The communitarian argument relies on the idea that is good for the whole is necessarily good for its parts [47]. Communitarians view individuals' identities and the meaningfulness of their lives as indelibly tied to the well-being of their community. Clinical research in a developing nation to be deemed ethical requires community engagement, so that the research can contribute to the social value. Thus, on this view, public health interventions are good for individuals simply because they benefit the community as a whole. It thus encourages a cooperative way of thinking about public health interventions. Its main shortcoming, however, is that it assumes too tight a connection between individuals and the communities to which they belong, thereby incurring the potential for abuses of less privileged individuals within certain communities in the name of communal well-being [48]. It is unfortunately not always the case that the interests of individuals and the interests of their communities coincide in this convenient way. Rather, such interests often come apart, and can come into conflict in ways that require us to address yet again the questions: how much can we ask of individuals for the sake of others, of which individuals can we ask sacrifices for the sake of the community, and why? There is a conceptual distance between what is good for particular individuals, what is good for all individual members of a community, and what is good for the community [8, 49]. Thus, there can sometimes be direct trade-offs between what is good for the community and what is good for particular individuals within it. Notwithstanding these difficulties, this is certainly a strategy worth giving serious consideration as a possible avenue for the justification of public health interventions, particularly in some contexts where there is a strong sense of community solidarity [3, 50].

3. Aspect of justice and fairness in public health

Whether social justice is viewed as a side constraint on the beneficence-based foundation of public health, or as foundational in its own right, there is broad agreement that a commitment to improving the health of those who are systematically disadvantaged is as constitutive of public health as is the commitment to promote health generally (Powers and Faden 2006, Institute of Medicine's Committee for the Study of the Future of Public Health [50-52].

In this regard, there is an intimate connection between public health and the field of health and human rights. Many in public health accept that there is a fundamental right to health, as codified in the United Nations Universal Declaration of Human Rights or otherwise, although there is less agreement about the justification for such a right or what precisely the right entails [24]. A key question for public health ethics is on whom the duties generated by a right to health fall. Since so many of these duties require collective action. The governments are obvious candidates, but so, too, are other social institutions in the private sector as well as those global in structure that bear on the right to health [8, 35]. A failure on the part of these institutions to ensure the social conditions necessary to achieve a sufficient level of health is an injustice that on the view of many violates a basic human right. Note that as a basic human right, the claims of the right to health are not in any fundamental respect restricted to national borders but rather fall on the human community [9].

When inequalities in health exist between socially dominant and socially disadvantaged groups, they are all the more important because they occur in conjunction with other disparities in well-being and compound them [1, 15]. Reducing such inequalities are specific priorities in the public health goals of national and international institutions.

One of the most difficult challenges for public health ethics emerges when moral function conflicts with the injunction to improve, if not maximize, aggregate or collective health outcomes [39]. Although the health of the world's most desperately poor can in many cases be improved by extremely cost-efficient interventions like basic childhood immunizations and vitamin supplementation, reducing other unjust inequalities in health can consume significant resources.

Another challenge in social justice for public health ethics emerges when the health needs of systematically disadvantaged groups conflict with other dimensions of well-being as well as with considerations of collective efficiency. Targeting a public health program to poor and minority communities can sometimes both serve social justice concerns and be efficient if, for example, the health problem the intervention targets occurs disproportionately in these groups [7, 42]. At the same time, however, if the health problem is itself associated with stigma or shame, targeting the poor and minorities may reinforce existing invidious stereotypes, thereby undermining another critical concern of social justice, equality of social respect. In such cases, public health authorities must decide whether a commitment to social justice requires foregoing an efficient, targeted program in favor of a relatively inefficient, universal program that also may produce less improvement in health for the disadvantaged group (thus failing to narrow unjust inequalities) in order to avoid exacerbating existing disrespectful social attitudes [19].

Some formal methods, including most notably cost-utility analysis, rely on what are referred to as summary health measures in which mortality and diverse morbidities are combined in a single metric such as a quality-adjusted or disability-adjusted life year. These measures, and the formal methods that employ them, sometimes rely on assessments of what may be only vague individual preferences for trade-offs between different states of health or different kinds of benefits. Moreover, they make morally problematic assumptions including, for example, whether to differentially value years saved in different stages of life and about how to disvalue specific disabilities [34]. Depending on how these and other assumptions are determined and specified, summary health measures have been criticized as being ageist or not ageist enough, as discriminating unfairly against people with disabilities, as failing to capture the moral uniqueness of life-saving, as treating as commensurable qualitatively different losses and benefits, and as failing to take adequate account of the claims of those who are most disadvantaged [14, 50].

3.1. Burden distributions in ethical research

Another appeal that can be used to defend certain public health interventions that impose unequal burdens on different members of a population relies on considerations of fairness. The basic premise of this line or argument would be that burdens have to be roughly equivalent for everyone [23]. The same could be said for certain public health "burdens," understood as both the burdens of disease and disability and the burdens of public health interventions. Based on considerations such as a particular group's likelihood to contract a certain disease, and their overall health status, other parts of the population can legitimately be asked to "contribute," as it were, in order to make the distribution of disease burdens more equitable [9, 50]. For example, part of the rationale for requiring child immunization prior to enrollment in school is that this is a way to ensure that low-income children, who are generally less healthy than other children, have access to the needed vaccines [44]. Another example of public health interventions that appear to be guided by this justification is rubella vaccination of children for the sake of pregnant women and their fetuses [50]. This reasoning can help explain why individuals are sometimes asked to bear public health burdens that do not directly benefit them. However, the question of how far we can go in redistributing health-related burdens will likely continue to plague any proponent of this justificatory strategy. Moreover, questions about the plausibility of viewing health-related burdens as subject to distribution in this manner may also arise [6, 17].

3.2. Paternalism

Paternalism is classically understood as interfering with the liberty of action of a person, against his/her will, to protect or promote his/her welfare is as controversial as the harm principle is uncontroversial (Dworkin 2005). Few public health interventions are justified exclusively or even primarily on unmediated, classic paternalistic grounds, although many more public health programs may have paternalistic effects. By contrast, other classes of arguments that are sometimes described as paternalistic, including soft paternalism, weak paternalism, and libertarian paternalism, are evoked more frequently [19, 21].

Soft and weak paternalism are usually interpreted as interchangeable, though they have sometimes been taken to denote different concepts [14, 46]. A common interpretation defines this kind of paternalism as interferences with choices that are compromised with regard to voluntariness or autonomy. Though a person might voice or hold a preference different from the one that is sought for him, his preference is not entitled to robust respect if it is formed under conditions that significantly compromise its autonomy or voluntariness, such as cognitive disability or immaturity and, in very limited cases, ignorance or false beliefs [20]. Adaptive preferences are also considered compromised with regards to autonomy: sometimes, individuals modify their preferences in order to be able to adapt to difficult, unjust, or undesirable circumstances [32]. Such preferences also do not have the same standing as preferences formed under normal conditions and are therefore viewed as subject to interference [32].

Libertarian paternalism defends interventions by planners (such as public health authorities) in the environmental architecture in which individuals decide and act in order to make it easier for people to behave in ways that are in their best interests (including their health), provided two conditions are satisfied [5, 31]. First, individuals are steered by these interventions in ways that make them better off, as judged by themselves. Thus, in libertarian paternalism there is no attempt to contravene the will of individuals, in contrast to what some hold to be a necessary feature of paternalism. Second, the interventions must not overly burden individuals who want to exercise their freedom in ways that run counter to welfare. In this sense, libertarian paternalism claims to be liberty-preserving, hence libertarian.

A key conceptual question about paternalism is whether the interference with individual liberty must be against the person's will [3]. If this feature is a necessary condition of paternalism, then libertarian paternalism is inappropriately titled. From the standpoint of public health ethics, however, whether libertarian paternalism is appropriately titled is less important than the moral issues it raises and how it is justified [1, 52].

3.3. Mutual benefit

Finally, there is a more pragmatic reason to attend to public health in the developing world. Beyond claims of justice, morality, and common decency, we live in a world where mobility and interaction within and across countries is very high. Diseases such as SARS, H1N1, and drug-resistant TB, as well as less headline-grabbing ailments such as cholera and malaria, are not neatly contained within one national boundary. Citizens of all countries would benefit from improving public health in the developing world. Contributing to the availability and improvement of medical, sanitary, and other health-related resources for those who live in poverty and deprivation is ultimately good for us all, whether we are in the habit of traveling around the world or not [7]. There is also the need for understanding the emerging diseases and those poverty related diseases that is of major economic concerns [36, 52].

4. Research for low income ecomomies

Medical research is sometimes undertaken in the low income economies in order to further the understanding and treatment of diseases, not primarily for the benefit of those in the developing world, but rather for the benefit of citizens of the developed world. In such cases, participants and their communities might well claim that they are entitled to share in the benefits of the research [9, 16]. However, compensation to participants and their communities is often non-existent or not nearly in line with the potential benefits their participation will bring to those fortunate enough to have been born in a different geographical location [6, 36]. Note that this is a different issue from the question of whether researchers working on indigenous diseases in the developing world have a duty to provide medical care or other ancillary services to their research subjects [5, 21].This is less a question of justice as of research ethics more generally.

4.1. Uneven research focus

Much medical research is focused on diseases that affect less than 10% of the world's population, while millions die every year from diseases that potentially could be prevented or more easily treated if only enough research and other medical resources were devoted to them [1, 20]. Given the sheer numbers of people who needlessly die every day from such neglected but widespread diseases, and given that the developed world clearly has the resources to change that state of affairs, justice claims arguably also arise in this context [22, 35].

4.2. The legal compensatory claims

Many poor, underdeveloped countries that are massively underserved when it comes to public health resources continue to suffer from the direct and indirect effects of historical, unjust harms perpetrated by many of the world's wealthiest countries such as colonialism, war, occupation, and other forms of violent economic exploitation [36, 43]. In many cases, harms are more recent or are continuing, for example the diamond wars in Sierra Leone and other African countries as well as the more general on-going exploitation of local natural resources. Both the historical effects and the persistent effects of such violence and exploitation on public health in those countries ground additional justice-based claims against the wealthy nations to reduce the profound inequalities in health that exist between the world's poor and advantaged people [8, 26].

4.2.1. The role of the ethics committee

There are many synonymous for committees that review and approve biomedical research protocols to safeguard the dignity, rights, safety and well being of actual or potential research participants (WHO, 2000; Tedlock, 1983).Terminologies such as Independent Ethics Committee (IEC), Institutional Review Boards (IRB), Institutional Ethics Committee (IEC), National Ethics Committee (NEC) and Ethics Review Boards (ERB) are interchangeably used. The two WHO guidelines have addressed in details the description of what ERB are, or are intended to be, recommended compositions, what ethical review entails, how they should operate, reach decisions and communicate those decisions. Other publications have provided ethical framework for evaluating whether proposed research is ethical (CIOMS, 2008, Emmanuel et al., 2000; Amdur and Elizabeth, 2002. It is important therefore to look at the different roles of stakeholders in ethical research.

Responsibilities of the participants

The greatest role of ERB is to ensure that research that is conducted among the communities is ethical. Also important to this obligation is to ensure that in its basic setup, composition, operations and follow up activities are such that the mandate of protecting research participants is carried out effectively.

Research and legal liability

Legal liability claims against health professionals were traditionally confined to those who engaged in clinical practice. However, in recent years an increasing number of civil claims have emerged in the health research realm. In this regard, three trends have emerged: (1) the types of legal claims have diversified; (2) the number and types of defendants named in such lawsuits have increased beyond researchers; and (3) class action lawsuits are increasingly being lodged on behalf of groups of research subjects (Mello et al., 2003). While the overwhelming number of research-related lawsuits has arisen in affluent countries, the filing of multi-jurisdictional lawsuits against drug maker, Pfizer, in relation to its Trovan drug trial in Nigeria illustrates that developing countries are also becoming battlegrounds from lawsuits against those involved in research. This work outlines the liability risks of researchers, host institutions, research ethics committees, consulting bioethicists, and research sponsors through a review of sample cases involving these parties.

There exist a number of liabilities in the ethical conduct of research involving all the stakeholder that can be outline as follows:

Research liability

This involves civil claims against researchers which in the early days centered around the notion of informed consent If we consider the case of Wess versus Solomon (1989), the heirs of a subject who died while a volunteer in a non therapeutic study successfully sued the investigator and his university-affiliated hospital. The judge found the principal investigator and hospital, through its research ethics committee responsible for not disclosing a rare fatal complication caused by fluorescent dye and not adequately screening the subject who suffered from undisclosed hypertropic cardiomyopathy.

Research ethics committee liability

Research ethics committee (RECs) or Institutional Review Boards (IRBs), are responsible for assessing human research protocols for conformity to ethical principles (Zlotnik Shaul, 2002). RECs liability has been recognized as far back as in the 70s, when the US National Commission for the protection of Human Subjects of Biomedical and Behavioral research published a report captioned *Report and Recommendation: Institutional Review Board* (NCPHSBBR, 1978).The principles state that one who undertakes to protect others must act responsibly. IRB members could be liable if they did not exercise reasonable care in carrying out their review. This may occur if their approval led to a research activity and injuries that would not have occurred if a reasonable person, confronted with the same information would have placed conditions on the research that would have prevented the injury. Therefore an injured can possibly press charges for negligence by the IRB members in assessing the risks and benefits of proposed research, or in approving consent procedures not necessarily likely to assure legally effective consent.

4.2.2. Institutional liability

Institutional liability arises from the Common Law doctrine of vicarious liability, which holds superiors accountable for the wrongs of their subordinates (Amir, 2009). Amir JA. Research and Legal Liability. Acta Tropica, 2009;112S:S71-S75).An illustrated case is that in the US of Berman versus Fred Hutshinson cancer centre (2002) where the husband of a research participant (Hamilton) died in a chemotherapy trail brought filed a law suit against the Fred Hutchinson Cancer Centre alleging that his wife's consent to participate in the study was not informed because the institution failed to disclosed the following:

That the researchers had no idea whether the relevant drugs would have any protective effect against organ damage; Hamilton would not receive the planned dosage of the drug if she were unable to ingest the oral version of the drug; seven prior protocol participants had died, one of whom had suffered serious organ damage; and there were alternative treatments that were less risky and were reporting a significantly higher cure rate. In summary Berman argued that his diseased wife did not give informed consent to participate in the trial as she was not informed that an experimental drug to prevent lethal side effects of chemotherapy was not available was not available in the intravenous form. After trying to swallow the pills, the participant vomited the pills and died. The trial court handling the case ruled that the Fred Hutchinson Cancer Research Centre's failure to disclose the unavailability of the intravenous form of the drug invalidated Hamilton's consent to participate in the trial.

Bioethicist liability

The bioethicist liability case can be exemplified in the Robertson case where the plaintiffs' alleged that the consulting bioethicist in the matter was careless, negligent and reckless for the following: failing to exercise reasonable care under all of the circumstance, in accordance with the accepted bioethical practice; failing to follow and abide by by the guidelines set forth by various governmental agencies and acting negligently.

Sponsor laibility

The most high profile lawsuit filed against a study sponsor are those lodged against the US pharmaceutical firm, Pfizer, y the Nigerian plaintiffs and authorities. The lawsuits arose from a 1996 drug study conducted by Pfizer in the Northern State of Kano during a meningitis epidemic. In the US case of Abdullahi versus Pfizer Inc (2003), the plaintiffs, parents of the child participants in the trial, alleged the use of the drug TROVAN on children with meningitis was done without the parental informed consent and resulted in nearly a dozen dying, and others being left with brain damage, paralysis and slurred speech. In January 2009, the US Court of Appeals for the Second Circuit in New York overturned a lower court's finding that the cases brought by the plaintiffs could not be heard in the United States (Perlroth, 2009). In April 2009, Pfizer reportedly settled the case for $75 million (Howden, 2009).However, the settlement of the US case did not affect other pending cases against Pfizer in Nigeria such as the $7 billion case lodged by the Nigeria Federal Government in June 2007 and a $2 billion case lodged by the Kano State Government (Sturcke, 2007).The Pfizer case is significant for various reasons. To begin with, it illustrates that research participants in the developing countries are gaining increasing awareness of their rights and are prepared to act accordingly. The second point is that research conducted by US sponsors of research in developing countries is actionable against those sponsors in the US. Thirdly, research liability lawsuits may also be brought by government authorities, even though they were not the affected parties. Lastly, liability suits may be filed concurrently in different countries and a judgment or settlement in one country does not affect pending cases elsewhere. Some countries require sponsors and investigators to obtain insurance coverage for trial participants for trial-related injuries as a prerequisite to trial commencement. The Pfizer case demonstrates that it is important for sponsors and investigators to have insurance cover clinical drug testing trials.

There exist other potential areas of law suit given the increase in multi-country, multi-national collaborations. Potential lawsuits are emerging from legal issue with material transfer agreement, data sharing agreement and intellectual property rights. The use and storage of biological materials/samples, particularly those exported for storage and analysis to institutions in sponsor countries for use such as to determine biomarkers that confer protective immunity where capacity to conduct such analysis is not available in host countries in the developing countries. Solutions to solving such potential problems involve signing contractual agreements, memoranda of understanding such as data sharing agreement (DSA), Material Transfer Agreement (MTA), entered into between the disputing parties. Such agreements should be negotiated between all relevant stakeholders before any clinical research can commence, and that a dispute resolution mechanism are jurisdictional issues are prospectively determined in the case of any foreseeable dispute.

4.3. Contribution of International Research Integrity (IRI) in public health research promotion

National Science Foundation NSF implementation of Section 7009 of the America Creating Opportunities to Meaningfully Promote Excellence in Technology, Education, and Science (COMPETES) Act requires that the Authorized Organizational Representative complete a certification at the time of proposal submission that the institution has a plan to provide appropriate training and oversight in the responsible and ethical conduct of research to undergraduates, graduate students, and postdoctoral researchers who will be supported by NSF to conduct research. Additional information on NSF's responsible conduct of research (RCR) policy is available in the Award and Administration Guide, Chapter IV.B [46]. While training plans are not required to be included in proposals submitted to NSF, institutions are advised that they are subject to review upon request.

With the increasing globalization of science and engineering research and education, and the associated issues related to the responsible conduct of research within a global context, NSF recognizes that projects involving international partners may present special risks and challenges. Maintaining high standards of ethical and scientific integrity helps to maintain public trust in the research enterprise. An increasing number of authors have pointed to the importance of mentoring and education in relation to the responsible conduct of science in preventing transgressions of scientific integrity. Just like in clinical research and biomedicine, epidemiologists and other public health researchers have the responsibility to exhibit and foster the very highest standards of scientific integrity [46]

The following resources are provided to assist in developing training and oversight plans for the responsible and ethical conduct of research in an international context and to understand the codes of conduct in other countries. NSF does not provide content or endorse these sites' content, but provides them as possible resources.

4.4. National institute of health in public health research clinical excellence

The National Institute for Health and Clinical Excellence (NICE) is a special health authority of the English National Health Service (NHS), serving both English NHS and the Welsh NHS. It was set up as the National Institute for Clinical Excellence in 1999, and on 1 April 2005 joined with the Health Development Agency to become the new National Institute for Health and Clinical Excellence (still abbreviated as NICE). NICE carries out assessments of the most appropriate treatment regimes for different diseases. This must take into account both desired medical outcomes (i.e. the best possible result for the patient) and also economic arguments regarding differing treatments. NICE have set up several National Collaborating Centres bringing together expertise from the royal medical colleges, professional bodies and patient/carer organizations which draw up the guidelines [47]. The centres are the National Collaborating Centre for Cancer, the National Clinical Guidelines Centre for Acute and Chronic Conditions, the National Collaborating Centre for Women and Children's Health, and the National Collaborating Centre for Mental Health. The National Collaborating Centre then appoints a Guideline Development Group whose job it is to work on the development of the clinical guideline. This group consists of medical professionals, representatives of patient and carer groups and technical experts. They work together to assess the evidence for the guideline topic (e.g. clinical trials of competing products) before preparing a draft guideline. There are then two consultation periods in which stakeholder organizations are able to comment on the draft guideline. After the second consultation period, an independent Guideline Review Panel reviews the guideline and stakeholder comments and ensures that these comments have been taken into account. The Guideline Development Group then finalizes the recommendations and the National Collaboration Centre produces the final guideline. This is submitted to NICE who then formally approve the guideline and issues this guidance to the NHS [47].

4.5. Institute of tropical medicine and hygiene in public health research ethics

The London School of Hygiene and Tropical Medicine is an institution promoting research in public health through the introduction of research training courses which aim at equipping students with skills needed to appreciate and analyze public health problems in developing countries, and to design and evaluate actions to improve public health. The course considers issues of global health, development and the provision of health services from a multidisciplinary perspective. All the public health students are expected to have a substantial experience of planning or implementation of public health programmes, of teaching or research, in developing countries. Graduates from this course work in global health, health service management, in health programmes in developing countries, in international and national NGOs, and in research. In addition to MSc Public Health in Developing Countries. By the end of the course students should be able to: demonstrate knowledge and understanding of theory and practice in the core public health disciplines (epidemiology, statistics, social sciences, health policy and health economics; demonstrate specialized knowledge and skills in other areas relevant to public health from a wide range of options (e.g., primary health care, medical anthropology, epidemiology and control of malaria, and population studies); apply these skills to identify and assess public health problems in developing countries and evaluate actions designed to improve public health; formulate public health strategies and approaches to public health problems appropriate to a given culture and environment; and apply appropriate research skills for evaluation and use of research findings.

4.6. World Health Organization (WHO) in public health research ethics

Health ethics has been an integral part of the activities of many units and departments at WHO for many years and is addressed not only within the Department of Ethics and Social Determinants (ESD) and throughout the organization. ESD works collaboratively with staff from all departments and the regional offices to identify, design, and carry out projects addressing the ethics of health care, public health, and biomedical science. This encompasses projects that originate in the department and those on which it provides advice and assistance to activities located in other clusters and in regional offices. In October 2002, the World Health Organization launched its Ethics and Health Initiative to provide a focal point for the examination of the ethical issues raised by activities throughout the organization, including the regional and country offices, and to develop activities regarding a wide range of global bioethics topics, from organ and tissue transplantation to developments in genomics, and from research with human beings to fair access to health services.

Work in ethics and health is now carried out by the Department of Ethics and Social Determinants in the Innovation, Information, Research and Evidence cluster at headquarters. This department is involved in a wide range of ethics activities, both on its own initiative and in response to the needs of other parts of WHO. The specific projects, many of which link different departments and involve experts from outside the organization, evolve in response to changes in the field.

4.7. NEPAD in promoting public health research in Africa

The New Partnership for Africa's Development (NEPAD) is a socio-economic development programme of the African Union (AU) whose express objective is to stimulate Africa's development by bridging existing gaps in Infrastructure (Energy, Water and Sanitation, Transport and ICT); Agriculture and Food Security; Human Resource Development, especially Health/Education, Youth and Training, Social Affairs; Science, Technology and Innovation; Trade, Industry/Market Access and Private Sector Development; Environment/Climate Change and Tourism; Governance/Public Administration, Peace and Security; Capacity

Development, and Gender Development. The implementation of these programmes is based on the AU/NEPAD principles of African leadership and the ownership of the continent's development agenda and process, as well as a commitment to good political, economic and corporate governance. African leaders have explicitly recognized that socio-economic transformation of the continent cannot be achieved without increased investments in science, technology, and innovation. To that end, the leaders have initiated a number of concrete actions geared towards promoting the continent's scientific and technological development. The actions include the creation of the African Ministerial Council on Science and Technology (AMCOST) and its subsidiary bodies -- the NEPAD Office of Science and Technology, and the AU Commission for Human Development, Science and Technology. These institutions have collectively developed a comprehensive strategy and action plan -- Africa's Science and Technology Consolidated Plan of Action -- adopted at the second African Ministerial Conference on Science and Technology in Dakar, Senegal, in September 2005. The main goals of Africa's Science and Technology Consolidated Plan of Action (CPA) are to strengthen Africa's capacities to develop, harness and apply science, technology, and innovation to achieve millennium development goals (MDGs), as well as mobilizing the continent's expertise and institutions to contribute to the global pool of science and technological innovations. Key to these goals is the promotion of transnational Research and Development (R&D) programmes

4.7.1. Technological trends and Innovation systems in public health delivery in Africa

There is need for a common and shared understanding of what can be done in order to tap science, technology and innovation tools to address Africa's current huge burden of disease. First, African countries and institutions have to show the qualities of leadership necessary for generating and utilizing technology and innovations in health in order to address diseases that are peculiar to this continent. It is evident that many of these diseases are not being addressed by the global scientific community for reasons which need no enumerating here. This can only be Africa's responsibility. Secondly, Africa needs to position itself strategically with regard to shaping and driving a new research and innovation agenda necessary for disease treatment and diagnosis. Today, the continent does not have access to relevant health innovation tools that are widely available around the world. Worse still, Africa is not a key player in the public health research and innovation enterprises. Inequality in science, technology and health innovation capacity in Africa is evident in the extent of the disease burden in many countries. Consequently, the current global funding arrangements for public health, including for global pandemics like HIV/AIDS and neglected diseases, must go beyond merely treating the symptoms through the provision of treatment but should also focus on building requisite health research and development [53] infrastructure on the continent. Thirdly, new continental initiatives must focus on shifting the apparent successes in health innovations to product development and product delivery. It is evident that while promising innovations have been developed in Africa and/or for Africa's specific diseases, not many investments are taking place in product development and product delivery. It is therefore important to address this shortcoming in the context of the Africa health strategies for NEPAD and the AU.

Finally, Africa must take advantage of the wide pool of scientific knowledge and technology tools available globally. This means that, on the one hand, individual countries and continental institutions must invest in technology prospecting in order to exploit existing and relevant health technologies and products. On the other hand, Africa must invest in setting up or transforming research institutions that are not only knowledge-based but also oriented towards product development. There is an immediate need to strengthen African institutions, especially universities and schools of medicine, by increasing funding and revising the curricula. Thus the issue of how science, technology and innovation can alleviate Africa's burden of disease.

4.7.2. Ethics in European Union research

Public attitudes towards science and technology are overwhelmingly positive. The confidence generated by messages such as 'scientifically tested' or 'scientifically proven' is testament to society's support of scientific endeavour. It also highlights the social responsibility that accompanies research. As science advances and evolves, and the relationship between science and society gets better explanations, new challenges are created for the scientific community. Nowadays, there are more scientists than ever before. On a regular basis, exciting research opportunities spring into existence. Grant driven projects and non funded projects are larger, more complex, and more expensive. The role that science plays in our lives continues to gain more significance and recognition in importance, and society, in turn, has a stake in science. Consequently, the relationship between science and society continues to change and intensify in the pursuit of progress [54].

Excellence in science means addressing ethical concerns - to improve the quality of the science itself, but also to highlight the importance of its outcomes to the wider community. The EU's commitment to ethics in research is reflected in explicit requirements, and more specifically in the evaluation of project proposals. Ethics may be context-dependent, but any research team's approach to ethical matters is taken as an indication of the honesty and the clarity of its proposal. While there are rarely clear-cut answers when it comes to ethics, some areas are excluded from EU funding by definition. These are human cloning for reproductive purposes, altering the genetic heritage of human beings, and creating human embryos only to conduct research or obtain stem cells [54].

5. Conclusion

The population of low income economies are highly vulnerable in medical research. The fundamental ethical principles need to have its place in the global public health research sectors. With the increase research in finding new investigational products, developing new disease diagnostics techniques puts the human population into a vulnerable position vis a vis participation into clinical research trials. It is therefore imperative for the public health sector to place more emphasis in the implementation of research that is ethical. By so doing the fundamental principle of morality, autonomy and respect for others, beneficence, non-maleficence and justice shall be practicable and sustainable as within the universal declaration of Helsinki. The public health sector in both developing and developed nations has a duty to set up a working platform that may reduce the 10/90 gap that has remained static in the sub-Saharan Africa. Medical research should be undertaken in the low income economies in order to further the understanding and treatment of poverty related diseases, primarily for the benefit of those in the developing world, not rather for the benefit of citizens of the developed world. Ethics is therefore a non negotiable principle and policy in Public Health Clinical Research practice. It is also evident with increasing clinical research that there shall be more potential legal issues. This calls for more scrutiny in the institutions that be in regulating the ethical framework in the conduct of human research. Those implicate in research should ensure that they are fully versed with their legal rights and obligations associated with the research they are engaged in, and also in tuned with the import and export regulations relevant to biological material transfer, data sharing as the shortcoming of these regulation are potential points for legal liability.

Acknowledgements

We wish to acknowledge the special financial grant from the Ministry of Higher Education of Cameroon, the EDCTP Grant award to the National Ethics Committee of Cameroon, and the financial support from the University of Bamenda. All contributed to the research and processing of this invited write-up by the Publisher.

Author details

C. N. Fokunang[1,2], E. A. Tembe-Fokunang[1], P. Awah[3], M. Djuidje Ngounoue[2,4], P. C. Chi[2], J. Ateudjieu[1,5], R. Langsi[6], Lazare Kaptue[2] and O. M. T. Abena[1]

1 Faculty of Medicine and Biomedical Sciences, University of Yaounde 1, Centre Region, Cameroon

2 Cameroon National Ethics Committee (CNEC), Yaoundé, Cameroon

3 Faculty of Arts and Modern Letters, University of Yaoundé 1. Ipas, Chapel Hill, North Carolina, United States

4 Faculty of Sciences, University of Yaoundé 1, Centre Region, Cameroon

5 Faculty of Sciences, University of Dschang; Division of Health Operations Research, Ministry of Public Health Cameroon, Cameroon

6 Health Division, University of Bamenda, Cameroon

References

[1] Barrett DH, Bernier RH, Sowell AL. Strengthening public health ethics at the centers for disease control and prevention.; Centers for Disease Control and Prevention Public Health Ethics Committee Steering Group. Journal Public Health Management Practice. 2008:.14(4):348-53.

[2] Beauchamp, T.L., Childress, J.F. Principles of Biomedical Ethics, 5th edition Oxford University Press.2001 p.133.

[3] Beauchamp, T. The concept of paternalism in biomedical ethics. In Beauchamp, T. Standing on principles. New York: Oxford University Press. 2010: (pp. 101–119).

[4] Beecher, H.K., Ethics and Clinical Research. New England Journal of Medicine.1966: 274, 1354.

[5] Belsky, L., and Richardson, H. S. Medical researchers' ancillary clinical care responsibilities. *British Medical Journal*, 2004: 328(7454), 1494–1496.

[6] Benatar, S. R. Reflections and recommendations on research ethics in developing countries. Social Science and Medicine, 2002: 54(7), 1131–1141.

[7] Bernheim, R.G., Melnick, A. Principled leadership in public health: integrating ethics into practice and management. Journal Public Health Management Practice. 2008: 14(4):358-66.

[8] Bernheim, R.G. Public health ethics: the voices of practitioners.J Law Med Ethics. 2003:31(4 Suppl):104-9.

[9] Beskow, L.M., Namey, E.E., Cadigan, R.J., Brazg, T., Crouch, J., Henderson, G.E., Michie M., Nelson, D.K., Tabor, H.K., Wilfond, B.S. Research participants' perspectives on genotype-driven research recruitment. Journal of Empirical Research for Human Research Ethics.2011: 6(4):3-20.

[10] Bhan, A., Jerome, A., Singh, R., Upshur, E.G., Grand Challenges in global health: engaging civil society organizations in biomedical research in developing countries. PLoS Med, 2007:. 4 (9), e272, www.plosmedicine.org.

[11] Bhutta, Z.A., Ethics in international health research:a perspective from the developing world. Bulletin WHO, 2002: 80:114-120.

[12] Buchanan, D. R. Autonomy, paternalism, and justice: Ethical priorities in public health. American Journal of Public Health, 2008: 98(1), 15.

[13] Büken NO, Büken E.The legal grounds regarding clinical trial in Turkey.Medical Law. 2011: 30 (4) : 591-611.

[14] Cadigan, R.J., Michie, M., Henderson, G., Davis, A.M., Beskow, L.M.. The meaning of genetic research results: reflections from individuals with and without a known genetic disorder.J Empirical Research and Human Research Ethics. 2011: 6(4):30-40.

[15] Cambon-Thomsen, A., Rial-Sebbag, E., Knoppers, B.M..Trends in ethical and legal frameworks for the use of human biobanks.European Respiratory Journal; 2007 : 30(2):373 82.

[16] Childress, J. F., Faden, R. R., Gaare, R. D., Gostin, L. O., Kahn, J., Bonnie B. Public health ethics: Mapping the terrain. *The Journal of Law, Medicine & Ethics*, (2002:. 30(2), 170–178.

[17] Chilengi, R. An ethics perspective on responsibilities of investigators, sponsors and research participants. Acta Tropica, 2009: 112S:S53-S62.

[18] Cohen, J. T., Neumann, P. J., & Weinstein, M. C. Does preventive care save money? Health economics and the presidential candidates. *The New England Journal of Medicine*, 2008: 358(7), 661–663.

[19] Council for International Organizations of Medical Sciences (CIOMS). International Guidelines for Biomedical Research Involving Human Subjects. Geneva. CIOMS. 2002. pp.112.

[20] Emanuel, E., Wendler, D., Killen, J., and Grady, C. What makes clinical research in developing countries ethical? the benchmarks of ethical research. The Journal of Infectious Diseases, 2004. 189(5), 930–937.

[21] Fineberg, H.VShattuck Lecture. A successful and sustainable health system--how to get there from here.North England Journal of Medicine 2012: 366(11):1020-1027.

[22] Gafni, A. Willingness-to-pay as a measure of benefits: Relevant questions in the context of public decisionmaking about health care programs. *Medical Care*. 1991: 29(12), 1246–1252.

[23] Gitau-Mburu, D. Should public health be exempt from ethical regulations? Intricacies of research versus activity.East Africa Journal of Public Health., 2008: (3):160-162.

[24] Gollust, S.E., Baum, N.M., Jacobson, P.D. Politics and public health ethics in practice: right and left meet right and wrong.Journal of Public Health Management Practice. 2008: 14(4):340-347.

[25] Goodman, E. P. (2006). Stealth marketing and editorial integrity. *Texas Law Review*, 85, 83–152.

[26] Harper, I.. Translating ethics: researching public health and medical practices in Nepal., Canadian Journal of Public Health. 2006: 97 (5) : 402-424

[27] Horstkötter D, Berghmans R, de Ruiter C, Krumeich A, de Wert G. "We are also normal humans, you know?" Views and attitudes of juvenile delinquents on antisocial

behavior, neurobiology and prevention. International Journal of Law and Psychiatry. 2012:.35(4):289-97.

[28] Huddle TS. 2012. Honesty is an internal norm of medical practice and the best policy.American Journal of Bioethics. 12(3):15-27..

[29] Hyder, A. A., and Merritt, M. W. Ancillary care for public health research in developing countries. *Journal of the American Medical Association*, 2009: 302(4), 429.

[30] International Conference on Harmonization (ICH) Guidelines for Good Clinical Practice, 1996. Available freely on the websites and other sources.

[31] Jefferson, A.L., Carmona, H., Gifford, K.A., Lambe, S., Byerly, L.K., Cantwell, N.G., Tripodis, Y., Karlawish, J. Clinical Research Risk Assessment Among Individuals With Mild Cognitive Impairment. American Journal of Geriatrics and Psychiatry. 2012: 30. 12-30

[32] Jones, M. M., & Bayer, R. Paternalism & its discontents: Motorcycle helmet laws, libertarian values, and public health. *American Journal of Public Health*, 2007:. 97(2), 208–217.

[33] Joyce, G.F., Carrera, M.P., Goldman, D.P., Sood, N., Physician prescribing behavior and its impact on patient-level outcomes.American Journal of Management Care. 2011: 17(12):62-71.

[34] Kass, N. E. An ethics framework for public health. *American Journal of Public Health*, 2001:. 91(11), 1776–1782.

[35] Kilama, W.L). The 10/90 gap in sub-Saaran Africa: Resolving inequities in health Research. Acta Tropica., 2009:112S:S8-S15.

[36] Kost, R.G., Lee, L.M., Yessis, J., Coller, B.S., Henderson, D.K. Assessing research participants' perceptions of their clinical research experiences.; Research Participant Perception Survey Focus Group Subcommittee. Clinical Translational Science. 2011:. 4(6):403-413.

[37] Krech R..Working on the social determinants of health is central to public health. Journal Public Health Policy. 2012: 33(2):279-84.

[38] Lavery, J.V., Harrington, L.C., Scott, T.WEthical,social, and cultural considerations for the site selection for research with genetically modified mosquitoes. American Journal of Tropical Medicine and Hygiene. 2008: 79 (3), 312-318.

[39] London AJ, Kimmelman J, Carlisle B. Research ethics. Rethinking research ethics: the case of postmarketing trials.Science 4; 2012: 336(6081):544-555.

[40] Nicholas, J. Next steps in clinical trial redesign. Journal of National Cancer Institute. 2012:. 18;104(2):90-2.

[41] New Partnership for Africa's Development (NEPAD). Science, Technology and Inno-
      vation for Public Health in Africa. In : Fetson Kalua, Abolade Awotedu, Leonard
      Kamwanja and John Saka editions: 2009, pp 213.www.nepadst.org.

[42] Nyika, A., Kilama, W., Chilengi, R., Tangwa, G., Tindana, P., Ndebele, P., Ikingura,
      J., Composition, training needs and independence of ethics review committees across
      Africa: are the gate-keepers rising to the emerging challenges? Journal of Medical
      Ethics, 2009:. 35, 189-193.

[43] Omonzejele, P.FIs the codification of vulnerability in international documents a suffi-
      cient mechanism of protection in the clinical research ethics context? Medical Law.
      2011: 30(4):497-515.

[44] Reichert, T. A., Sugaya, N., Fedson, D. S., Glezen, W. P., Simonsen, L., & Tashiro, M.
      (2001). The japanese experience with vaccinating schoolchildren against influenza.
      The New England Journal of Medicine, 344 (12), 889–896.

[45] Sade, R.M. Why physicians should not lie for their patients. American Journal of Bio-
      ethics.(2012:.12(3):17-9.

[46] Steven S C, Amyre B, Angus D. Ethics and Scientific Integrity in Public Health, Epi-
      demiological and Clinical Research. Public Health Reviews, 2009, Vol. 34, No 1.

[47] Sorenson, C; Drummond, M; Kanavos, P; McGuire, A. *National Institute for Health and
      Clinical Excellence (NICE): How does it work and what are the implications for the U.S.?*.
      National Pharmaceutical Council. Retrieved 2009-09-18.

[48] Tangwa, G.B., Ethical principles in health research and review process. Acta Tropica,
      2009:. 112S:S2-S7.

[49] Thomas, J.C., MacDonald, P.D., Wenink, E., Ethical decision making in a crisis: a case
      study of ethics in public health emergencies. : Journal Public Health Management
      Practice; 2009. 15 (2):E16-21.

[50] Thomas, J. C., Sage, M., Dillenberg, J., and Guillory, V. J. A code of ethics for public
      health. *American Journal of Public Health*, 2002: 92(7), 1057–1059.

[51] Wikler, D., and Brock, D. W. Population-level bioethics: Mapping a new agenda. In
      Dawson, A., and Verweij, M, *Ethics, prevention, and public health*, New York: Oxford
      University Press. 2007: p 78.

[52] World Medical Association Declaration of Helsinki, Available at http://
      www.wma.net/e/policy/17-c-e.html. Ethical principles for Medical Research Involv-
      ing Human Subjects. 52nd WMA General Assembly, Edinburgh, Scotland.

[53] Andanda P, Awah P, Ndebele P, Onigbogi O, Udatinya D and Mwondela M.The eth-
      ical and legal regulation of HIV-vaccine research in Africa: lessons from Cameroon,
      Malawi, Nigeria, Rwanda and Zambia, African Journal of AIDS Research 2011, 10(4):
      451–463 ISSN 1608–5906 EISSN 1727–9445

[54] Http://Cordis.europa.eu/fp7/ethics-en.htm/

[55] Abdullahi v Pfizer Inc., 77 Fed.Appx. 48 (2d Cir. 2003.

[56] Anderlik, MR. Legal Liability for Bioethics Involved in Research. Health Law and
      Policy   Institute.   http://www.law.uh.edu/healthlaw/perspectives/Research/
      001002Best.html/>(assessed 03/09/2012.

[57] Berman v Fred Hutchinson Cancer Centre Case No C01-0727L (BJR), August 8, 2002.
      United States District Court Western District of Washington at Seattle. Accessible:
      http://biotech.law.Isu.edu/research/wa/Berman_v_Hutchinson.pdf/   (accessed
      03/09/2012.

[58] Mello MM., Joffe S. Compact versus contract-industry sponsor's obligations to their
      research subjects. Ann. Intern. Med; 2003:43:231−561.

[59] Perlroth N. Pfizer's Nigerian Plaintiffs Get Day In Court, January, 2009 http://
      www.forbes.com/2009/01/pfizer-nigeria-trovan-business-healthcare-0130_tro-
      van.html/ accessed 03/09/2012.

[60] Robertson v McGee. No 01CV00G0H (M) (ND Okla filed January 29, 2001). Sherman,
      Silverstein, Kohl, Rose and Podolsky Law Offices.http://www.sskrplaw.com/gene/
      robertson/complaint.html/ (accessed 03/09/2012).

[61] Weiss v Solomon. A.Q.no 312.1989.http://www.commonlaw.uottawa.ca/index.php?
      option=com_docmans&task=doc_download&gid=1644/ (accessed 03/09/2012)

[62] Zlotnik Shaul R.Reviewing the reviewers: the vague accountability of research ethics
      committees. Crit. Care; 2002; 6 (2):12-22.

[63] National Commission for the Protection of Human Subjects of Biomedical and Be-
      havioural Research subjects(NCPHSBBRS). Protection of Human Subjects: Institu-
      tional Review Boards. Fed Regist; 1978; 43:231-561.

Chapter 9

Contribution of Biomedical Research Ethics in Public Health Advances

CN Fokunang, EA Tembe-Fokunang,
M. Djuidje Ngounoue, P.C. Chi, J Ateudjieu,
Awah Pascal, G. Magne, N.M. Ndje, O.M.T. Abena,
D. Sprumont and Kaptue Lazare

Additional information is available at the end of the chapter

1. Introduction

The term research refers to a class of activities designed to develop or contribute to generalizable knowledge. Generalizable knowledge consists of theories, principles or relationships, or the accumulation of information on which they are based, that can be corroborated by accepted scientific methods of observation and inference [1]. In the present context "research" includes both medical and behavioral studies pertaining to human health. Generally "research" is usually modified by the adjective "biomedical" to indicate that the reference is to health-related research [1, 2].

Progress in medical care and disease prevention depends upon an understanding of physiological and pathological processes or epidemiological findings, and requires at some time research involving human subjects. The collection, analysis and interpretation of information obtained from research involving human beings contribute significantly to the improvement of human health [3].

Research involving human subjects includes patient care (clinical research) and that undertaken on patients or other subjects, or with data pertaining to them, solely to contribute to generalizable knowledge (non-clinical biomedical research) [4]. Research is defined as "clinical" if one or more of its components is designed to be diagnostic, prophylactic or therapeutic for the individual subject of the research. Invariably, in clinical research, there are also components designed not to be diagnostic, prophylactic or therapeutic for the subject;

examples include the administration of placebos and the performance of laboratory tests in addition to those required to serve the purposes of medical care [5].

Advances in biomedical science and technology, and their application in the practice of medicine, are provoking some anxiety among the public and confronting society with new ethical problems. Society is expressing concern about what it fears would be abuses in scientific investigation and biomedical technology [1, 5]. This is understandable in view of the meth-odology of biomedical experimental research. Investigation begins with the construction of hypotheses and these are then tested in laboratories and with experimental animals. For the findings to be clinically useful, experiments must be performed on human subjects, and, even though carefully designed, such research entails some risk to the subjects [6]. This risk is justified not by any personal benefit to the researcher or the research institution, but rather by its benefit to the human subjects involved, and its potential contribution to human knowledge, to the relief of suffering or to the prolongation of life [7].

Society devises measures to protect against possible abuses. The first international code of ethics for research involving human subjects — the Nuremberg Code — was a response to the atrocities committed by Nazi research physicians, revealed at the Nuremberg War Crimes Trials [8]. Thus it was to prevent any repetition by physicians of such attacks on the rights and welfare of human beings that human-research ethics came into being. The Nuremberg Code, issued in 1947, laid down the standards for carrying out human experimentation, emphasizing the subject's voluntary consent. In 1964 the World Medical Association took an important step further to reassure society: it adopted the Declaration of Helsinki, most recently revised in 1989, which lays down ethical guidelines for research involving human subjects. In 1966 the United Nations General Assembly adopted the International Covenant on Civil and Political Rights, which entered into force in 1976, and which states (Article 7): "No one shall be subjected to torture or to cruel, inhuman or degrading treatment or punishment. In particular, no one shall be subjected without his free consent to medical or scientific experimentation ". It is through this statement that society expresses the fundamental, human value that is held to govern all research involving human subjects — the protection of the rights and welfare of all human subjects of scientific experimentation.

In the late 1970s, in view of the special circumstances of developing countries in regard to the applicability of the Nuremberg Code and the Declaration of Helsinki, the Council for Inter-national Organizations of Medical Sciences (CIOMS) and the World Health Organization (WHO) undertook a further examination of these matters, and in 1982 issued *Proposed International Guidelines for Biomedical Research Involving Human Subjects*. The purpose of the *Proposed Guidelines* was to indicate how the ethical principles that should guide the conduct of biomedical research involving human subjects, as set forth in the Declaration of Helsinki, could be effectively applied, particularly in developing countries, given their socioeconomic circumstances, laws and regulations, and executive and administrative arrangements [9].

Certain areas of research do not receive special mention in the guidelines; they include human genetic research, embryo and fetal research, and fetal tissue research. These represent research areas in rapid evolution and in various respects controversial.

The mere formulation of ethical guidelines for biomedical research involving human subjects will hardly resolve all the moral doubts that can arise in association with such research, but the guidelines can at least draw the attention of investigators, sponsors and ethical review committees to the need to consider carefully the ethical implications of research protocols and the conduct of research, and thus conduce to high scientific and ethical standards of research.

Given the different perceptions and priority views in the debate over the value and role of biomedical research, it is believed that the biomedical community must take stock and recommit its efforts to diseases that have a major effect on the population. This requires a re-evaluation of funding priorities, open interactions among researchers, and creating a more effective relations among stakeholders, government, foundations and institutions of higher learning. There is also the need for a shift in paradigm in biomedical research towards poverty related diseases and emerging diseases to reduce the 90/10 gap [6, 30].

2. International declarations and guidelines for ethical framework

The first international document on the ethics of research, the Nuremberg Code, was promulgated in 1947 as a consequence of the trial of physicians who had conducted atrocious experiments on unconsenting prisoners and detainees during the Second World War. The Code, designed to protect the integrity of the research subject, sets out conditions for the ethical conduct of research involving human subjects, emphasizing the human subject's "voluntary consent" to research.

To give the Universal Declaration of Human Rights, adopted by the United Nations General Assembly in 1948, legal as well as moral force, the General Assembly of the United Nations adopted in 1966 the International Covenant on Civil and Political Rights, of which Article 7 states " *No one shall be subjected to torture or to cruel, inhuman or degrading treatment or punishment. In particular, no one shall be subjected without his free consent to medical or scientific experimentation.* "

The Declaration of Helsinki, promulgated in 1964 by the World Medical Association, is the fundamental document in the field of ethics in biomedical research and has had considerable influence on the formulation of international, regional and national legislation and codes of conduct. The Declaration, revised in Tokyo in 1975, in Venice in 1983, and again in Hong Kong in 1989, is a comprehensive international statement of the ethics of research involving human subjects. It sets out ethical guidelines for physicians engaged in both clinical and non- clinical biomedical research, and provides among its rules for informed consent of subjects and ethical review of the research protocol [10].

The publication in 1982 of *Proposed International Guidelines for Biomedical Research Involving Human Subjects* was a logical development of the Declaration of Helsinki. As stated in the Introduction of that publication, the Guidelines were intended to indicate how the ethical principles embodied in the Declaration could be effectively applied in developing countries. The text explained the application of established ethical principles to biomedical research involving human subjects and drew attention to new ethical issues arising in the period that preceded its publication. The present publication, *International Ethical Guidelines for Biomedical Research Involving Human Subjects*, supersedes the 1982 *Proposed International Guidelines*.

CIOMS and WHO have continued to work together to provide ethical guidance for research involving human subjects. One important outcome of this cooperation has been *International Guidelines for Ethical Review of Epidemiological Studies*, published by CIOMS in 1991, intended to assist investigators and institutions as well as regional and national authorities in setting and maintaining standards for the ethical review of epidemiological studies [10].

2.1. Fundamental ethical principles

All research involving human subjects should be conducted in accordance with three basic ethical principles, namely respect for persons, beneficence and justice. It is generally agreed that these principles, which in the abstract have equal moral force, guide the conscientious preparation of proposals for scientific studies [11]. In varying circumstances they may be expressed differently and given different moral weight, and their application may lead to different decisions or courses of action. The present guidelines are directed at the application of these principles to research involving human subjects.

2.1.1. Respect for persons

Respect for persons incorporates at least two fundamental ethical considerations, namely:

a) respect for autonomy, which requires that those who are capable of deliberation about their personal choices should be treated with respect for their capacity for self-determination; and
b) protection of persons with impaired or diminished autonomy, which requires that those who are dependent or vulnerable be afforded security against harm or abuse [12].

2.1.2. Beneficence

Beneficence refers to the ethical obligation to maximize benefits and to minimize harms and wrongs. This principle gives rise to norms requiring that the risks of research be reasonable in the light of the expected benefits, that the research design be sound, and that the investigators be competent both to conduct the research and to safeguard the welfare of the research subjects. Beneficence further proscribes the deliberate infliction of harm on persons; this aspect of beneficence is sometimes expressed as a separate principle, non-maleficence (do no harm).

2.1.3. Justice

Justice refers to the ethical obligation to treat each person in accordance with what is morally right and proper, to give each person what is due to him or her. In the ethics of research involving human subjects the principle refers primarily to distributive justice, which requires the equitable distribution of both the burdens and the benefits of participation in research. Differences in distribution of burdens and benefits are justifiable only if they are based on morally relevant distinctions between persons; one such distinction is vulnerability [13].

"Vulnerability" refers to a substantial incapacity to protect one's own interests owing to such impediments as lack of capability to give informed consent, lack of alternative means of obtaining medical care or other expensive necessities, or being a junior or subordinate member of a hierarchical group. Accordingly, special provisions must be made for the protection of the rights and welfare of vulnerable persons [14].

2.1.4. Research involving human subjects includes the following areas

i. controlled trials of diagnostic, preventive or therapeutic measures in larger groups of persons, designed to demonstrate a specific generalizable response to these measures against a background of individual biological variation

ii. studies designed to determine the consequences for individuals and communities of specific preventive or therapeutic measures; and studies concerning human health-related behaviour in a variety of circumstances and environmentsstudies of a physiological, biochemical or pathological process, or of the response to a specific intervention, whether physical, chemical or psychological- in healthy subjects or patients;

iii. Research involving human subjects may employ either observation or physical, chemical or psychological intervention; it may also either generate records or make use of existing records containing biomedical or other information about individuals who mayor may not be identifiable from the records or information. The use of such records and the protection of the confidentiality of data obtained from those records are discussed in *International Guidelines for Ethical Review of Epidemiological Studies [15]*.

Research involving human subjects also includes research in which environmental factors are manipulated in a way that could affect incidentally-exposed individuals. Research is defined in broad terms in order to embrace field studies of pathogenic organisms and toxic chemicals under investigation for health-related purposes.

Research involving human subjects is to be distinguished from the practice of medicine, public health and other forms of health care, which is designed to contribute directly to the health of individuals or communities. Prospective subjects may find it confusing when research and practice are to be conducted simultaneously, as when research is designed to obtain new information about the efficacy of a drug or other therapeutic, diagnostic or preventive modality.

Research involving human subjects need to be conducted only by, or strictly supervised by, suitably qualified and experienced investigators and in accordance with a protocol that clearly states: the aim of the research; the reasons for proposing that it involve human subjects; the nature and degree of any known risks to the subjects; the sources from which it is proposed to recruit subjects; and the means proposed for ensuring that subjects' consent will be adequately informed and voluntary. The protocol should be scientifically and ethically appraised by one or more suitably constituted review bodies, independent of the investigators [16].

3. Consideration of some important ethical guidelines

3.1. Informed consent human participation in clinical research

3.1.1. Guideline 1: Individual informed consent

For all biomedical research involving human subjects, the investigator must obtain the informed consent of the prospective subject or, in the case of an individual who is not capable of giving informed consent, the proxy consent of a properly authorized representative [5, 13].

Informed consent is consent given by a competent individual who has received the necessary information; who has adequately understood the information; and who, after considering the information, has arrived at a decision without having been subjected to coercion, undue influence or inducement, or intimidation.

Informed consent is based on the principle that competent individuals are entitled to choose freely whether to participate in research. Informed consent protects the individual's freedom of choice and respects the individual's autonomy [17].

In itself, informed consent is an imperfect safeguard for the individual, and it must always be complemented by independent ethical review of research proposals. Moreover, many individuals, including young children, many adults with severe mental or behavioural disorders, and many persons who are totally unfamiliar with modern medical concepts, are limited in their capacity to give adequate informed consent [17]. Because their consent could imply passive and uncomprehending participation, investigators must on no account presume that consent given by such vulnerable individuals is valid, without the prior approval of an independent ethical-review body. When an individual is incapable of making an informed decision whether to participate in research, the investigator must obtain the proxy consent of the individual's legal guardian or other duly authorized representative [18].

When the research design involves no more than minimal risk- that is, risk that is no more likely and not greater than that attached to routine medical or psychological examination -and it is not practicable to obtain informed consent from each subject, the ethical review committee may waive some or all of the elements of informed consent [19]. Investigators should never initiate research involving-human subjects without obtaining each subject's informed consent, unless they have received explicit approval to do so from an ethical review committee.

3.1.2. Guideline 2: Essential information for prospective research subjects

Before requesting an individual's consent to participate in research, the investigator must provide the individual with the following information, in language that he or she is capable of understanding:

i.   that each individual is invited to participate as a subject in research, and the aims and methods of the research; -the expected duration of the subject's participation; -the benefits that might reasonably be expected to result to the subject or to others as an outcome of the research;

ii.   any foreseeable risks or discomfort to the subject, associated with participation in the research;

iii.   any alternative procedures or courses of treatment that might be as advantageous to the subject as the procedure or treatment being tested;

iv.   the extent to which confidentiality of records in which the subject is identified will be maintained;

v.   the extent of the investigator's responsibility, if any, to provide medical services to the subject;

vi.   that therapy will be provided free of charge for specified types of research-related injury;

vii.   whether the subject or the subject's family or dependants will be compensated for disability or death resulting from such injury; and

viii.   that the individual is free to refuse to participate and will be free to withdraw from the research at any time without penalty or loss of benefits to which he or she would otherwise be entitled [20].

3.1.3. Guideline 3: Obligations of investigators regarding informed consent

The investigator has a duty to:

1. communicate to the prospective subject all the information necessary for adequately informed consent;

2. give the prospective subject full opportunity and encourage- ment to ask questions;

3. exclude the possibility of unjustified deception, undue influence and intimidation;

4. seek consent only after the prospective subject has adequate knowledge of the relevant facts and of the consequences of participation, and has had sufficient opportunity to consider whether to participate;

5. as a general rule, obtain from each prospective subject a signed form as evidence of informed consent; and

6. Renew the informed consent of each subject if there are material changes in the conditions or procedures of the research [21].

3.1.4. Guideline 4: Inducement to participate

Subjects may be paid for inconvenience and time spent, and should be reimbursed for expenses incurred, in connection with their participation in research; they may also receive free medical services. However, the payments should not be so large or the medical services so extensive as to induce prospective subjects to consent to participate in the research against their better judgment ("undue inducement"). All payments, reimbursements and medical services to be provided to research subjects should be approved by an ethical review committee [21].

3.1.5. Guideline 5: Research involving children

Before undertaking research involving children, the investigator must ensure that:

i.   children will not be involved in research that might equally well be carried out with adults;

ii.   the purpose of the research is to obtain knowledge relevant to the health needs of children;

iii.   a parent or legal guardian of each child has given proxy consent;

iv.   the consent of each child has been obtained to the extent of the child's capabilities;

v.   the child's refusal to participate in research must always be respected unless according to the research protocol the child would receive therapy for which there is no medically- acceptable alternative;

vi.   the risk presented by interventions not intended to benefit the individual child-subject is low and commensurate with the importance of the knowledge to be gained; and

vii.   interventions that are intended to provide therapeutic benefit are likely to be at least as advantageous to the individual child-subject as any available alternative [22]..

3.1.6. Guideline 6: Research involving persons with mental or behavioural disorders

Before undertaking research involving individuals who by reason of mental or behavioural disorders are not capable of giving adequately informed consent, the investigator must ensure that:

i.   such persons will not be subjects of research that might equally well be carried out on persons in full possession of their mental faculties;

ii.   the purpose of the research is to obtain knowledge relevant to the particular health needs of persons with mental or behavioural disorders;

iii.   the consent of each subject has been obtained to the extent of that subject's capabilities, and a prospective subject's refusal to participate in non-clinical research is always respected;

iv.   in the case of incompetent subjects, informed consent is obtained from the legal guardian or other duly authorized person;

v.   the degree of risk attached to interventions that are not intended to benefit the individual subject is low and commensurate with the importance of the knowledge to be gained; and

vi.   interventions that are intended to provide therapeutic benefit are likely to be at least as advantageous to the individual subject as any alternative [23].

3.1.7. Guideline 7: Research involving prisoners

Prisoners with serious illness or at risk of serious illness should not arbitrarily be denied access to investigational drugs, vaccines or other agents that show promise of therapeutic or preventive benefit.

3.1.8. Guideline 8: Research involving subjects in underdeveloped communities

Before undertaking research involving subjects in underdeveloped communities, whether in developed or developing countries, the investigator must ensure that:

i.   persons in underdeveloped communities will not ordinarily be involved in research that could be carried out reasonably well in developed communities;

ii.   the research is responsive to the health needs and the priorities of the community in which it is to be carried out;

iii.   every effort will be made to secure the ethical imperative that the consent of individual subjects be informed; and

iv.   the proposals for the research have been reviewed and approved by an ethical review committee that has among its members or consultants persons who are thoroughly familiar with the customs and traditions of the community [24].

3.1.9. Guideline 9: Informed consent in epidemiological studies

For several types of epidemiological research individual informed consent is either impracticable or inadvisable. In such cases the ethical review committee should determine whether it is ethically acceptable to proceed without individual informed consent and whether the investigator's plans to protect the safety and respect the privacy of research subjects and to maintain the confidentiality of the data are adequate [25].

3.1.10. Guideline 10: Equitable distribution of burdens and benefits

Individuals or communities to be invited to be subjects of research should be selected in such a way that the burdens and benefits of the research will be equitably distributed. Special justification is required for inviting vulnerable individuals and, if they are selected, the means of protecting their rights and welfare must be particularly strictly applied [26].

3.1.11. Guideline 11: Selection of pregnant or nursing (breastfeeding) women as research subjects

Pregnant or nursing women should in no circumstances be the subjects of non-clinical research unless the research carries no more than minimal risk to the fetus or nursing infant and the object of the research is to obtain new knowledge about pregnancy or lactation. As a general rule, pregnant or nursing women should not be subjects of any clinical trials except such trials as are designed to protect or advance the health of pregnant or nursing women or fetuses or nursing infants, and for which women who are not pregnant or nursing would not be suitable subjects [27].

3.1.12. Guideline 12: Safeguarding confidentiality

The investigator must establish secure safeguards of the confidentiality of research data. Subjects should be told of the limits to the investigators' ability to safeguard confidentiality and of the anticipated consequences of breaches of confidentiality [28].

3.1.13. Guideline 13: Right of subjects to compensation

Research subjects who suffer physical injury as a result of their participation are entitled to such financial or other assistance as would compensate them equitably for any temporary or permanent impairment or disability. In the case of death, their dependants are entitled to material compensation. The right to compensation may not be waived [29]

3.1.14. Guideline 14: Constitution and responsibilities of ethical review committees

All proposals to conduct research involving human subjects must be submitted for review and approval to one or more independent ethical and scientific review committees. The investigator must obtain such approval of the proposal to conduct research before the research is begun. The provisions for review of research involving human subjects are influenced by political institutions, the organization of medical practice and research, and the degree of autonomy accorded to medical investigators. Whatever the circumstances, however, society has a dual responsibility to ensure that [30]

i.   all drugs, devices and vaccines under investigation in human subjects meet adequate standards of safety; and

ii.   the provisions of the Declaration of Helsinki are applied in all biomedical research involving human subjects.

3.2. Externally sponsored research

3.2.1. Guideline 15: Obligations of sponsoring and host countries

Externally sponsored research entails two ethical obligations:

i.   An external sponsoring agency should submit the research protocol to ethical and scientific review according to the standards of the country of the sponsoring agency, and the ethical standards applied should be no less exacting than they would be in the case of research carried out in that country.

ii.   After scientific and ethical approval in the country of the sponsoring agency, the appropriate authorities of the host country, including a national or local ethical review committee or its equivalent, should satisfy themselves that the proposed research meets their own ethical requirements.

3.2.2. Definition

The term "externally sponsored research" refers to research undertaken in a host country but sponsored, financed, and sometimes wholly or partly carried out by an external international or national agency, with the collaboration or agreement of the appropriate authorities, institutions and personnel of the host country.

Ethical and scientific review. Committees in both the country of the sponsoring agency and the host country have responsibility for conducting both scientific and ethical review, as well as the authority to withhold approval of research proposals that fail to meet their scientific or ethical standards. Special responsibilites may be assigned to review committees in the two countries when a sponsor or investigator in a developed country proposes to carry out research in a developing country. When the external sponsor is an international agency the research protocol must be reviewed according to its own independent ethical review procedures and standards [31].

Committees in the external sponsoring country or international agency have a special responsibility to determine whether the scientific methods are sound and suitable for the aims of the research, whether the drugs, vaccines or devices to be studied meet adequate standards of safety, whether there is sound justification for conducting the research in the host country rather than in the country of the external sponsoring agency, and that the proposed research does not in principle violate the ethical standards of the external sponsoring country or international organization [32].

Committees in the host country have the special responsibility to determine whether the goals of the research are responsive to the health needs and priorities of the host country. Moreover, because of their better understanding of the culture in which the research is proposed to be carried out, they have special responsibility for assuring the equitable selection of subjects and the acceptability of plans to obtain informed consent, to respect privacy, to maintain confidentiality, and to offer benefits that will not be considered excessive inducements to consent.

In short, ethical review in the external sponsoring country may be limited to ensuring compliance with broadly stated ethical standards, on the understanding that ethical review committees in the host country will have greater competence in reviewing the detailed plans for compliance in view of their better understanding of the cultural and moral values of the population in which the research is proposed to be conducted [33].

3.2.3. Research designed to develop therapeutic, diagnostic or preventive products

When externally sponsored research is initiated and financed by an industrial sponsor such as a pharmaceutical company, it is in the interest of the host country to require that the research proposal be submitted with the comments of a responsible authority of the initiating country, such as a health administration, research council, or academy of medicine or science.

Externally sponsored research designed to develop a therapeutic, diagnostic or preventive product must be responsive to the health needs of the host country. It should be conducted only in host countries in which the disease or other condition for which the product is indicated is an important problem. As a general rule, the sponsoring agency should agree in advance of the research that any product developed through such research will be made reasonably available to the inhabitants of the host community or country at the completion of successful testing. Exceptions to this general requirement should be justified and agreed to all concerned parties before the research begins. Consideration should be given to whether the sponsoring agency should agree to maintain in the host country, after the research has been completed, health services and facilities established for purposes of the study [34].

3.2.4. Obligations of external sponsors

An important secondary objective of externally sponsored collaborative research is to help develop the host country's capacity to carry out similar research projects independently, including their ethical review. Accordingly, external sponsors are expected to employ and, if necessary, train local individuals to function as investigators, research assistants, or data managers or in other similar capacities. When indicated, sponsors should also provide facilities and personnel to make necessary health-care services available to the population from which research subjects are recruited.[34]. Although sponsors are not obliged to provide health-care facilities or personnel beyond that which is necessary for the conduct of the research, to do so is morally praiseworthy. However, sponsors have an obligation to ensure that subjects who suffer injury as a consequence of research interventions obtain medical treatment free of charge, and that compensation is provided for death or disability occurring as a consequence of such injury. Also, sponsors and investigators should refer for health care services subjects who are found to have diseases unrelated to the research, and should advise prospective subjects who are rejected as research subjects because they do not meet health criteria for admission to the investigation to seek medical care. Sponsors are expected to ensure that research subjects and the communities for which they are recruited are not made worse off as a result of the research (apart from justifiable risks of research interventions) — for example, by the diversion of scarce local resources to research activities. Sponsors may disclose to the proper authorities in the host country information that relates to the health of the country or community, discovered in the course of a study [35].

External sponsors are expected to provide, as necessary, reasonable amounts of financial, educational and other assistance to enable the host country to develop its own capacity for independent ethical review of research proposals and to form independent and competent scientific and ethical review committees. To avoid conflict of interest, and to assure the independence of committees, such assistance should not be provided directly to the committees; rather funds should be made available to the host-country government or to the host research-institution [36].

Obligations of sponsors will vary with the circumstances of particular studies and the needs of host countries. The sponsors' obligations in particular studies should be clarified before research is begun. The research protocol should specify what, if any, resources, facilities, assistance and other goods or services will be made available during and after the research, to the community from which the subjects are drawn and to the host country.The details of these arrangements should be agreed by the sponsor, officials of the host country, other interested parties, and, when relevant, the community from which subjects are to be drawn. The ethical review committee in the host country should determine whether any or all of these details should be made a part of the consent process [36].

4. World medical association declaration of Helsinki

It is the mission of the physician to safeguard the health of the people. His or her knowledge and conscience are dedicated to the fulfillment of this mission. The Declaration of Geneva of the World Medical Association binds the physician with the words, "The health of my patient will be my first consideration," and the International Code of Medical Ethics declares that "A physician shall act only in the patient's interest when providing medical care which might have the effect of weakening the physical and mental condition of the patient."

The purpose of biomedical research involving human subjects must be to improve diagnostic, therapeutic and prophylactic procedures and the understanding of the etiology and pathogenesis of disease.

In current medical practice most diagnostic, therapeutic or prophylactic procedures involve hazards. This applies especially to biomedical research.

Medical progress is based on research which ultimately must rest in part on experimentation involving human subjects.

In the field of biomedical research a fundamental distinction must be recognized between medical research in which the aim is essentially diagnostic or therapeutic for a patient, and medical research, the essential object of which is purely scientific and without implying direct diagnostic or therapeutic value to the person subjected to the research. Special caution must be exercised in the conduct of research which may affect the environment, and the welfare of animals used for research must be respected.

Because it is essential that the results of laboratory experiments be applied to human beings to further scientific knowledge and to help suffering humanity, the World Medical Association has prepared the following recommendations as a guide to every physician in biomedical research involving human subjects. They should be kept under review in the future. It must be stressed that the standards as drafted are only a guide to physicians all over the world. Physicians are not relieved from criminal, civil and ethical responsibilities under the laws of their own countries [37].

4.1. Basic principles

1. Biomedical research involving human subjects must conform to generally accepted scientific principles and should be based on adequately performed laboratory and animal experimentation and a thorough knowledge of the scientific literature.

2. The design and performance of each experimental procedure involving human subjects should be clearly formulated in an experimental protocol which should be transmitted for consideration, comment and guidance to a specially appointed committee independent of the investigator and the sponsor, provided that this independent committee is in conformity with the laws and regulations of the country in which the research experiment is performed.

3. Biomedical research involving human subjects should be conducted only by scientifically qualified persons and under the supervision of a clinically competent medical person. The responsibility for the human subject must always rest with a medically qualified person and never rest on the subject of the research, even though the subject has given his or her consent.

4. Biomedical research involving human subjects cannot legitimately be carried out unless the importance of the objective is in proportion to the inherent risk to the subject.

5. Every biomedical research project involving human subjects should be preceded by careful assessment of predictable risks in comparison with foreseeable benefits to the subject or to others. Concern for the interests of the subject must always prevail over the interests of science and society.

6. The right of the research subject to safeguard his or her integrity must always be respected. Every precaution should be taken to respect the privacy of the subject and to minimize the impact of the study on the subject's physical and mental integrity and on the personality of the subject.

7. Physicians should abstain from engaging in research projects involving human subjects unless they are satisfied that the hazards involved are believed to be predictable. Physicians should cease any investigation if the hazards are found to outweigh the potential benefits.

8. In publication of the results of his or her research, the physician is obliged to preserve the accuracy of the results. Reports of experimentation not in accordance with the principles laid down in this Declaration should not be accepted for publication.

9. In any research on human beings, each potential subject must be adequately informed of the aims, methods, anticipated benefits and potential hazards of the study and the discomfort it may entail. He or she should be informed that he or she is at liberty to abstain from participation in the study and that he or she is free to withdraw his or her consent to participation at any time. The physician should then obtain the subject's freely-given informed consent, preferably in writing.

10. When obtaining informed consent for the research project the physician should be particularly cautious if the subject is in a dependent relationship to him or her or may consent under duress. In that case the informed consent should be obtained by a physician who is not engaged in the investigation and who is completely independent of this official relationship.

11. In case of legal incompetence, informed consent should be obtained from the legal guardian in accordance with national legislation. Where physical or mental incapacity makes it impossible to obtain informed consent, or when the subject is a minor, permission from the responsible relative replaces that of the subject in accordance with national legislation. Whenever the minor child is in fact able to give consent, the minor's consent must be obtained in addition to the consent of the minor's legal guardian.

12. The research protocol should always contain a statement of the ethical considerations involved and should indicate that the principles enunciated in the present Declaration are complied with.

4.2. Medical research combined with professional care (Clinical research)

1. In the treatment of the sick person, the physician must be free to use a new diagnostic and therapeutic measure, if in his or her judgment it offers hope of saving life, reestablishing health or alleviating suffering.

2. The potential benefits, hazards and discomfort of a new method should be weighed against the advantages of the best current diagnostic and therapeutic methods.

3. In any medical study, every patient — including those of a control group, if any — should be assured of the best proven diagnostic and therapeutic method.

4. The refusal of the patient to participate in a study must never interfere with the physician-patient relationship.

5. If the physician considers it essential not to obtain informed consent, the specific reasons for this proposal should be stated in the experimental protocol for transmission to the independent committee.

6. The physician can combine medical research with professional care, the objective being the acquisition of new medical knowledge, only to the extent that medical research is justified by its potential diagnostic or therapeutic value for the patient.

4.3. Non therapeutic research involving human subjects (Non-clinical biomedical research)

1. In the purely scientific application of medical research carried out on a human being, it is the duty of the physician to remain the protector of the life and health of that person on whom biomedical research is being carried out.

2. The subjects should be volunteers, either healthy persons or patients for whom the experimental design is not related to the patient's illness.

3. The investigator or the investigating team should discontinue the research if in his/her or their judgment it may, if continued, be harmful to the individual.

4. In research on man, the interest of science and society should never take precedence over considerations related wellbeing of the subject.

5. The phases of clinical trials of vaccines and drugs

5.1. Vaccine development

Phase I refers to the first introduction of a candidate vaccine into a human population for initial determination of its safety and biological effects, including immunogenicity. This phase may include studies of dose and route of administration, and usually involves fewer than 100 volunteers.

Phase II refers to the initial trials examining effectiveness in a limited number of volunteers (usually between 200 and 500); the focus of this phase is immunogenicity.

Phase III trials are intended for a more complete assessment of safety and effectiveness in the prevention of disease, involving a larger number of volunteers in a multicentre adequately controlled study [5].

5.2. Drug development

5.2.1. Phase I

Phase I refers to the first introduction of a drug into humans. Normal volunteer subjects are usually studied to determine levels of drugs at which toxicity is observed. Such studies are followed by dose-ranging studies in patients for safety and, in some cases, early evidence of effectiveness.

5.2.2. Phase II

Phase II investigation consists of controlled clinical trials designed to demonstrate effectiveness and relative safety. Normally, these are performed on a limited number of closely monitored patients.

5.2.3. Phase III

Phase III trials are performed after a reasonable probability of effectiveness of a drug has been established and are intended to gather additional evidence of effectiveness for specific indications and more precise definition of drug-related adverse effects. This phase includes both controlled and uncontrolled studies.

5.2.4. Phase IV

Phase IV trials are conducted after the national drug registration authority has approved a drug for distribution or marketing. These trials may include research designed to explore a specific pharmacological effect, to establish the incidence of adverse reactions, or to determine the effects of long-term administration of a drug. Phase IV trials may also be designed to evaluate a drug in a population not studied adequately in the premarketing phases (such as children or the elderly) or to establish a new clinical indication for a drug. Such research is to be distinguished from marketing research, sales promotion studies, and routine post-marketing surveillance for adverse drug reactions in that these categories ordinarily need not be reviewed by ethical review committees

In general, Phase I drug trials and Phase I and Phase II vaccine trials should be conducted according to the articles of the Declaration of Helsinki that refer to non-clinical research. However, some exceptions can be justified. For example, it is customary and ethically justifiable to conduct Phase I studies of highly toxic chemotherapies of cancer in patients with cancer, rather than in normal volunteers as prescribed in the Declaration of Helsinki, Article III.2. Similarly be ethically it may be ethically justifiable to involve HIV-seropositive individuals as subjects in Phase II trials of candidate vaccines [37].

Phase II and Phase III drug trials should be conducted according to the articles of the Declaration of Helsinki that refer to "medical research, combined with professional care (clinical research)". However, the Declaration does not to provide for controlled clinical trials. Rather, it assures the freedom of the physician "to use a new diagnostic and therapeutic measure, if in his or her judgment it offers hope of saving life reestablishing health or alleviating suffering" (Article II.1). Also in regard to Phase II and Phase III drug trials there are customary and ethically justified exceptions to the requirements of the Declaration of Helsinki. A placebo given to a control group, for example, cannot be justified by its "potential diagnostic or therapeutic value for the patient", as Article II.6 prescribes. Many other interventions and procedures characteristic of late-phase drug development have no possible diagnostic or therapeutic value for the patients and thus must be justified on other grounds; usually such justification consists of a reasonable expectation that they carry little or no risk and that t contribute materially to the achievement of the goals of the research [37].

Phase III trials of vaccines do not use "a new diagnostic and therapeutic measure" that offers "hope of saving life, reestablishing health or alleviating suffering" (clinical research). Yet administration of the vaccine is intended to be a benefit to the subject rather than the purely scientific application of medical research carried out on a being" (non-clinical biomedical research). Thus, Phase III vaccine-trials do not conform to either of the categories defined in the Declaration of Helsinki.

6. Advances in biomedical research in 2012

Biomedical research in the United States is a $100 billion enterprise, with approximately 65% supported by industry, 30% by government (predominately the NIH), and 5% by charities, foundations, or individual donors. Although total sponsorship tripled between the mid-1990s and mid-2000s [15], the rate of increase has fallen since 2003 and declined in real (inflation-adjusted) terms since 2007 [3, 17]. The number of new drugs entering human trials has also fallen during the past two decades, especially for new molecular entities and entirely new classes of drugs. In contrast, the number of approvals of medical devices by the Food and Drug Administration (FDA) has increased steadily each year [23]. Driven by demand, total medical spending on devices has increased at a rate that is several times that for health services and twice that for drugs [5, 30].

Since the mid-1990s, the United States has invested approximately 4.5% of its total health expenditures on biomedical research. In contrast, only 0.1% supports research in health services, comparative effectiveness, new care models, best practices, and quality, outcome, or service innovations [37]. This funding will increase to approximately 0.3% from appropriations in 2010 health legislation.

Misconceptions regarding the scientific process are common. Research is costly, capital-intensive, and collaborative. Researchers in both academic and industrial settings require access to much the same information, samples and tissue, instrumentation, and specialized technical skills. They also depend on one another as a source of new ideas. It is a paradox, during this decade of growing scrutiny of ties between academic institutions and companies, that academic investigators value their nonfinancial company ties (with access to technology or research materials) more than personal compensation or support of their laboratory [4, 19]. Moreover, the notion that "pure" (basic) and "applied" (clinical) research exist as distinct activities is belied by their source of sponsorship and the self-reports of how researchers actually spend their time [27]. Such multimode researchers are more productive, as judged by the number of publications, impact factor, success at winning peer-reviewed NIH funding, and number of patents. This reality was cited by a recent U.S. Federal Court opinion over-turning the patentability of several genes that predispose women to breast cancer. The court called for patenting practices that favor openness whenever basic discovery is inhibited [3, 20].

Sponsors have sought to improve their research productivity through the NIH Roadmap initiative (especially Clinical and Translational Science Awards) by encouraging alliances between companies and universities, alternative organizational models, and joint investment in costly facilities, such as imaging or gene sequencing [1, 23]. We reviewed the lessons from 70 such alliances from the mid-1960s through 2000 [5]. Although it is too soon to judge the success of the most recent models, in the main, earlier ones have not accelerated the pace of either discovery or clinical application. The sources of difficulty are idiosyncratic, but recurrent problems are a failure at inception to agree on intellectual-property provisions, excessive secrecy, and disagreements over research aims. In our view, the most salient reason for failure is the centralization of authority within large, inherently cautious bureaucracies in govern-ment, universities, foundations, and companies. Collectively, such factors inhibit scientists' creativity by disregarding the pluralism of ideas and the diversity of approaches that are necessary for innovation. Conversely, the most successful collaborations have found a balance between external direction and scientists' curiosity. Many of the most experienced observers from government, industry, and academia concur with this viewpoint [25, 31].

Economic forces are also relevant. In the United States, the gain in life expectancy between 1970 and 1990 added $2.4 trillion per year to the gross domestic product by 2000. Moreover, biomedical research bolsters employment, economic development, balance of trade, and exports. Studies from many countries show that investment in new technology of all types is the primary source of economic growth, especially when such investment is made by the private sector [2, 35]. In contrast, in areas in which public spending on technology is dominant, the rates of productivity and growth are lower. The differences are most marked in medical research [15, 44].

Despite these observations, some federal policymakers express doubt that scientific advance is a prerequisite for improved health. They favor predictable, low-cost public health measures and expanded access to basic care during the current decade of austerity [11, 26]. Other policymakers question whether spending on new devices and high-cost bioengineered drugs produce commensurate clinical value [7], 39. Such criticism is driven by estimates that new technology of marginal benefit (as measured by reduced disease burden or improved longevity) accounts for one half to two thirds of health care inflation in Western countries [31, 46] Even the commercial value of biomedical research is questioned by some companies, as is reflected by their reduced rates of research and development because of unfavorable returns as compared with marketing [1, 17], or mergers and acquisitions [6].

Other observers assert that social, educational, and macroeconomic factors are more important than medicine or public health practice in promoting a population's health [20]. They see technology as a distraction from enlightened social, tax, and regulatory policies. Debate over the goals has already begun [14, 22].

As a consequence, we believe that steps must be taken to reestablish public confidence in researchers and clinicians, along with their institutions. Measures are needed that go beyond those recommended by the Institute of Medicine [3] the Council of Medical Specialty Societies and the National Institute of Health. These reports emphasize remedies that focus primarily on competing interests without dealing with the opportunities. We are concerned that the recommendations overlook the potential for new models to foster productivity[52].

6.1. Seven remedies for consideration

The discontent arising from the current circumstances demands the consideration of sweeping changes in the way we conduct biomedical research. We believe that seven measures should be considered to reconcile competing goals. They require recognition of the multilayered sources of conflict, especially those based on different scientific aims and social values [15].

6.2. Improve data on clinical value

We must develop and apply better objective information about clinical value. This goal implies a higher standard for adopting new devices (including clinical trials similar to those for drugs) and better information on the effectiveness of existing drugs and devices, especially data that are available only from proprietary insurance databases. It is unlikely that provisions for comparative-effectiveness research in the 2010 health care legislation or the changes proposed by the FDA for device approval will be sufficient. New incentives are needed for private and government insurers to disclose clinical data to researchers, along with expanded access to device registries, easier access to data from Medicare and Medicaid, and development of more robust analytical techniques for ascertaining clinical value. Moreover, physicians and surgeons must commit to a new level of objectivity in judging clinical value, while resisting the influence of commercial potential or personal financial interests [13, 48].

6.3. Change the role of teaching hospitals

The roles of academic health centers and teaching hospitals must be modified to improve their ability to conduct early-stage (proof-of-concept) clinical trials. Here, entirely new models for interaction are required, probably involving freestanding independent institutes or autonomous units within academic centers, where patients come specifically for access to such early-stage studies and where the mutual expectations for investigators, companies, and patients are clear and unambiguous. This change will hasten the divergence between institutions that offer routine care (and that are managed to provide low-cost, reproducible high quality) and those with capability for scientific innovation (where early-stage investigations occur). Making these interactions effective and avoiding the shortcomings of past attempts will require new models of intellectual property, patents, and licensing by moving these aspects farther down the chain of discovery [5]. Two very different approaches should be tried: creating patent pools involving multiple companies and universities [19] and a renunciation of patenting in return for more latitude to conduct high-risk laboratory experimentation and initial clinical trials [26]. It is likely that only some of the 130 academic health centers will choose to undertake such changes.

6.4. Develop new models for collaboration and financing

In asserting the need for an increase of total spending on biomedical research and the need to foster the diversity of scientific approaches, consideration should be given to new models of collaboration and cooperation. Such measures would allow the NIH to concentrate on basic biomedical science and large, multi-institutional projects, where its scale can be most valuable, while providing offset to industry's declining investment in research. These models might include the following [6, 52].

6.5. Create a new class of bonds

States and the federal government might issue bonds to support innovation in biomedical science and health services, with preference given to high-risk research and diseases important to public health. Such bonds have long been used to support athletic facilities, airports, and roads. They provide a mechanism for private investment to meet public needs [18].

6.7. Defer patents to later in the discovery chain

In return for new sources of funding and greater latitude to conduct high-risk research, the new entities would forgo claims to patents or other intellectual property and place positive and negative findings immediately in the public domain.

Emphasizing new incentives, creating new entities, and mobilizing additional funding sources avoid the risk of disrupting productive research relationships currently found in universities, established research institutes, and the NIH. The measures also allow new laboratories to attract the best talent, while providing a route to enhance the productivity of research and its early clinical application [25].

6.8. Establish biomedical innovation trusts

The formation of new nonprofit, public–private partnerships, biomedical innovation trusts, could enable individuals and corporations to receive immediate federal tax credits for contributions to support research in high-priority diseases. Such trusts might be administered by decentralized new foundations or new regional public entities and be directed at particular diseases, universities, freestanding laboratories, or small companies. Similar tax incentives have been used historically to preserve land, create parks, and build factories [31, 54].

6.9. Use incentives to promote pluralism

To enhance the diversity of scientific approaches and innovation in its application, preference in funding might be given to new research institutes or entities, rather than existing universities or companies.

6.10. Renew professional commitments

All physicians must renew their commitment to professionalism and their duty to their patients. This will not be easy in an age when commercial values are paramount and the competition of the marketplace drives personal and institutional financial decisions. Yet, without such a recommitment, no safeguards will prevent an inexorable loss of trust in our institutions and us. Professionalism, as interpreted today, means not a return to paternalism, but objectivity in judgment on behalf of the patient, with open communication and an absence of bias [37]. It must be translated into action by a blanket proscription of product promotion in any guise.

6.11. Focus on cost-effective targets

We must recognize that new technology creates value to the general economy and has many clinical benefits but that it also usually spurs new clinical costs. Observers who are the most critical of medicine believe we have failed to recognize that historical compromise. In an era in which many favor public-policy goals to ensure a basic level of care for all citizens and a reduction in the rate of increase of aggregate health care spending, the technological imperative will surely be challenged with greater stridency. This requires incentives for researchers to focus on diseases that are common, cannot currently be prevented or effectively treated, are expensive, and have a major effect on the patients' health [2, 13]. Such choices among diseases are onerous but inescapable [47, 60].

6.12. Adopt realistic research goals

We must embrace a new realism about the difficulty of the scientific process and what can (and cannot) be expected from it. We must not overpromise. Such realism will not be popular with patient advocacy groups, the press, politicians, benefactors, or company investors. Each of these groups has a vested interest in overstating their case. Yet to do otherwise runs the risk of eroding the trust on which so much depends. Paradoxically, a commitment to realism may itself have a positive effect on the scientific process by reducing the pressure to promote findings prematurely and by fostering openness [13, 51].

6.13. Redefine the terms of conflict

Finally, we in medicine must recognize that those who have a public health perspective or who see social and economic factors as paramount will not be sympathetic to increasing the technology-driven momentum of the past 60 years. Inevitably, we face growing conflict over individual choice, access to the latest drug or device, the true cost of technology over a lifetime, perceptions of value, and preferences for competition versus regulation. Such tensions have long been implicit. They are now explicit. Not everyone believes biomedical research is essential [8].

7. Promotion of biomedical research in Sub Saharan Africa (SSA)

7.1. Setting the policies by SSA and stakeholders to prioritize funding for health research

The African heads of state during this decade have embarked on the need for poverty disease control supported by health research. In the Abuja Declaration of 2000, the heads of state pledged their commitments to apply strategies needed to improve on malaria control. They also called for additional resources to stimulate the development of malaria vaccines appropriate for Africa and to provide similar incentives for other anti-malaria technologies [39-41]. In addition the African Union has set a target of allocating 15% of national budget to the health sector, and 2% of health budget to finance health research. The AU countries reportedly agreed to allocate 1% of their countries GDP to research. In its 2008 report, the Global Forum for Health Research only list Liberia to have surpassed the set goal of allocating 15% of its national budget to the health sector by 2003; the report listed Burkina Faso, Central African Republic, Gabon, Gambia, Namibia, Niger and Tanzania to be just over 12%. Before then many of these countries invested very little in health systems. From this report, few low and middle income countries collect and report data on investments in health research [42, 53].

Since the 90s, there are only a few institutions enabling developing country scientists to undertake health research. The situation has since changed significantly, in terms of their allocations. There are currently a number of government agencies that support research, such as World Bank, European Union, World Health Organization (WHO), World Health Organization/Special Programme for Research and Training in Tropical Diseases (WHO/TDR), European Developing Countries Clinical Trials Partnership (EDCTP), Kenya Medical Research Institute (KEMRI), African Malaria Network (AMANET), Drug for neglected Diseases Initiatives (DNDI), National Institute of Health (NIH), Japanese Internatioanl cooperation (JICA), Department for International Development (DFID),), United Nation Development Programme (UNDP), Danish International Development Agency, Dutch Ministry of Foreign Affairs (DGIS), International Development Research Centre (IDRC), Swiss Development Cooperation (SDC), Swedish International Development cooperation agency (SIDA), United State Agency for International Development (USAID) and many other unlisted. Some private philanthropic support to health has been very beneficial in promoting health and reducing the 10/90 gap in sub-Saharan Africa. These include the Bill and Melinda Gates Foundation, EXXON Mobil, Rockefeller Foundation, Wellcome Trust, BH Billiton to name but a few. There are other self financing bodies supporting health research such as the Medical Research Council (MRC) of UK, National Institute of Health (NIH), GlaxoSmithKline (GSK), Pfizer, Norvatis and the United States Department of Defence (DOD) [58-60]

7.2. Major agencies promoting biomedical research and capacity building in Sub-Saharan Africa (SSA)

7.2.1. European Developing Countries Clinical Trials Partnership (EDCTP)

The European Developing Countries Clinical Trials Partnership (EDCTP) was created in 2003, as a European response to the global health crisis caused by malaria. HIV/AIDs and tuberculosis, three poverty-related diseases. EDCTP involves 15 members of the European Union, plus Norway, and Switzerland in partnership with the scientific community and policy makers from sub-Saharan Afica (SSA). The EDCTP started off with a five-year budget of €200 million; member states and the private sector were expected to each contribute a similar sum. EDCTP aims at accelerating the development of new or improved drugs, vaccines and microbicides, against HIV/AIDs tuberculosis and malaria, with a focus on phases II and III clinical trials in SSA. In its work, EDCTP supports clinical trials that combine capacity building and networking, in such a way that the developed human and infrastructure capacity is utilized to conduct multicenter trials, often spanning different SSA countries [52].

The impressive performance of EDCTP is reflected in is 2008 annual report when 21 projects were approved for funding, 27 project contracts worth €54 million were signed. The founding of CANTAM (Central Africa Network of Tuberculosis, HIV/AIDs and Malaria) with EDCTP support, in a research neglected area of Africa is worth mention www.edctp.org. With regard to promoting research and capacity building of researchers and research institutions in SSA, there is no doubt that none compares any closer to WHO/TDR, (the special Programme for Research and Training on Tropical Diseases) which is an independent global programme of scientific collaboration that helps to coordinate support of global efforts to combat major diseases of the poor and the disadvantaged [30].

7.2.2. World Health Organization/special programme for research and training in Tropical Diseases (WHO/TDR),

WHO/TDR was established in 1975, and therefore preceded by a decade and a half the work of the Commission on Health Research for Development, whose members included the founding Director of WHO/TDR. WHO/TDR is soibsired by UNICEF, UNDP, World Bank and WHO; it also receives funding from other agencies across the globe [61].

At the start WHO/TDR restricted its activities to addressing what were by then major neglected diseases, namely malaria, bancroftian filariasis, onchocerciasis, leprosy, leishmaniasis, and African and American trypanosomiasis. Dengue, intestinal helminthes, sexually transmitted infections and tuberculosis were added later. In its early years WHO/TDR made unequaled contributions not only to research on these diseases, but also contributed immensely to capacity building of research leaders in Africa today benefitted from WHO/TDR sponsorship. WHO/TDR also contributed financially and strategically to the development of many new tools and strategies against diseases of poverty. http://apps.who.int/tdr/.

7.2.3. The Kenya Medical Research Institute (KEMRI)

KEMRI established in 1979, operates 10 research centres across the country and employs over 200 national researches and another 500 technical staff. KEMRI has an annual budget of nearly

USD 40 million (of which one-half is Government of Kenya contribution). Several international research teams contribute another 45% KEMRI carries out national ethics review. Major achievements of KEMRI include; national policy basis for control of malaria, tuberculosis, leprosy and leishmaniasis, established surveillance and rapid response systems for major disease outbreaks, improved diagnostics such as KEMRI Hep-cell kit for Hepatitis, particle Agglutination (PA) kit for HIV, and HLA tissue typing techniques [42]

KEMRI successfully collaborated with the Government of Japan to establish global training centres for control of parasitic and infectious diseases. The KEMRI Institute of Tropical Medicine and Infectious Diseases, founded in collaboration with local Jomo Kenyatta University of Agriculture and Technology offers training at MSc and PhD levels. KEMRI founded the African Health Sciences Congress and African Health Journal. www.kemri.org/ (accessed 01/07/12). the progress made by KEMRI since its inception are attributable TO: (i) effective n-s and s-s collaboration (ii) implementation of innovative planning and initiatives, (iii) focused local capacity development and (iv) commitment of the national authorities to strengthen health research and development[23].

7.2.4. African Malaria Network Trust (AMANET)

AMANET has its origins in the African Malaria Vaccine Testing Network (AMVTN) which was established in 1995 with the primary goal of preparing African malaria research institutions to participate in malaria vaccine trials, in 2002, AMANET was registered as a Trust in Tazania and became the Legal successor of AMVTN. This change enabled AMANET to carry out holistic capacity strengthening of trial sites and Centres, and to take on legal responsibilities including sponsorship of trials. The change also signaled the network's commitment and interest in a wider range of malaria interventions, although malaria vaccine development would remain its main focus [29].

The mission of ANANET s to promote capacity strengthening and networking of malaria R&D in Africa, where it has provided institutions with support for essential infrastructure improvement, short-term training to over one thousand health researchers, and uniquely postgraduate degree training in preparation for participation in malaria vaccine development AMANET is funding over 40 projects across SSA, and is well known in Africa for its networks in vaccine trials, bioethics and the Afro-immunoassay network. AMANET also sponsors several blood stage malaria vaccine trials across Africa and has hosted the multilateral initiative on Malaria (MIM) since January 2006 [23]. AMANET Research Ethics capacity strengthens Grant: supported by the Gates foundation where identification of specific gaps in the ethical review process followed by a capacity building programme tailor-made for the identified gaps. A total of 32 ECs have been surveyed in Africa and benefitted from the capacity strengthening sub grants and training activities (www.amanet-trust.org): The south African Research Training initiative (SARETI); based at the University of Kwazulu-Natal and Pretoria University in South Africa, providing training inEthics to African researchers and ERC members. (www.whsph.up.ac.za/sareti/sareti/sareti.htm): The international Research Ethics Network for Southern Africa (IRENSA); based at the University of cape Town, running short term training programmes for mid-career African scientist and embers of Ethics Committees (www.irensa.org):The Training and Resources in research Ethics Evaluation (TRREE) for Africa, which focuses on development or research ethics educational programmes for e-learning and provision of e-resources [23].

7.2.5. Drugs for Neglected Diseases Initiative (DNDI)

DNDI was established in 2003 is a not-for-profit drug development organization, focused on improving the health and quality of life of people suffering from neglected diseases. DNDI was founded by Médicins Sans Frontières (MSF) with five public sector organizations, viz Kenya Medical Research Institute, Indian Council of Medical Research, Malaysian Ministry of Health, Oswaldo Cruz Fondation, Institute Pasteur France, and WHO/TDR as observer. DNDi support covers basic science, as well as preclinical and clinical research, focusing on human African trypanosomiasis, leishmaniasis, chaga's disease, and malaria. In 2007 DNDi in partnership with Sanofi Aventis, completed trial of a combination of Artesunate with Amodiaquine (ASAQ), as a patent free drug against malaria. DNDi is also responsible for the HAT Platform which addresses Human African Trypanosomiasis (HAT) which is truly a neglected disease; there is very limited clinical research activity geared to improving its treatment or diagnosis, and it is endemic only in remote areas. The HAT platform was therefore established through a partnership of the five most affected countries (the Sudan, Democratic Republic of Congo, Uganda, Republic of Congo, and Angola) in collaboration with DNDi and the Swiss Tropical Institute, and other partners to build and strengthen clinical trial capacity including the search for appropriate diagnostics for HAT. In 2008, the HAT Platform received a US$68.2 million grant from the Bill & Melinda Gates Foundation for this purpose[23].

7.2.6. The Japanese chemical giant Sumitomo Chemical Company

They undertook R&D that led to production of Olyset Nets which incorporate an insecticide (permethrin) into the actual fibers of the net, and releases it slowly over a number of years. Olyset nets are guaranteed to last at least five years; they never need retreatment, are tear-resistant, ash proof, provide maximum ventilation; they inhibit mosquito (Anopheles spp.) biting, they repel, knockdown and kill mosquitoes. Olyset nets were the first long-lasting insecticidal net (LLIN) to be submitted and fully registered by the WHO Pesticide Evaluation Scheme (WHOPES) www.olyset.net/.[23]

In 2003 through a PPP a royalty-free technology transfer was undertaken under which Sumitomo Chemical Company would further develop Olyset nets, which eventually led to setting up a factory in Arusha, Tanzania, that was officially launched in early 2008; it aimed at producing 51 million units during 2009, employing 6000 people in Arusha alone, and supporting over 20,000 others. The factory in Arusha is now a 50/50 joint venture between Sumitomo Chemical Company and A to Z textile Mills, a Tanzania company. Another factory is being set up in Nigeria that will bring global production to more than 60 million nets annually, www.olyset.net/olysetnet/manurfacturinginafrica/ (accessed 06.07.12).

7.2.7.Medical research council UK

The MRC supports and advances medical research in three main ways: through their research facilities, by funding research centres in partnership with universities, and by providing research grants and career awards to scientists in UK universities and hospitals. Supporting scientists. Around 5,700 research staff are supported by the MRC, either employed directly in our institutes and units or funded through grants and fellowships. It spends about £86m on training awards for postgraduate students and fellows in 2011/12, including those in the MRC's own institutes and units[59].

The MRC expects valuable data arising from MRC-funded research to be made available to the scientific community with as few restrictions as possible so as to maximize the value of the data for research and for eventual patient and public benefit. Such data must be shared in a timely and responsible manner.The MRC believes that data sharers should receive full and appropriate recognition by funders, their academic institutions and new users for promoting secondary research. New studies that result from this data-sharing should meet the high standards of all MRC research regarding scientific quality, ethical requirements and value for money. It should also add recognizable value to the original dataset. Such research is often most fruitful when it is a collaboration between the new user and the original data creators or curators, with the responsibilities and rights of all parties agreed at the outset. Data arising from MRC-funded research must be properly curated throughout its life-cycle and released with the appropriate high-quality metadata. This is the responsibility of the data custodians, who are often those individuals or organisations that received MRC funding to create or collect the data[55].

Research fish (formerly known as MRC e-Val) gathers outputs, outcomes and impacts arising from MRC-funded research. MRC e-Val is an online survey designed to gather feedback from MRC-funded researchers about the results of their work. The aim is to compile accurate information about the outputs of MRC research and to capture impact as it occurs. This information will then be used to communicate the benefits of MRC funding; support evaluations of the economic, social and academic impact of MRC research; and provide evidence for strategy development. Information was sought across the whole MRC portfolio from all MRC researchers that had held MRC support since 2006 (approximately 3000 principal investigators) [60]. A full set of responses was submitted for 2541 Awards. This represents 83% of Awards that were invited to complete MRC e-Val as shown in figure 1.

8. Use of animal in biomedical research

8.1. Using animals in research: Benefits and ethical consideration

In 1780, Jeremy Bentham, an English Philosopher, first initiated the arguments of ethics in the vicinity of protection and treatment against animal by stating that animals should be treated equally as humans and they should not be neglected because they can not speak nor express their emotions [38]. In 1859, Darwin's theory on evolution placed human and animals on the same physical and emotional continuum. From late 19th century till now, a number of animal rights advocates have presented various arguments against animal uses in biomedical research. Using animals in the discovery of scientific knowledge is not only subject to the prosperity of mankind but also that of all species on earth:

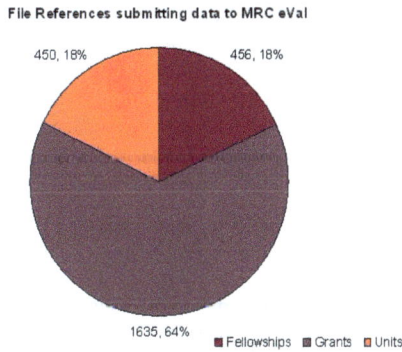

Figure 1. Representation of 83% of Awards that were invited to complete MRC e-Val [51]

The welfare of animals used in research, testing and teaching is affected by a combination of a number of factors. It is the combined effect of biological factors, environmental factors and interactions with the researchers that determine the welfare of animals used for research or teaching purposes [39]. The various factors that affect the welfare of animals used in research have been outlined in table 1.

Biological factors	Environmental factors	Interaction with researchers or teachers
Age if the animals	Ventilation of the room where the animals are kept	Nature of handing (gentle or rough; pain or distress could be caused)
Sex of the animals	Room temperature	Frequency of research procedures could be stressful
Reproductive status of the animals	Relative humidity of the room	Duration of manipulations or procedures (e.g. a class of students using animals in 5-h practical). The same animals may be used by more than one class over a certain period of time
Genetic factors based on the genotype of the animals	Diet during breeding and experimentation	Management practices such as number tags castration, dehorning and tail docking
Stress of the animals	Water availability for the animals	
Physiological/metabolic state of the animals	Light cycle and quality in the room where the animals are kept	
	Noise in the vicinity of the room where the animals are kept Bedding in the cages	
	Size of cages and number of animals per cage	
	Transportation of animal	

Table 1. Types of independent factors that may affect welfare of animals used in research or teaching [46].

One of the strongest grounds of using animals in scientific research is the values of research toward animals and human beings. In the perspective of human health, many diseases such as small pox virus that our forefathers significantly suffered from have now been eradicated or controlled with the aid of biomedical research on animals. The use of animals in research is prevalent because they share at least 200 common illnesses and diseases with humans [38]. Animals are used in research or experimentation in place of human subjects for various reasons. Using animals in research affords the scientist to monitor reactions to stimuli and other variables in complex organs and tissue, while allowing the scientist to minimize environmental variables. Animals are used in scientific research to further science in many arenas. They are used most often in the following cases: Disease Treatment, Prevention, Treatment of Injuries, Basic Medical Testing, and Medical Diagnosis. Animals in research have made possible many scientific breakthroughs that humans benefit from each day such as in; Vaccinations, Anesthesia, Antibiotics, Numerous medical treatments for various diseases. Animals provide the scientist with unique possibilities especially using animals for medical research [39, 40].

When experimenting with new drugs for the treatment of disease it would be virtually impossible to isolate a human the way an animal can be isolated. All mammals share the same systems, there are variants but they are far outweighed by the likeness that humans and animals share. There are just certain testing that can not be accomplished without the use of live organs and tissue. There is no way to duplicate a complex disease in a culture, nor to enable a computer to completely analyze the effects of drugs on a system. Animals play a vital role in medical research [40-42].

8.1.2. Some facts about animal biomedical research

85 % of the animals used in research are rodents - rats and mice that have been bred for laboratory use. Most laboratory tests on animals are simple single type tests - change in diet, drawing a simple blood sample, administering a drug, Animals are given anesthetics if a procedure is going to be invasive in any way. Dogs, cats and non-human primates account for only 3 out of 1000 subjects in experimentation. Humans are still the largest group that is used for research and experimentation and beats out all other lab animals when it comes to testing [44].

A criterion which all scientists must follow is known as the three R's. The three R's in research refer to the following: Refinement, Reduction, and Replacement. Refinement of testing must be arranged so that animal distress is minimal. The scientist must reduce the number of animals used in the experimentation whenever possible and if possible, replace animals with other adequate research methods. There are animal restrictions in place to insure that animals are not used when not necessary[45]. When there are other viable models to conduct research those methods supposed to be used instead of using an animal subject. Only the minimal number of animals is to be used as subjects in an experiment or research project. Unnecessary research and experimentation is considered unethical and use of animals is not supported. The use of animals in research is heavily regulated[46]. The care is mandated through regulatory guidelines and there are heavy damages and fines assessed when these regulations are not followed. The regulations dictate how the animals will be housed and treated to include veterinary care, pain management and other measures to make sure the animals do not suffer throughout the course of the experiment. The scientist needs to get permission from an ethical committee, which have a full description of the project, before starting any research on animals, to ensure for minimum of suffer among the animals [47-49].

8.1.2.1. Replacement

Animals should be replaced in experiments by less sentient alternatives such as invertebrates or in vitro methods whenever possible.

8.1.2.2. Refinement

If animal experiments can not be avoided protocols should be refined to minimize any adverse effects for each individual animal. Appropriate anaesthesia and analgesia should be used for any surgical intervention. Humane endpoints should be used whenever possible. Staff should be well trained, and housing should be of a high standard with appropriate environmental enrichment. Animals should be protected from pathogens[50, 51].

8.1.2.3. Reduction

The number of animals should be reduced to the minimum consistent with achieving the scientific objectives of the study, recognizing that important biological effects may be missed if too few animals are used. Alternatively, methods should be found to obtain more information from each experiment, thus speeding up the pace of research. This can be achieved by careful control of variation and by appropriate experimental design and statistical analysis [52]..

The use of animals in medical research remains essential. However, in accordance with the law, scientists must avoid using animals wherever possible. If applying for funding for studies involving animals, researchers must give sound scientific reasons for using them and explain why there are no realistic alternatives [52, 55] Around 30 per cent of the research we fund involves animals. Some of the key players involved in one way or another in promoting the implementation of the 3 Rs and the dissemination of information about alternatives to animals in research and teaching are illustrated in table 2.

Organization	Web site address
European centre for the Validation of Alternative Methods (ECVAM)	http://ecvam.jrc.it/index.htm(Accessed on 04 June 2009).
Interagency Coordinating Committee on Validation of Alternative methods (ICCVAM) in the USA	http://iccvam.niehs.nih.gov/(Accessed on 04 June 2009).
National interagency Center for the Evaluation of Alternative Toxicological methods (NICEATM) which provides support to the ICCVAM	http://ntp.niehs.nih.gov/ntpweb/index.cfm?objectid =7182FF48-BDB7-CEBA-F8980E5DD01A1E2D (accessed on 04 June 2009)
Norwegian Reference Centre for laboratory Animal Science and Alternatives that maintains the NORINA database containing guidelines on use of animals in	

Organization	Web site address
research as well as audiovisual aids and other teaching materials.	
Alternative to Animal Testing Web Site (Alweb) developed by the John Hopkins Centre for Alternatives to Animal Use	Htt://www.altweb.org (accessed on 04 June 2009)
InterNICHE which promotes humane use of animals in education	www.interniche.org (accessed on o4 June, 2009)
The Netherlands Centre for Alternatives to Animal Use	www.nca-nl.org (accessed on 04 June 2009)
Australian and New Zealand Council for the Care of Animals in Research and teaching (ANZCCART)	anzccart@adelaide.edu.au (Accessed on 04 June 2009).

Table 2. some organizations involved in promoting implementation of the 3Rs [53].

9. Conclusion

Ethical consideration in biomedical research has created a great impact in improving clinical trial research initiatives in both low income economies and industrialized nations. However the lack of scientific expertise and the slow response of scientists, sponsors to ethical questions involving some clinical projects has had a negative effect in the promotion of ethics in biomedical research initiatives. These considerations will require decades of reorientation of our biomedical research efforts. The failure to resolve ethical conflicts be it politically motivated, policy-related, or personal (scientist bias), claims of legitimately competing priorities has limited progress in biomedical research and has encouraged new regulatory constraints in new product development. The IRBs should therefore build a solid working framework, advance capacity building strategies and implement a synergy working platform to promote biomedical and clinical research geared to promote science contribution to human development.

It is also of importance to recognize the contribution of animals used in biomedical research to the good health of humans as well as animal, as moral agents, human beings should always make efforts to ensure that animals are treated humanely in research and teaching.

Efforts should be made to uphold the principles of 3Rs, which ensures that researchers should replace animals with other alternatives whenever possible, and if not possible then the number of animals used should be reduced to the minimum possible sample size as regards to the required statistical power, and refine the methodologies in order to minimize any harm that may be caused by the experimental procedures. It is a welcome idea for the creation of animal ethics committee, and the development of credible national ethics and legal framework, capacity building of research on humane treatment of experimental animals and dialogue among the different stakeholders concerned with the welfare of animal implicated in research.

Special effort have been made to identify some key players in the promotion of biomedical research and their responsibilities, and all the guidelines indicated in this study are intended to protect research participants, and uphold the fundamental ethical principles.

Although there are many action put in place to resolve the 10/90 gap and much has been achieved, the gap still persist. There is the need for more investments towards strengthening of capacities in health research and institutions in sub-saharan Africa to bridge the 10/90 gap. There is also the need to find better ways of translating health research results conducted within the framework of fundamental ethical principles into action and policy implementations.

Acknowledgements

The authors wish to thank the Council for International Organizations of Medical Sciences (CIOMS), the World Health Organization (WHO) for the free accessible document that facilitated the preparation of this document. International Ethical Guidelines for Biomedical Research Involving Human Subjects of Geneva 1993 that was very useful for the preparation of this document. The national ethics committee of Cameroon for the technical support in putting together this writes up. The Ministry of Higher Education is also acknowledged for the research allowance that supported processing charge of the manuscript.

Author details

CN Fokunang[1,2,3], EA Tembe-Fokunang[1], M. Djuidje Ngounoue[2], P.C. Chi[2], J Ateudjieu[2], Awah Pascal[4], G. Magne[2], N.M. Ndje[2], O.M.T. Abena[1], D. Sprumont[5] and Kaptue Lazare[2]

*Address all correspondence to: charlesfokunang@yahoo.co.uk

1 Faculty of Medicine and Biomedical Sciences, University of Yaoundé 1, Cameroon

2 Cameroon National Ethics Committee (CNEC), Yaoundé, Cameroon

3 Faculty of Health Sciences, University of Bamenda, Bambili, Cameroon

4 Department of Philosophy, Faculty of Arts and Social Sciences, University of Yaoundé 1, Cameroon

5 Chaire de Droit de la Santé, University of Neuchatel, Switzerland

References

[1] Barrett DH, Bernier RH, Sowell AL .Strengthening public health ethics at the centers for disease control and prevention.; Centers for Disease Control and Prevention Public Health Ethics Committee Steering Group. Journal Public Health Management Practice. 2008; 14(4):348-53.

[2]   Beauchamp, T.L., Childress, J.F. Principles of Biomedical Ethics, 5th edition Oxford University Press. 2001.

[3]   Beauchamp, T. The concept of paternalism in biomedical ethics. In Beauchamp, T. Standing on principles. New York: Oxford University Press 2010; pp. 101–119).

[4]   Beecher, H.K. Ethics and Clinical Research. New England Journal of Medicine. 1966. 274, 1354.

[5]   Benatar, S. R. (2002). Reflections and recommendations on research ethics in developing countries. Social Science and Medicine, 54(7), 1131–1141.

[6]   Bernheim, R.G., Melnick, A. Principled leadership in public health: integrating ethics into practice and management. Journal Public Health Management Practice.2008; 14(4):358-66.

[7]   Beskow, L.M., Namey, E.E., Cadigan, R.J., Brazg, T., Crouch, J., Henderson, G.E., Michie M., Nelson, D.K., Tabor, H.K., Wilfond, B.S. Research participants' perspectives on genotype-driven research recruitment. Journal of Empirical Research for Human Research Ethics.2011; 6(4):3-20.

[8]   Bhutta, Z.A., (2002). Ethics in international health research:a perspective from the developing world. Bulletin WHO, 80:114-120.

[9]   Buchanan, D. R. Autonomy, paternalism, and justice: Ethical priorities in public health. American Journal of Public Health, 2008; 98(1), 15.

[10] Cadigan, R.J., Michie, M., Henderson, G., Davis, A.M., Beskow, L.M. The meaning of genetic research results: reflections from individuals with and without a known genetic disorder.J Empirical Research and Human Research Ethics. 2011; 6(4):30-40.

[11] Chilengi, R. An ethics perspective on responsibilities of investigators, sponsors and research participants. Acta Tropica, 2009; 112S:S53-S62.

[12] Council for International Organizations of Medical Sciences (CIOMS) .International Guidelines for Biomedical Research Involving Human Subjects. Geneva.CIOMS; 2002; pp.112.

[13] Department of Health. Tackling health inequalities: 10 years on, Publication No. 291444, London: Crown.2009.

[14] Emanuel, E., Wendler, D., Killen, J., and Grady, C. What makes clinical research in developing countries ethical? the benchmarks of ethical research. The Journal of Infectious Diseases,2004; 189(5), 930–937.

[15] Fineberg, H.V.Shattuck Lecture. A successful and sustainable health system--how to get there from here. North England Journal of Medicine. 2012; 15; 366(11):1020-7.

[16] Gitau-Mburu, D. Should public health is exempt from ethical regulations? Intricacies of research versus activity.East Africa Journal of Public Health. 2008; (3):160-2.

[17] Gollust, S.E., Baum, N.M., Jacobson, P.D. Politics and public health ethics in practice: right and left meet right and wrong. Journal of Public Health Management Practice. 2008. 14(4):340-7.

[18] Huddle TS. Honesty is an internal norm of medical practice and the best poli-cy.American Journal of Bioethics.2012; 12(3):15-27.

[19] Hyder, A.A., Merritt, M., Ali, J., Tran, N.T., Subramaniam, K., Akhtar, T. Integrating ethics, health policy and health systems in low- and middle-income countries: case studies from Malaysia and Pakistan. Bulletin World Health Organization.2008; 86 (8): 606-611.

[20] International Conference on Harmonization (ICH) Guidelines for Good Clinical Prac-tice,1996. Available freely on the websites and other sources.

[21] Jefferson, A.L., Carmona, H., Gifford, K.A., Lambe, S., Byerly, L.K., Cantwell, N.G., Tripodis, Y., Karlawish, J. Clinical Research Risk Assessment among Individuals with Mild Cognitive Impairment. American Journal of Geriatrics and Psychiatry. 2012; 30. 12-30.

[22] Joyce, G.F., Carrera, M.P., Goldman, D.P., Sood, N., Physician prescribing behavior and its impact on patient-level outcomes American Journal of Management Care. 2011; 1;17(12):e462-71.

[23] Kilama, W.L. The 10/90 gap in sub-Saaran Africa: Resolving inequities in health Re-search. Acta Tropica 2009; 112S:S8-S15.

[24] Kost, R.G., Lee, L.M., Yessis, J., Coller, B.S., Henderson, D.K. Assessing research par-ticipants' perceptions of their clinical research experiences; Research Participant Per-ception Survey Focus Group Subcommittee. Clinical Translational Science.2011; 4(6): 403-13.

[25] Krech R.Working on the social determinants of health is central to public health. Journal Public Health Policy.2012; 33(2):279-84.2012.10.

[26] Lavery, J.V., Harrington, L.C., Scott, T.W. Ethical , Social, and Cultural considera-tions for the site selection for research with genetically modified mosquitoes. Ameri-can Journal of Tropical Medicine and Hygiene, 2008; 79 (3), 312-318.

[27] London AJ, Kimmelman J, Carlisle B . Research ethics. Rethinking research ethics: the case of post-marketing trials. Science 2012; 4; 336(6081):544-5.

[28] Nicholas, J. Next steps in clinical trial redesign. Journal of National Cancer Institute. 2012; 18;104(2):90-2.

[29] Nuffield Council on Bioethics. Public health: Ethical issues. Cambridge: Cambridge Publishers, 2007, p212.

[30] Nyika, A., Kilama, W., Chilengi, R., Tangwa, G., Tindana, P., Ndebele, P., Ikingura, J., Composition, training needs and independence of ethics review committees across

Africa: are the gate-keepers rising to the emerging challenges? Journal of Medical Ethics, 2009: 35, 189-193.

[31] Omonzejele, P.FIs the codification of vulnerability in international documents a sufficient mechanism of protection in the clinical research ethics context? Medical Law. 2011: 30(4):497 515.

[32] Reiter-Theil, S., Agich, G.J., Research on clinical ethics and consultation. Introduction to the theme. Medical Health Care Philos. 2008; 11(1):3-5.

[33] Sade, R.M. Why physicians should not lie for their patients. American Journal of Bioethics. 2012:12(3):17-9.

[34] Tangwa, G.B., Ethical principles in health research and review process. Acta Tropica, 2009. 112S:S2-S7.

[35] Thomas, J.C., MacDonald, P.D., Wenink, E., Ethical decision making in a crisis: a case study of ethics in public health emergencies : Journal Public Health Management Practice; 2009. 15, (2):E16-21.

[36] Wikler, D., and Brock, D. W. Population-level bioethics: Mapping a new agenda. In Dawson, A., and Verweij, M, Ethics, prevention, and public health, 2007. p. 78. New York: Oxford University Press.

[37] World Medical Association Declaration of Helsinki, Available at http://www.wma.net/e/policy/17-c-e.html. Ethical principles for Medical Research Involving Human Subjects. 52nd WMA General Assembly, Edinburgh, Scotland. www.dndi.org (accessed 04.08.12).

[38] Blakemore C: Misguided thinking on animals. Nature 1989;339:414.

[39] Bowman P: Institutional animal care and use committee review of wildlife field research. Lab Animal 1989;18:28-30.

[40] Britt D: Ethics, ethical committees and animal experimentation. Nature 1984;311:503-506.

[41] Dawkins MS: From an animal's point of view: Motivation, fitness, and animal welfare. Behav Brain Sci 1990;13:1-61.

[42] Duggan JM: Resource allocation and bioethics. Lancet 1989;1:772-773.

[43] Fox MW: A call for common understanding of animal welfare, animal rights, and animal well-being. J Am Vet Med Assoc 1990;196:832-833.

[44] Good RA: The value of animal research. Science 1990;248:538

[45] Harvard University's Office of Government and Community Affairs: The Animal Rights Movement in the United States: Its Composition, Funding Sources, Goals, Strategies and Potential Impact on Research. Clarks Summit, PA, Society for Animal Rights, Inc., 1982..

[46] Hoff C: Immoral and moral uses of animals. New England Journal of Medicine 1980;302:115-118.

[47] Lutts RH: The Nature Fakers: Wildlife, Science and Sentiment. Golden, CO, Fulcrum Publishing, 1990.

[48] Markell DL: The case for revising our laws on animal experimentation. International Journal for the Study of Animal Problems 1981;2:87-95.

[49] Meischke HRC, Begbie RA: Philosophical and moral aspects of the use of animals in experimentation. Australian Veterinary Association Yearbook 1981;232-237.

[50] Miller HB, Williams WH: Ethics and Animals. Clifton,NJ, Humanic Press, 1983..

[51] National Research Council: Use of Laboratory Animals in Biomedical and Behavioral Research. Washington, D.C., National Academy Press, 1988..

[52] Thelestam M, Gunnarsson A: The ethics of animal experimentation. Proceedings of the second CFN symposium held in Stockholm, Sweden, August 12-14, 1985. Acta Physiologica Scandinavica 1986;128:269pp.

[53] National Commission for the Protection of Human Subjects of Biomedical and Behavioural Research subjects (NCPHSBBRS). Protection of Human Subjects: Institutional Review Boards. Fed Regist; 1978; 43:231-561.

[54] ICH-GCP E6. International Conference on Harmonization Guidance: Good Clinical Practices. Global Medical Education and Development. 1997. Available at http// www.icr-global.org.

[55] Lavery VJ, Grady C, Wahl RE, Emmanuel JE. Ethical issues in International Biomedical Research: A case book, Oxford University Press, 2007.

[56] United Nation. Universal Declaration of Human Rights. Available at http:// www.un.org/en/document/udhr/.1948.

[57] World Health Organization. Operational Guidelines for ethics committees that review biomedical research, available at http://apps.who.int/tdr/svc/publications/training-guideline-publications/operational-guidelines-ethics-biomedical-research, 2000.

[58] Shemdoe GS. Introduction to intellectual property rights for investigator in health research and institutional intellectual property policy. Acta Tropica 2009; 112S:S80-S83.

[59] Kilama W. From Research to control: Translating research findings into health policies operational guidelines and health products. Acta Tropica, 2009; 112S:S91-S101.

[60] World Medical Association. Declaration of Helsinki. Ethical principles for research involving human subjects. Adopted by the 52 nd WMA General Assembly, Seoul, South Korea, 2008.

[61] Amir JA. Research and Legal Liability. Acta Tropica, 2009;112S:S71-S75).

Chapter 10

Mental Health and Social Capital:
Social Capital as a Promising Initiative to Improving the Mental Health of Communities

Emma Bassett and Spencer Moore

Additional information is available at the end of the chapter

1. Introduction

Mental illness is a growing public health concern and has been estimated to impact up to 450 million people across the globe [1]. In countries with particularly high prevalence rates, more than a third of the population will meet the criteria for some form of mental illness during their lifetime [2]. Mood and anxiety disorders tend to have the highest prevalence rates and it has been projected that major depressive disorder will be the second leading disease burden worldwide by 2020 [3]. Mental illness often has chronic effects that can last a life-time and negatively impacts individuals' quality of life at home, work, school, and in social settings [4].

The identification of specific factors that improve or worsen one's mental health is beneficial when aiming to understand onset and course of illness and also for preventing declines in mental health that may sequentially lead to clinical-level cases. Recognizing the key contributors to mental health is a crucial step in enhancing the efficiency of health promotion initiatives. Social capital has been identified as an upstream determinant of mental health and may be particularly beneficial when taking a population health approach. Social capital refers to the material, informational and affective resources to which individuals and, potentially, groups have access through their social connections [5]. It has been proposed that high levels of social capital result in improved mental well-being in both individuals and communities and that enhancing the social resources of groups may allow for improvement in overall population mental health.

To determine social factors that contribute to mental health and to identify who is at greatest risk, there is a need to understand how social capital may help or hinder mental well-being and to examine how predictive factors vary between groups. This chapter will begin by describing the development of social capital, the debates that exist within the current social capital literature, and the ways in which social capital may be connected to health related outcomes. Next, the current literature will be examined in greater detail through the conduction of a systematic search of recently published studies. Findings of these studies, limitations in the current literature and suggestions for future research directions will be outlined. Lastly, public health implications and support for incorporating social capital into population-based mental health promotion programs will be discussed.

2. The development of social capital

Social capital is most often associated with concepts such as trust, norms, power, relationships, and networks and although it is relatively new to health and social sciences research as a whole, its separate components have been studied for centuries [6]. At the basis of social capital is the notion that people invest in social relations with expected returns [7]. While theorists tend to agree upon this underlying understanding, the specific definitions and measurements used in the social capital literature are often disputed [7]. In fact, discrepancies in the definition have existed since the very first attempts to define social capital beginning in the late 1980s and early 1990s. Bourdieu, Coleman, and Putnam are often referred to as early theorists of social capital, and their approaches have influenced the ways in which social capital is viewed in the field of health sciences today [7,8]. Bourdieu was interested in the distribution of social capital within society and explained that like economic or cultural capital, social capital was unequally distributed among individuals and groups [7,8]. Coleman's approach to social capital was similar to Bourdieu's in that they both emphasized the importance of examining social networks. Rather than considering structural measures of social networks, as Bourdieu and Coleman suggested, Putnam focused on relational factors including norms of trust and reciprocity [7]. Despite advances in social capital, there has tended to be a divide between those who follow approaches that are more in line with Putnam's work and those who support Bourdieu or Coleman's definitions of social capital. These approaches have led to two somewhat divergent dimensions of social capital. The first dimension can be labelled 'communitarian', and the second 'network'.

2.1. Debates within the literature

2.1.1. Communitarian versus network approaches to social capital

A central debate within social capital research is whether social capital is a communitarian- or network-driven phenomenon. Communitarian approaches to social capital typically include psychosocial or cognitive constructs (e.g.,perceptions of trust or cohesion) as well as indicators of community participation [8]. Putnam's definition, which focuses on community-level communitarian social capital, has been the most dominant in health sciences to date. In his definition, social capital encompasses five main principles: (1) 'community networks'; the number and density of voluntary, state, and personal networks, (2) 'civic engagement';

the amount of participation in civic networks, (3)'local civic identity'; the degree to which there is a sense of belonging, solidarity, and equality between community members, (4)'reciprocity and cooperation norms'; the degree to which there is a sense of obligation to help others, as well as feelings that others will reciprocate in the future, and (5) 'community trust'; the degree of trust held by individuals within the network [6,10]. Although community networks are included in this definition, Putnam and others who follow a communitarian approach typically focus on the latter four components. A network approach, as represented in the work of Bourdieu, defines social capital as resources that are accessed within social networks for the benefit of individuals or groups [11]. Network approaches to social capital measure directly how and to whom individuals are connected within their social structures by investigating the size, range, and diversity of individuals' social connections, and the resources potentially available within those networks. Although researchers typically adhere to one or the other of these two approaches, some recent studies have sought to compare communitarian and network measures within their work to understand better the potential mechanisms linking social capital to health [5,12]. An approach that includes the incorporation of both communitarian and network dimensions of analysis in studies of social capital is supported throughout this chapter. A more comprehensive approach to social capital will provide researchers and health professionals with a greater understanding of how cognitive, participatory, and network-related elements may work together to influence health outcomes. Understanding the range of social capital processes that may influence health is challenging if social capital dimensions are examined separately.

Critiques of the communitarian approach

Although the communitarian approach to social capital is the most visible in health research today, researchers have expressed several concerns about its prominence. First, the predominance of communitarian approaches in public health research has been largely due to the ways in which social capital was initially translated and cited in the field of public health [8]. Early leading papers on social capital focused on communitarian aspects of social capital, which has resulted in less attention to actual network dimensions [8]. Furthermore, network measures have appeared only recently in the social capital literature, whereas cognitive measures of trust and perceived cohesion appeared early on. Ease of measurement may be a second factor contributing to the uptake of the communitarian approach. The inclusion of network measures in research centred on social capital may give a more complete picture of the association of social capital and mental health outcomes than currently found in the literature.

Second, communitarian measures have often been labelled as proxy, or indirect, measures of social capital since they do not directly assess a person's or group's access to resources [5]. Hence, the communitarian approach has often been criticized for measuring concepts that more closely relate to theories of social cohesion than social capital [7,11]. For example, perceptions of trust may be more suited to measure social cohesion than an individual's general access to resources. Network measures may be advantageous in deciphering the types of resources accessible to individuals and groups within social networks.

A third critique of the communitarian approach lies in its supposed inability to address issues of inequality and power [8]. Other forms of capital (i.e., economic and human) have historically addressed these issues and it seems appropriate that social capital should do the same. Although social capital has been criticized for falling short in this regard, it may not be the concept itself that is ill suited to address distributions and inequalities in social capital within and between societies, but the communitarian measures that are often used. Network measures may offer clearer insights into inequality due in part to the measure's capacity to compare and contrast the types of resources accessed by certain individuals and groups.

2.1.2. Dimensions and levels of social capital

Debates within the social capital literature also concern the levels and dimensions of analysis. Dimensions of social capital include the aforementioned approaches of psychosocial, participation, and network. In terms of the levels of analysis, researchers sometimes differ in their opinions as to whether social capital should be measured with individual- or ecological-level measures. Table 1 provides examples of common individual- and ecological-level measures of social capital according to each dimension. At an ecological level, social capital measures are meant to reflect group and neighbourhood levels of connectivity [6, 14]. Ecological measures capture elements of the community that are often not measurable through individual-level data [13] and are often derived from aggregating individual-level measures. It has been suggested that aggregate data is a proxy measure of exogenous characteristics and more direct measures of neighbourhoods must be created to address this issue [15]. Multilevel studies are increasingly used to assess associations between social capital and health outcomes, and have the benefit of being able to disentangle individual- and neighbourhood-level characteristics [14].

Dimension	Level	
	Individual	Ecological (area)
Cognitive/Psychosocial	Trust, Perceptions	Community trust, Social cohesion
Participation	Participation	Area participation
Network	Ego networks	Network structures

Table 1. Dimensions and levels of analysis in social capital.

Another debate that has arisen from social capital research has been whether social capital is a concept that should be assessed generally or within certain environments, such as within neighbourhoods. General social capital would represent an individual's general levels of trust towards others, their overall participation in associations, and resources obtained from their entire social networks. Others postulate that although social capital may be measured generally, it can also be assessed in more specific contextual environments [16]. For instance, examining social capital both inside and outside individual's neighbourhoods allows for identifying where people are accessing valued resources [12]. Knowledge of whether the benefits of social capital for health arise from network sources within or outside the neighbourhood may be important for research and health promotion purposes. Neighbourhood social capital may be measured at an individual-level and is most commonly measured through self-report. With regards to each dimension of social capital, psychosocial measures assess perceived neighbourhood cohesion or trust in neighbours; participation measures would assess involvement in neighbourhood associations; and network measures would examine resources accessed within the neighbourhood. Both general- and neighbourhood-specific measures of social capital are being included in health research to gain a more well-rounded understanding of how and where individuals access their resources.

3. General overview: Social capital and health

3.1. Mechanisms linking social capital to health

Research on social capital has examined a range of health outcomes which have included health-related behaviours, as well as physical and mental illnesses. Social capital may influence health outcomes within neighbourhoods through mechanisms that include: (1) rapid promotion and diffusion of health information, (2) ensuring that health behaviours and norms are adopted, and (3) minimizing opportunities for negative health behaviours [17]. These mechanisms more closely relate to the communitarian rather than the network approach to social capital due to their focus on norms and social cohesion. Several broad areas of physical health are associated with social capital in the communitarian sense, and include mortality and life expectancy, self-rated health, cardiovascular disease, cancer, obesity, diabetes, and infectious disease [18].

High levels of social capital at group, neighbourhood, and network levels has been shown to provide individuals with increased resources in terms of finance, care, and transportation which in turn is found to benefit overall health [19]. The measurement of individual resource access via social connections, along with the emotional support received from these connections, are said to reinforce physical and mental health [19]. For example, those with large social networks may have greater access to social support, which in turn leads to better health [16]. Furthermore, those who have access to network members leading healthy lifestyles may turn to these connections for information which may in turn reinforce positive health behaviours [16]. Researchers have highlighted the benefits of network capital by relating those to the potential positive health benefits that may result from a person's or a group's greater access to informational, material, and socially supportive types of resources. Health-related outcomes that have been shown associated with network components of social capital include self-rated health and obesity [5,12,20]. Thus, research indicates important associations between social capital and health outcomes using both communitarian and network measures. As research moves forward, it is important to understand how both dimensions may work together to influence health outcomes.

3.2. Social capital and mental health

A general search of the social capital and mental health literature show that studies of depression occupy a central part of the literature. The high prevalence rates of depression and the ease of measuring depression through short questionnaires likely contribute in part to prominence of research on depression and social capital. Most studies of social capital and depression have used communitarian measures of social capital, such as trust and participation. Several studies have shown individual-level generalized trust to be inversely related to depressive symptoms [13,21-25]. In studies measuring perceived neighbourhood trust, higher trust in neighbours has also been shown to be a protective factor of depression [22,25]. Studies using indicators of community participation and volunteer work to measure social capital have not shown social capital to be related to depression [22]. While individual-level studies have lent some support for the relationship between depression and social capital, the measures of social capital used in these studies are problematic since they tend to include only communitarian measures such as trust and participation.

Less research has examined social capital and mental health using formal social network data. Analyses that have examined social networks and depression have shown that individuals who report being socially isolated within their social networks are more likely to have depression than those who report more network ties [22,25-28]. Using a resource generator to measure access to specific types of resources within individual's neighbourhoods, researchers did not find any association of social capital with depression over a six-month period [25]. Another study found that women with core neighbourhood ties reported fewer depressive symptoms when compared to women with both neighbourhood and non-neighbourhood core ties, demonstrating the importance of examining neighbourhood connectivity and mental health [29]. One research group [30] conducted a particularly comprehensive study which investigated the spread of depression through social networks. Individuals with several core ties and those who were located centrally within their networks had lower rates of depression [30]. It was found that depressive symptoms do spread within social networks and individuals with depression are more likely to have close ties that also suffer from depression [30]. In fact, having close ties with depression doubled the probability that the respondent will develop depressive symptoms themselves [30]. Initial findings thus demonstrate that both network and communitarian components of social capital may be associated with depressive symptoms, and such relationships require further exploration.

Further research on social capital and other forms of mental illness, including major depression, is needed. On an international level, anxiety disorders typically have even higher prevalence rates than mood disorders with lifetime estimates of approximately 16.6% [31-32]. Anxiety disorders include generalized anxiety, post-traumatic stress, specific phobias, obsessive-compulsive, panic, and social anxiety disorders [32]. Almost half of those diagnosed with depression are also diagnosed with an anxiety disorder [31]. Yet, research studies examining social capital as a potential determinant of anxiety disorders (and other forms of mental illness) are largely understudied. Again, research has tended to focus on communitarian dimensions when examining anxiety. Initial studies suggest inverse associations between psychosocial dimensions of social capital with anxiety symptoms and post-traumatic stress disorder [33-35]. When network and participation items were measured together in one scale, "structural" social capital was also shown to be negatively associated with anxiety symptoms [34]. More research is needed that examines formal network data in relation to various mental illnesses.

4. Systematic review of literature

4.1. Rationale and objectives

Earlier reviews of social capital and mental health have shown inconsistent results in the association between social capital and mental health [6]. Inconsistencies in the measures of social capital make it difficult to compare studies and to draw common conclusions from the literature. To summarize recent findings on social capital and mental health, we performed a systematic literature review. Compiling and comparing results allows for researchers and health professionals to determine which dimensions of social capital may be most important when examining important mental health outcomes. Gaps within the literature may also be discovered through this process. The main research questions underlying our review were (1) how has social capital been measured in recent studies of social capital and mental health (e.g., psychosocial, participation, or network measures)?; (2) what are the main findings from these studies?

4.2. Methods

Search Procedure. The literature review search was conducted in PubMed; a database that includes access to various health-related articles and journals. Search terms included "social capital AND mental health", "social capital AND mental illness", "social capital AND depression", "social capital AND depressive symptoms", "social capital AND anxiety", and "social capital AND schizophrenia". Search criteria specified that terms were included in the titles of research papers and that articles were published within the last 5 years. After abstracts were gathered, studies that did not in fact examine direct associations between social capital and depressive symptoms, and articles that were not obtainable in English were excluded.

4.3. Results

Search Results. PubMed yielded 31 articles. The majority of articles (n = 16) were derived from the "social capital AND mental health" search. No articles were found with "social capital AND mental illness" or "social capital AND anxiety" searches. The search "social capital AND depression" yielded 10 articles, "social capital AND depressive symptoms" resulted in 4 articles found, and "social capital AND schizophrenia" generated 1 article. Of these articles, 3 were not available in English and 7 did not look at direct associations between social capital and mental health. The final article count included in analyses was 21 [16,21-22,25,33-49].

Mental Health and Social Capital: Social Capital as a Promising Initiative to
Improving the Mental Health of Communities

285

Table Information. Table 2 includes summary information for each of the 21 studies. In-formation obtained from each study included: citation number, country of study, study design, sample, measures of social capital, dimension/s of social capital measured, mental health outcome, dimension/s of social capital associated with outcome, and main study findings. In order to compare the findings of studies measuring similar dimensions of so-cial capital, "dimension of analysis" and "social capital dimensions associated with out-come" categories were created. Dimensions of analysis include psychosocial, participation, and network dimensions discussed previously. In many instances, researchers did not use these terms, but may have used 'cognitive' instead of 'psychosocial', or 'structural' instead of 'participation'. In these cases, we re-classified the terms to correspond with one of our defined dimensions (ie. 'cognitive' became 'psychosocial'). Terms used in the "measures of social capital" and " study findings" were consistent with those used in the original re-search articles.

Descriptive Results. Studies took place in 11 countries across the globe. Most studies meas-ured social capital and mental health outcomes in the general adult population. However, three studies examined social capital and mental health in adolescents, and three examined associations in older adults. Although several studies were cross-sectional in design, seven were longitudinal or prospective cohort studies. The majority of studies examined depres-sion or depressive symptoms as a mental health outcome (n = 15). Other mental health out comes examined included anxiety (n = 2), post-traumatic stress disorder (PTSD) (n = 2), schizophrenia (n = 1), psychological distress (n = 1), and self-rated mental health (n = 4). Var-ious social capital measures were used in study analyses. Consistent with previous litera-ture, psychosocial (n= 17) and participation (n= 9) dimensions were most frequently measured in conjunction with mental health.

Social Capital and Mental Health Findings

Psychosocial dimensions and mental health. Eleven studies examining the direct associa-tion between psychosocial dimensions of social capital and depression or depressive symp-toms found that social capital was inversely associated with symptoms. Similar inverse associations were found for studies that included PTSD, anxiety, self-rated poor mental health, and psychological distress as mental health outcomes (N = 7).

Participation dimensions and mental health. Studies reported mixed results when examin-ing direct associations between participation dimensions and mental health outcomes. Of the 3 studies examining participation in relation to depression or depressive symptoms, none found participation in local contexts to be associated with decreased risk of experienc-ing depressive symptoms. On the other hand, participation was associated with self-rated mental health status in three additional studies.

Network dimensions and mental health. Results of studies examining network dimensions of social capital in association with mental health outcomes were inconsistent. Two of the four studies found network capital to be inversely associated with depressive symptoms. Network dimensions were not examined in relation to other mental health outcomes.

Study	Country of Study	Study Design	Sample	Social Capital (constructs measured)	Social Capital Dimension Measured*	Mental Health Outcome (measure)	Dimension Associated with Outcome?*	Main Findings
16.	USA	Cross-sectional, multilevel	N=497, adults.	Structural Network Capital (reach, range and diversity; Resource Network Capital (embedded employment, transportation, and educational resources)	N	Depressive symptoms (CESD-7)	N = yes	Network density (B = -.54), voluntary organization integration (B = -.34), access to mainstream individuals (B = -.13) and access to transportation resources (B = -.48) associated with decreased symptoms. Network social capital was mediator between neighbourhood disadvantage and symptoms.
21.	Sweden	Cross-sectional	N=7757, students aged 13-18.	Psychosocial (general trust) and Neighbourhood social capital (neighbourhood cohesion, reciprocity, safety and cleanliness)	PS	Depression (Depression self-rating scale, DSRS)	PS = yes	Neighbourhood social capital (B = -.10) and general social trust (B = -.20) negatively associated with depression.
22.	USA	Prospective study	N=724, adults.	Cognitive (trust in neighbours, sense of belonging, mutual aid); Structural (volunteer work, community participation)	PS & P	Major depression (CIDI-SF)	PS = yes P = no	Those with neighbourhood trust less likely to develop major depression during follow-up (OR=0.43). After excluding participants with depression at baseline, associations became non-significant. Structural dimensions not associated with depression.
25.	England	Longitudinal, six-month prospective cohort study	N=158, adults.	Network resources (Resource Generator-UK: access to 27 resources and skills)	N	Depression (HAD-D)	N = no	Social capital not independently associated with depression.
33.	England	Cross-sectional survey, multilevel	N=232, adults.	Community social capital (SA-SCAT), structural (know individuals holding certain job titles, participation) and cognitive (ie. trust).	PS, N, & P	Post-traumatic stress as indicator of disaster mental health (PTSD	PS = yes P&N = no	High cognitive social capital negatively associated with posttraumatic stress (B=-.36). Structural social capital not directly associated with PTSD.

Mental Health and Social Capital: Social Capital as a Promising Initiative to
Improving the Mental Health of Communities

287

					Checklist – Civilian version).		
34.	England	Cross-sectional N=232, adults.	Cognitive (trust, mutual help, reciprocity) Structural (community linkages) (SA+SCAT+15 item questionnaire)	PS & N	PTSD (PTSD Checklist Civilian Version) anxiety and depression (Hopkins Symptom Checklist-25)	PS = yes (mental health) P&N = yes (anxiety)	Cognitive social capital negatively associated with PTSD (B=-.28), anxiety (B=-.13) and depression (B=-.26) and structural social capital was positively associated with anxiety (B=.13).
35.	USA	Cross-sectional N=205, adult women.	Trust (neighbourhood trust, trust in people) Volunteering	PS & P	Depressive symptoms (Items from PHQ9, K10, CIDI-SF), anxiety symptoms (CIDI-SF, K10)	PS&P = yes	Social capital negatively associated with depression (B=-.41) and anxiety (B=-.41). Social capital mediated the association between acculturation and depression and anxiety symptoms.
36.	Mexico	Longitudinal N=2611, adults ages 65-74.	Social capital (groups and networks, trust and solidarity, collective action and cooperation, information and communication, social cohesion and inclusion, empowerment and political action)	PS, N & P	Depressive symptoms (Geriatric Depression Scale). Incidence assessed at 11-month follow-up.	PS&P&N = yes	Higher social capital at baseline associated with lower incidence rates of depressive symptoms in women only (OR=.73).
37.	Ireland	Cross-sectional survey N=5992, adults.	Trust	PS	Self-reported mental health	PS = yes	Those from rural areas more likely to report high trust and poorer mental health.
38.	Finland	Cross-sectional N=1102, adults ages 65 and older.	Cognitive social capital (social support, trust, help from neighbours)	PS	Self-reported depression (CIDI-SF) and Psychological distress (General Health Questionnaire)	PS = yes	Cognitive social capital (difficult access to help from neighbours) associated with depression. Not having people to count on, lack of concern from others, and mistrust towards others associated with psychological distress.
39.	Sweden, Finland	Cross-sectional N=6838, adults aged	Psychosocial (trust in friends and neighbours);	PS & N	Depression (Geriatric	PS = yes N = yes	Low structural capital, measured by infrequent

		65, 70, 75, and 80.	structural (frequency of social contact with friends and neighbours)		Depression Scale-4)			contact with friends (OR=1.53) and neighbours (OR=1.33) associated with depression. Mistrust between friends (OR = 2.01), but not neighbours, associated with increased symptoms.
40.	Japan	National cross-sectional survey, multilevel	N=5956, adults.	Cognitive (trust); structural (membership in sports, recreation, hobby or cultural groups).	PS & P	Self-reported mental health (SF-36).	PS = yes P = yes	Social capital associated with mental health at individual and ecological levels. Cognitive (B= 9.56) and structural social capital (B=8.72) at the ecological level associated with better self-rated mental health.
41.	South Korea	Cross-sectional survey, multilevel	N=5934, adults.	Participation (individual-level participation in organizations); cognitive social capital(individual-level perceived helpfulness); contextual social capital (derived from individual measures)	PS & P	Mental health (self-rated 8-item scale).	PS = yes P = yes	Organizational participation (B=0.151) and cognitive social capital (B=.237) positively associated with mental health. Contextual level of social capital not associated.
42.	USA	Cross-sectional, survey	N=155, adults.	Religious social capital (religious involvement/use of spiritual leader for personal problems); group participation(membership in various groups); social trust(general trust, trust in other homeless, trust in service providers, trust in community leaders); bridging social capital(close ties different to themselves)	PS, N & P	Depression (CESD)	PS = yes P = no N = no P&PS=yes	Higher religious social capital (B = - .21) and higher trust (B = -.18) negatively associated with symptoms. Bridging social capital and group participation not associated.
43.	Germany	Cross-sectional, online survey	N=328, adults.	Perceived social capital at work (Social Capital in Organizations Scale:	PS	Depressive symptoms (German	PS = yes	Lower levels of perceived workplace social capital

Mental Health and Social Capital: Social Capital as a Promising Initiative to
Improving the Mental Health of Communities

289

				cohesion, trust, values, and support)		version of World Health Organization Five-Item Well-Being Index)			associated with depressive symptoms (OR=.76)
44.	England	Cross-sectional, survey	N=16459, adults.	Neighbourhood-level social capital (social cohesion, trust and social disorganization)	PS	Incidence of schizophrenia (ICD-10 F20). Incidence estimated using local data.	PS = yes		Association between social cohesion and trust and schizophrenia was u-shaped. Compared with neighbourhoods with medial levels of social cohesion and trust, incidence rates significantly higher in neighbourhoods with low (IRR 2.0) and high (IRR 2.5) cohesion and trust.
45.	Finland	Prospective cohort study, multilevel	N=33577, adults.	Workplace social capital (trust, norms, cohesion between other employees and employer)	PS	Depression (self-reported physician-diagnosed and recorded antidepressant prescriptions)	PS = yes		Odds for depression 20-50% higher for employees with low compared to high social capital. Aggregate-level social capital not associated with subsequent depression.
46.	Finland	Longitudinal cohort study	N=25763, adults.	Vertical social capital (trust and reciprocity between employee and employer); horizontal social capital (trust, reciprocity and norms among coworkers)	PS	Depression (self-reported physician-diagnosed and recorded antidepressant prescriptions)	PS = yes		Odds for new physician-diagnosed depression and antidepressant treatment were 30-50% higher for employees with low compared to high vertical and horizontal workplace social capital.
47.	England	Longitudinal, multistage	N=15770, adolescents.	Community social capital (parental involvement at school, sociability, involvement in activities outside the home)	P	Mental health (General Health Questionnaire-12)	P = yes		Adolescent sociability associated with decreased psychological distress only in boys (OR=.64).
48.	South Africa	Cross-sectional	N=16800 adults ages 15 and over.	Neighbourhood-level social capital (aggregated: support and reciprocity, association activity, collective norms, safety);	PS & P	Depressive symptoms (CESD-10)	PS = yes P = no		Compared to those with high neighbourhood-level social capital, those with moderate (B = 0.82) and low (B=0.89) social capital more likely to report symptoms. Compared to those with

			Individual-level trust and civic participation					high trust, moderate trust associated with increased symptoms (B=0.83). No associations found for participation.
49.	China	Longitudinal	N=5164, adolescents and their parents.	Family social capital (frequency have dinner with parents, home alone, go out with unfamiliar friends, parents check homework); Community social capital (perceived safety, neighbourhood ties, neighbourhood cohesion)	PS	Depressive symptoms (CESD)	PS = yes	Higher community social capital associated with lower levels of adolescent depressive symptoms (B=-.97). Family social capital mediated effects of contextual factors on adolescent depressive symptoms. Female adolescents reported more depressive symptoms as result of lower availability of family social capital.

*PS = psychosocial, P = participation, N = network.

Table 2. Search findings of social capital and mental health literature. Studies published within last 5 years.

Composite social capital and mental health. Five studies used scale or composite scores which included two or more dimensions of social capital. When measures of participation and network dimensions of social capital were assessed together, social capital was found to be positively associated with anxiety symptoms. On the other hand, these dimensions were not associated with post-traumatic stress disorder or depressive symptoms. Psychosocial and participation dimensions were also used as composite measures of social capital (N = 2). The fusion of both dimensions is consistent with a communitarian approach to social capital. Both studies found communitarian social capital to be inversely associated with depressive symptoms. Communitarian dimensions were also inversely associated with anxiety symptoms. Lastly, when all three dimensions of social capital were included as a social capital composite score, social capital was negatively associated with depressive symptoms in older adults.

4.4. Discussion

In this literature review, the diverse measurement of social capital in recent studies of mental health and social capital was investigated, and key findings of these studies were highlighted. The first objective of this review was to examine how social capital is currently being measured in the mental health literature. Studies of communitarian social capital were dominant. Psychosocial dimensions of social capital were included in most studies, and participation dimensions were second-most common. Network measures were least common. Yet, with network components increasingly recognized as a core construct of social capital in research on social capital and physical health outcomes [5], it is important that researchers and health professionals also consider network capital in studies of mental health.

Measurement of the psychosocial, participation, and network dimensions of social capital were often inconsistent. Psychosocial measures included a broad range of cognitive and so-cio-relational characteristics. Despite variations within psychosocial measurement, results consistently found psychosocial social capital to be associated with various mental health outcomes including depression, anxiety, PTSD, psychological distress, and self-reported mental health. Such findings speak to the magnitude of impact that psychosocial character-istics likely have on one's mental health. Measures of participation across studies tended to assess similar constructs and may allow for greater cross-comparison between studies. When examined as a separate dimension, participation was not associated with depressive symptoms. Comparing studies on psychosocial and participatory social capital with those that examined network social capital and mental health is difficult. Studies used various net-work measures and many failed to conduct comprehensive analyses of social networks and resources. For example, some studies investigated social networks as a complementary com-ponent to the participation dimension of social capital, but did not exclusively focus on this dimension of social capital as a potential key contributor to mental health. Nevertheless, net-work dimensions of social capital were inversely associated with depressive symptoms in two studies, lending support to the notion that network capital plays an important role in mental health outcomes. No studies in the current search observed network social capital in relation to health outcomes other than depression. More rigorous measurement of network connections and resources is needed to understand how network dimensions of social capi-tal may be associated with mental health outcomes.

4.5. Limitations and strengths of current literature review

There are a few limitations to the current literature review. First, search terms were limited to titles of studies. This was to ensure that the articles included in the review focused pri-marily on social capital and mental health outcomes; yet other studies that examined direct associations may have been missed. Second, articles that were not included in the PubMed database may have been left out from the final list of studies. Third, while common mental illnesses were included in search terms in hopes of capturing a larger range of articles than yielded by general 'mental health' and 'mental illness' searches, studies that examined out-comes other than depression, anxiety, schizophrenia, or general mental health in relation to social capital may have been missed. Researchers who conduct future literature reviews may wish to expand search results to include terms in abstracts or key terms, conduct searches in various databases, and expand searches to include a wider range of mental health outcomes.

This literature review has several strengths. To our knowledge, this is the most recent re-view of the social capital and mental health literature. Mental health research is an ever-growing field and social capital is increasingly examined as a potential contributor to well-being. Consequentially, reviews are needed to inform researchers of other works being conducted in an accessible and informative manner. This literature review has also worked towards drawing common conclusions from diverse studies that previously seemed incomparable. This was done by grouping social capital measures into the three most common dimensions of analysis and comparing findings across various mental health outcomes. As far as we are aware, this is the first review of the social capital literature to compare studies in such a manner. Previous review works have focused on individual- and ecological- levels of social capital in attempts to tease out measurement debates [13], however there has also been a need to understand how dimension of social capital is portrayed in the public health field. Lastly, another major strength of conducting this literature review lies in the implications that can be drawn from it. Several gaps within the literature have been highlighted throughout this review process and directions for future research and health promoting programs can be inferred from these gaps. These points will be expanded upon in the following sections.

5. Limitations in current research and suggested future directions

Having compiled and evaluated the literature, it is apparent that more research, particularly from a network perspective, is needed to understand how social capital contributes to mental health. With several debates surrounding the definition and measurement of social capital, it is evident that researchers must work towards building a consensus. An all-inclusive approach that considers psychosocial, participation, and network dimensions may be particularly beneficial when examining mental health outcomes, since it will allow for clearer depictions of contributing factors to the illness. Furthermore, discrepancies of measurement within each dimension must also be addressed. This might be achieved by building a consensus on the definition of social capital. Once social capital is uniformly defined, gold-standard measures of each dimension can be developed and standardized.

Furthermore, an overwhelming number of studies derived from the literature search measured depression or depressive symptoms as the primary mental health outcome. There is a need to understand how social capital, and its separate dimensions, relate to other relevant mental health issues. For example, other social determinants, including socioeconomic status and gender, have been outlined as potential contributors to anxiety spectrum disorder, and more research is needed to examine how social capital might impact one's risk for experiencing anxiety [50]. Co-morbid mental and physical illness may also be necessary to investigate in future studies of social capital. Current research suggests that social capital may have differential effects on different mental illnesses; however co-morbid illnesses within individuals are largely unexplored [34].

Another potential limitation to the current literature is that results are typically generalizable only to others experiencing symptoms of mental illness. Most studies have not conducted formal clinical diagnoses of the mental health outcome of interest, but have relied on brief questionnaires to assess symptomatology. Elevated symptoms may sometimes correspond with a diagnosable illness, however it has not yet been proven that current study results are applicable to those with clinical-level syndromes.

Having established some preliminary associations between social capital and mental health, more research is needed to determine how social capital may impact mental illness in different groups. Initial research suggests that social capital is an important predictor of mental illness at many different life stages. For example, social capital has been found to be associated with depressive symptoms in children, middle-aged, and older adults [21,36,49]. Studies on gender, social capital and health should be advanced. Recent studies suggest important differences in social capital and mental health between men and women. For example, although social capital has been found to be associated with depressive symptoms in both women and men, women may be more prone to experiencing negative mental health consequences in response to decreased levels of psychosocial and network dimensions of social capital in some instances [51]. Further research is needed to examine group differences between social capital and mental health outcomes.

Lastly, some lingering uncertainty exists when attempting to understand the causal relation between social capital and mental health. While cross-sectional studies have many advantages in terms of brevity and reduced resource load and are helpful when gaining an initial understanding of associations, longitudinal studies within the current area of research is a logical next step. Of the longitudinal studies conducted to date, there is some support that suggests social capital may in turn influence mental health [36,47,49]. Programs that promote mental health also seem to follow this rationale by first altering social constructs with hopes of in turn improving mental well-being. Such efforts will be discussed shortly. While the current evidence points to social capital as a potential contributor to mental health, there is a need for long-term longitudinal studies to ease existing uncertainties. Longitudinal investigations of the relationships between social capital and mental health may help identify specific causal directions, and will inform health professionals when developing tailored community programs.

6. Public health implications

Understanding the role that social capital may play in mental health has broader public health implications in terms of treatment and prevention programs. Several studies included in the literature review emphasized the practical public health implications of their findings [21,33,3-36,38,48]. As well as benefitting the general population, increasing social capital may also be used to address mental health issues faced by vulnerable groups including post-disaster victims, ethnic minorities, women, adolescents, older adults, homeless individuals, and those living in disadvantaged neighbourhoods [21,33,35,38,42,51]. Enhancing social capital within vulnerable groups may be achieved by increasing social skills and developing networks [52]. With increased social capital, it was expected that sequential improvements in mental health might be observed [52]. Since various groups are found to face differential barriers to achieving positive mental well-being, it has been suggested that intervention programs be tailored to specific groups of interest [53].

Determinants at individual, social, organizational and community levels must be considered when creating programs aimed at improving population-level mental health. While individual-level intervention programs may be beneficial in aiding those who require critical mental health care, population-based approaches may be most effective when prevention of mental illness and promotion of mental well-being in broader populations is the goal. Social capital is advantageous in that it can be applied at individual and group levels. From an organizational standpoint, it has been suggested that increased social capital between fellow co-workers and between employees and employers may be one potential outlet for improving mental health [45]. Social capital may also be used to foster positive mental well-being at the community level. Because social capital can be measured within neighbourhoods, programs have the potential to be designed from a community or group perspective. These programs may foster a sense of trust and cohesion within broader groups, while also developing community resources to maximize social capital within a given area. This may allow for the improvement or maintenance of positive mental health of larger population-level groups.

Countries across the globe have recognized the potential for social capital to be used as a health promoting mechanism. The improvement of social capital in communities (and its cognitive, network, and resource components), has recently been outlined as an important health promotion initiative in countries including Canada, Australia, and the United Kingdom. The Victorian Government suggest that social capital can be fostered by emphasizing community development, which can be improved by defining community-level goals, mobilizing resources, and developing plans to address collective problems [54]. European initiatives to improve the mental health of population include action goals such as promoting mental health in schools and the workplace, supporting mentally healthy aging and reducing disadvantage [55]. Goals such as these can be accomplished by promoting social inclusion, implementing community development programs, and encouraging social, cultural, economic and political contribution of individuals in society [55]. Through the development of social capital within communities, inequality issues in health and well-being and the ways in which groups come together to promote health can be directly addressed [54].

Canadian initiatives do not yet typically include the term 'social capital' within their mental health initiatives, as does the U.K.; however health promoting goals have included several of its key concepts for decades. For example, in 1986, efforts to improve mental well-being in its population, the Ottawa charter for mental health promotion strived to (1) build health public policy, (2) create supportive environments, (3) strengthen community action, (4) develop personal skills, and (5) reorient health services [56]. Each goal incorporates fundamental concepts of social capital by emphasizing the importance of building connections within social networks, developing health promoting resources and behaviours within communities, and fostering cohesion between individuals and groups. As social capital gains increased recognition in research and public health fields, the use of social capital within health initiatives are likely to become more common. Until then, it is promising that countries recognize the value in its individual components when outlining health promotion goals.

Mental Health and Social Capital: Social Capital as a Promising Initiative to
Improving the Mental Health of Communities

295

7. Concluding thoughts

Previous and recent evidence strongly suggests that social capital is a key contributor to mental health outcomes. Psychosocial components are consistently shown to be associated with symptoms of depression, anxiety, post-traumatic stress, psychological distress and self-rated mental health. Participation dimensions of social capital may be important for self-rated mental health, but do not seem to be associated with depressive symptoms. Network components on the other hand have been shown associated with depressive symptoms in some instances but have not been examined in relation to other forms of mental illness. More research is needed to establish associations between dimensions of social capital and various mental health outcomes. There remains important gaps within the literature that must be addressed. Nevertheless, social capital is a promising tool that can be used for policy and intervention purposes. Enhancing social capital of communities is thought to contribute to improved mental, and potentially physical, well-being of populations across the globe. With further research, the creation of health promoting programs, changes in policy, and increased knowledge translation between these realms, social capital may be a promising mechanism to improving mental well-being and preventing mental illness.

Author details

Emma Bassett[1*] and Spencer Moore[2]

*Address all correspondence to: 5eb29@queensu.ca

1 School of Kinesiology and Health Studies, Queen's University, Kingston Ontario, Canada

2 School of Kinesiology and Health Studies, Queen's University, Kingston Ontario, Canada

References

[1] World Health Organization. Investigating Mental Health. Switzerland: Nove; 2003. www.who.int/mental_health/media/investing_mnh.pdf

[2] Bulletin of the World Health Organization. Cross-national Comparisons of the Prevalences and Correlates of Mental Disorders. WHO International Consortium in Psychiatric Epidemiology 2000;78(4) 413-426.

[3] Moussavi S, Chatterji S, Verdes E, Tandon A, Patel V, Ustun B. Depression, chronic diseases, and decrements in health: results from the world health surveys. The Lancet 2007;370 851-858.

[4]   Government of Canada. The human face of mental health and mental illness in Cana-
      da.   http://www.phac-aspc.gc.ca/publicat/human-humain06/pdf/human_face_e.pdf
      (accessed 20 August 2012).

[5]   Moore S, Daniel M, Paquet C, Dubé L, Gauvin L. Association of individual network
      social capital with abdominal adiposity, overweight and obesity. Journal of Public
      Health, 2009;31(1) 175-183.

[6]   Whitley R, McKenzie K. Social capital and psychiatry: review of the literature. Har-
      vard Review of Psychiatry 2005;13(2) 71-84.

[7]   Lin, N. Building a network theory of social capital. Connections 1999;22(1) 28-51.

[8]   Moore S, Shiell A, Hawe P, Haines V. The privileging of communitarian ideas: cita-
      tion practices and the translation of social capital into public health research. Ameri-
      can Journal of Public Health 2005;85(8) 1330-1337.

[9]   Portes A. The two meanings of social capital. Sociological Forum 2000;15(1) 1-12.

[10] Putnam R. Making democracy work: civic traditions in modern Italy. Princeton, NJ:
      Princeton University Press; 1993.

[11] Carpiano RM. Toward a neighbourhood resource-based theory of social capital for
      health: can Bourdieu and sociology help? Social Science & Medicine 2006;62 165-175.

[12] Moore S, Bockenholt U, Daniel M, Frohlich K, Kestens Y, Richard L. Social capital
      and core network ties: a validation study of individual-level social capital measures
      and their association with extra- and intra-neighborhood ties, and self-rated health.
      Health & Place 2011;17(2) 536-544.

[13] De Silva MJ, McKenzie K, Harpham T, Huttly SR. Social capital and mental illness: a
      systematic review. Journal of Epidemiology and Community Health 2005;59 619-627.

[14] Poortinga W. Social capital: an individual or collective resource for health? Social Sci-
      ence & Medicine 2005;62 292-302.

[15] Diez-Roux AV. Neighborhoods and health: where are we and were do we go from
      here? Revue D'Epidemiologie et de Sante Publique 2007;55 13-21.

[16] Haines VA, Beggs JJ, Hurlbert JS. Neighborhood disadvantage, network social capi-
      tal, and depressive symptoms. Journal of Health and Social Behavior 2011;52(1)
      58-73.

[17] Kawachi I, Kennedy BP, Glass R. Social capital and self-rated health: a contextual
      analysis. American Journal of Public Health 1999;89(8) 1187-1193.

[18] Kawachi I, Subramanian SV, Kim D., editors. Social Capital and Health. New York:
      Springer; 2008.

[19] Nakhaie R, Arnold R. A four year (1996-2000) analysis of social capital and health status of Canadians: the difference that love makes. Social Science & Medicine 2010;71 1034-1044.

[20] Verhaeghe PP, Pattyn E, Bracke P, Verhaeghe M, Van De Putte B. The association between network social capital and self-rated health: pouring old wine in new bottles? Health & Place 2012;18(2) 358-365.

[21] Aslund C, Starrin B, Nilsson KW. Social capital in relation to depression, muskoskeletal pain, and psychosomatic symptoms: a cross-sectional study of a large population-based cohort of Swedish adolescents. BMC Public Health 2010;10 715-725.

[22] Fujiwara T, Kawachi I. A prospective study of individual-level social capital and major depression in the United States. Journal of Epidemiology and Community Health 2008;62 627-633.

[23] Sund ER, Jorgensen SH, Jones A, Krokstad S, Heggdal M. The influence of social capital on self-rated health and depression – the Nord-Trondelag health study (HUNT). Norwegian Journal of Epidemiology 2007;17(1) 59-69.

[24] Veenstra G. Location, location, location: contextual and compositional health effects of social capital in British Columbia, Canada. Social Science & Medicine 2005;60 2059-2071.

[25] Webber M, Huxley P, Harris T. Social capital and the course of depression: six-month prospective cohort study. Journal of Affective Disorders 2011;129 149-157.

[26] Berkman LF. The role of social relations in health promotion. Psychosomatic Medicine 1995;57 245-254.

[27] Bruce ML, Hoff RA. Social and physical health risk factors for first-onset major depression disorder in a community sample. Social Psychiatry and Psychiatric Epidemiology 1994;29 165-171.

[28] Walters K, Breeze E, Wilkinson P, Price GM, Bulpitt CJ, Fletcher A. Local area deprivation and urban-rural differences in anxiety and depression among people older than 75 years in Britain. American Journal of Public Health 2004;94(10) 1768-1774.

[29] Bassett E, Moore S. Social capital and depressive symptoms: the association of psychosocial and network dimensions of social capital with depressive symptoms in Montreal, Canada. Unpublished manuscript 2012.

[30] Rosenquist JN, Fowler JH, Christakis NA. Social network determinants of depression. Molecular Psychiatry 2011;16 273-281.

[31] Anxiety and Depression Association of America. Facts and Statistics. http:// www.adaa.org/about-adaa/press-room/facts-statistics (accessed August 22 2012).

[32] Somers JM, Goldner EM, Waraich P, Hsu L. Prevalence and incidence studies of anxiety disorders: a systematic review of the literature. Canadian Journal of Psychiatry 2006;51(2) 100-113.

[33] Wind TR, Komproe, IH. The mechanisms that associate community social capital with post-disaster mental health: a multilevel model. Social Science & Medicine 2012; http://dx.doi.org/10.1016/j.socscimed.2012.06.032.

[34] Wind TR, Fordham M, Komproe IH. Social capital and post-disaster mental health. Global Health Action 2011;4. Doi: 10.3402/gha.v4i0.6351.

[35] Valencia-Garcia D, Simoni JM Alegria M, Takeuchi DT. Social capital, acculturation, mental health, and perceived stress to services among Mexican American women. Journal of Consulting and Clinical Psychology 2012;80(2) 177-185.

[36] Bojorquez-Chapela I, Manrique-Espinoza BS, Mejia-Arango S, Solis MM, Salinas-Rodriguez A. Effect of social capital and personal autonomy on the incidence of depressive symptoms in the elderly: evidence from a longitudinal study in Mexico. Aging and Mental Health 2012;16(4) 462-471.

[37] Fitzsimon N, Shiely F, Corradino D, Friel S, Kelleher CC. Predictors of self-reported poor mental health at area level in Ireland: a multilevel analysis of deprivation and social capital indicators. The Irish Medical Journal 2007;100(8) suppl 49-52.

[38] Forsman AK, Nyqvist F, Wahlbeck K. Cognitive components of social capital and mental health status among older adults: a population-based cross-sectional study. Scandinavian Journal of Public Health 2011;39(7) 757-765.

[39] Forsman AK, Nyqvist F, Schierenbeck I, Gustafson Y, Wahlbeck K. Structural and cognitive social capital and depression among older adults in two Nordic regions. Aging and Mental Health 2012;16(6) 771-779.

[40] Hamano T, Fujisawa Y, Ishida Y, Subramanian SV, Kawachi I, Shiwaku K. Social capital and mental health in Japan: a multilevel analysis. PLoS One 2010;5(10):e13214.

[41] Han S, Lee HS. Individual, household and administrative area levels of social capital and their associations with mental health: a multilevel analysis of cross-sectional evidence. International Journal of Social Psychiatry 2012; DOI: 10.1177/0020764012453230.

[42] Irwin J, Lagory M, Ritchey F, Fitzpatrick K. Social assets and mental distress among the homeless: exploring the roles of social support and other forms of social capital on depression. Social Science & Medicine 2008;67(12) 1935-1943.

[43] Jung J, Ernstmann N, Nitzsche A, Driller E, Kowalski C, Lehner B, et al. Exploring the association between social capital and depressive symptoms: results of a survey in German information and communication technology companies. Journal of Occupational and Environmental Medicine 2012;54(1) 23-30.

Mental Health and Social Capital: Social Capital as a Promising Initiative to
Improving the Mental Health of Communities

299

[44] Kirkbride JB, Boydell J, Ploubidis GB, Morgan C, Dazzan P, McKenzie K, et al. Testing the association between the incidence of schizophrenia and social capital in an urban area. Psychological Medicine 2008;38(8) 1083-1094.

[45] Kouvonen A, Oksanen T, Vahtera J, Stafford M, Wilkinson R, Schneider J, et al. Low workplace social capital as a predictor of depression: the Finnish Public Sector Study. American Journal of Epidemiology 2008;167(10) 1143-1151.

[46] Oksanen T, Kouvonen A, Vahtera J, Virtanen M, Kivimaki M. Prospective study of workplace social capital and depression: are vertical and horizontal components equally important? Journal of Epidemiology and Community Health 2010;64(8) 684-689.

[47] Rothon C, Goodwin L, Stansfeld S. Family social support, community "social capital" and adolescents' mental health and educational outcomes: a longitudinal study in England. Social Psychiatry and Psychiatric Epidemiology 2012;47(5) 697-709.

[48] Tomita A, Burns JK. A multilevel analysis of association between neighborhood social capital and depression: evidence from the first South African National Income Dynamics Study. Journal of Affective Disorders 2012; http://dx.doi.org/10.1016/j.jad. 2012.05.066

[49] Wu Q, Xie B, Chou CP, Palmer PH, Gallaher PE, Johnson CA. Understanding the effect of social capital on the depression of urban Chinese adolescents: an integrative framework. American Journal of Community Psychology 2010;45(1-2) 1-16.

[50] Averina M, Nilsson O, Brenn T, Brox J, Arkhipovsky V. et al. Social and lifestyle determinants of depression, anxiety, sleeping disorders and self-evaluated quality of life in Russia: a population-based study in Arkhangelsk. Social Psychiatry and Psychiatric Epidemiology 2005;40(7) 511-518.

[51] Bassett E, Moore S. Perceived neighbourhood cohesion mediates the association between neighbourhood disadvantage and depressive symptoms in Montreal women but not men. Unpublished manuscript 2012.

[52] Dutt K, Webber M. Access to social capital and social support among South East Asian women with severe mental health problems: a cross-sectional survey. International Journal of Social Psychiatry 2010;56(6) 593-605.

[53] Berry HL. Social capital elite, excluded participators, busy working parents and aging, participating less: types of community participators and their mental health. Social Psychiatry and Psychiatric Epidemiology 2008;43(7) 527-537.

[54] State government of Victoria. Social capital & community development. Victorian State Government, Department of Health, Australia 2011. http:// www.health.vic.gov.au/healthpromotion/what_is/social_cap.htm (accessed 15 August 2012).

[55] Jané-Llopis E, Anderson P. Mental Health Promotion and Mental Disorder Prevention. A policy for Europe. Nijmegen: Radboud University Nijmegen; 2005.

[56] Public Health Agency of Canada. Ottawa Charter for Health Promotion: An International Conference on Health Promotion, 17-21 November 1986, Ottawa, Canada. http://www.phac-aspc.gc.ca/ph-sp/docs/charter-chartre/index-eng.php (accessed 16 August 2012).

Chapter 11

Communicating, Motivating and Teaching the Significance of Public Health

Claudia Marin-Kelso

Additional information is available at the end of the chapter

1. Introduction

Teaching public health represents a challenge for all health educators, as it includes a wide variety of important subjects that can be general, broad or specific and technical. Keeping students' attention is a difficult task when introducing purely theoretical concepts or subjects that for some, can be obvious, but are the building blocks of public health practice. Pretending to create a "hands on effect" is not an easy task for any health educator. More so, if your students come from different backgrounds, as those interested in Public Health. This chapter intends to address aspects of public health, such as skill sets needed, using technology and strategies to teaching public health, as well as, mentoring students to generate action. Each section will include examples and proposed exercises for the teacher to use in the classroom.

2. Significance of teaching public health

When does a health problem become a public health problem? That's the first question I asked myself when I was in the middle of my medical training. And, while everybody else was thinking about how to do well the semiology oral examination, I was thinking, how I could help not just one, but many people.

Theories in health education vary and they support themselves with behavioral change theories that are no less important, however, these theories are not discussed here due to length and the specific topic of this chapter. This section of the chapter emphasizes the importance of public health's applicability to one's practice, communities, governments and life in general.

After years of public health teaching experience I have come to identify that in order for public health students to understand what public health means and what they can do with it, they first have to learn basic definitions of the subject, a little bit of history, view the complexity of individuals and communities and their determinants of health and be up to date with the health priorities of their community and the world. In short, public health is exciting and challenging!

Public Health is one of those areas that appears to many, as a general science that is "out there" but not necessarily considered the way to go when choosing a career. In the medical world, it is way more attractive (financially speaking) to go further in your clinical training than explore fields related to community health. Public Health is all around us, it encompasses so many areas in which varied professionals can serve and contribute.

One of the earliest definitions of Public Health in the modern world was given by Charles-Edward Winslow in 1920, when he defined it as "the science and art of preventing disease, prolonging life and promoting health through the organized efforts and informed choices of society, organizations, public and private, communities and individuals"[1]. From all the definitions found, this one succinctly describes the subject with its dimensions, determinants and participants. Thereafter you can find other definitions that include terms of functionality, and community participation and involvement that you may relate too, helping facilitate your teaching style and syllabus.

In teaching public health it is very important to transfer not only knowledge but experiences to the students that can lead them to take action in their communities and will show them a breadth of possible areas that can be developed working in the public health field. Some of these include: Child and Maternal Health, Biostatistics, Behavioral Medicine, Environmental Health or Environmental Epidemiology, Epidemiology, Global Health, International Health, Health Care Services Delivery, Preventive Medicine, Public Policy, Health Care Organization amongst others.

Academic training requires students to consider all aspects of a topic, from a range of view-points. It also requires students to state general claims and then prove each claim by providing solid evidence from a range of sources. [2] Giving practical examples allows students to grasp the intricacies of public health challenges and how to face them.

Another recommendation in having people interested and involved in Public Health is to teach them some history. The best way to know what something is, is to know where it comes from. I always recommend to begin your public health teaching activities by exploring some of the history of public health, areas or public health, origins in the different civilizations, examples of actions that were public health efforts but were not considered as such until a definition of public health came out, the relationships of public health with other scientific disciplines, the process of emergence of key concepts, the influence on demographic, health, social, cultural and economic context and the role of public health in society. [3]

As a public health educator it is important to use a variety of teaching methods to meet individual preferences of your students. Possible methods to be used are discussed later.

Some of the best results in public health education are achieved by stimulating research the theory and practice of health education; supporting high quality performance standards for the practice of health education and health promotion; advocating policy and legislation affecting health education and health promotion; and developing and promoting standards for professional preparation of health education professionals [4].

Public health differs from clinical medicine by emphasizing prevention and keying interventions to multiple social and environmental determinants of disease; clinical medicine focuses on the treatment of the individual [4]. The best way to approach a health issue is by integrating both clinical assessment with public health perspective. A health professional can no longer treat his patients symptoms of pathology, but he has to view, analyze and treat all the other determinants of health that surround that individual ensuring a better outcome for the patient.

With the creation and updates of the program "Healthy People", by the United States Department of Health and Human Services, a vision was delineated of where public health wants to be, and it changed the way of planning, organizing and acting in public health. Health promotion and disease-prevention goals were set. It also has analyzed and transformed the determinants of health; including areas to fulfill one's needs and describe all the areas that affect individuals' health.

Determinants of health (as seen in figure 1) have evolved, encompassing five dimensions that need to be studied and understood by public health students. There are personal, social, economic, and environmental factors that influence health status, and those can be summarized as follows: Policymaking, Social factors, Health services, Individual Behavior and Biology and Genetics.

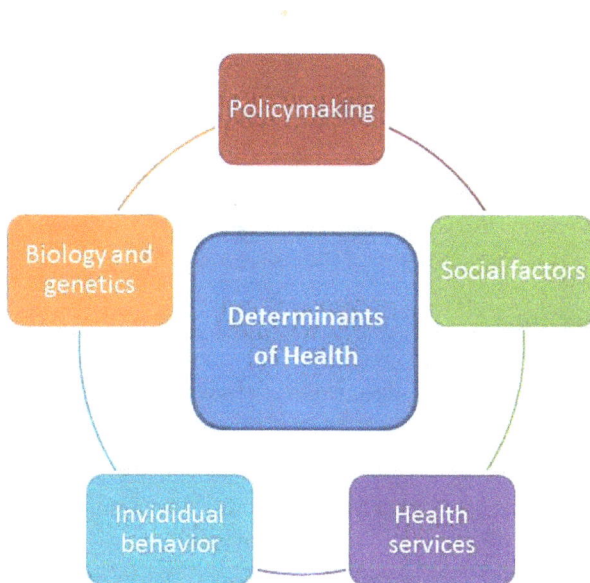

Figure 1. Determinants of Health

As it can be seen in the figure all five determinants are inter-related and each one can be targeted individually or as a group when working out a solution for a health problem.

Example: For the public health problem: "Motor-vehicle crashes among teen agers", one can analyze the problem by using the determinants of health. You can take one or several of the determinants to define what will you target in the intervention (Figure 2).

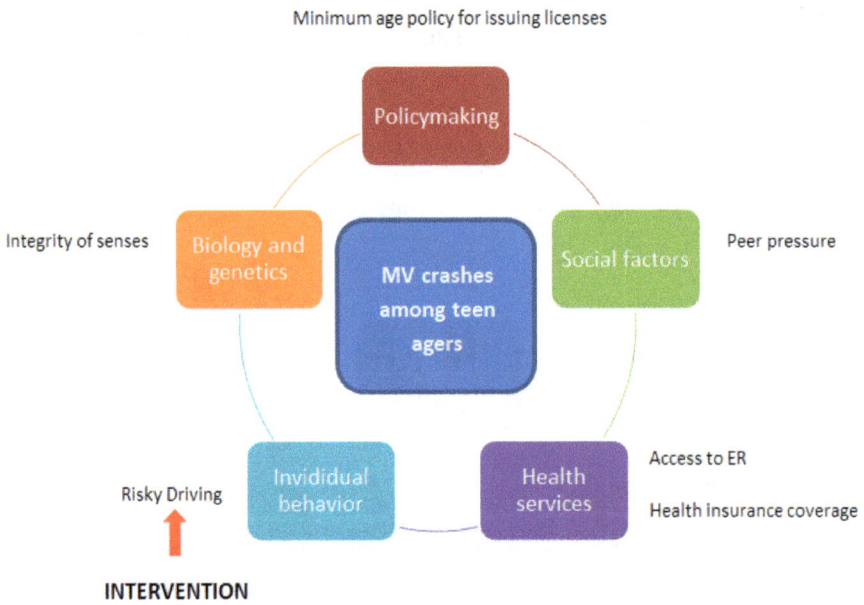

Figure 2. Assessment of Motor-vehicle crashes among teen agers using determinants of health

The world is changing fast. Often unclear is the impact that social, economic, and political change will have on health in general, on health inequities within countries or across the globe in particular. Action on the social determinants of health will be more effective if basic data systems, including vital registration and routine monitoring of health inequity and the social determinants of health are in place and there are mechanisms to ensure that the data can be understood and applied to develop more effective policies, systems, and programs [5]. This being said, education and training in social determinants of health are vital during teaching public health.

In conjunction with Healthy People 2020, we should ask ourselves two questions: "what makes some people healthy and others unhealthy?" and, "how can we create a society in which everyone has a chance to live long healthy lives?". In order to answer these questions, it is recommended to develop objectives that address the relationship between health status and biology, individual behavior, health services, social factors and policies; and emphasize an ecological approach to disease prevention and health promotion. An ecological approach focuses on both individual-level and population-level determinants of health and interventions [6].

Exercise 1	Exercise 1 Characteristics
1. Select a health problem 2. Ask your students to brainstorm and analyze the causes associated to the health problem according to the determinants of health 3. The students can analyze the problem from one or several determinants. 4. Moderate the discussion 5. Write on the board the related causes given by the students 6. Wrap up the discussion	**Type of exercise:** Brainstorming **Setting:** Classroom **Number of students recommended:** From 5 to 30 **Materials:** Bibliography resources, board, markers, eraser. **Duration:** 15 to 20 minutes. **Expected outcome:** Blackboard utilization with a health problem and its possible causes analyzed from each determinant of health.

Figure 3. Exercise 1 - Brainstorming

3. Who is interested in learning about public health?

People interested in public health come from a variety of backgrounds and with different educational levels (Technical, Professional, Masters, PhD). When teaching public health one has to be very well aware of this diversity to use the proper vocabulary, terms and information so it can reach those from non-health and health related backgrounds. Technical jargon should be utilized but only after being thoroughly introduced.

Traditionally, those interested in public health are health practitioners, especially physicians, nurses and social workers. However, I have worked with people from various backgrounds such as finances, administration, anthropology, information technology, biology, etc. actively working on public health. Some of them came into the public health arena by accident and some others because they truly liked it to begin with.

Public Health is a field easy to fall in-love with, challenging different backgrounds seeking the solutions and the outcomes expected for health problems. The recruitment of non-health professionals into public health is not so difficult, but we have an obligation as public health practitioners to promote and communicate that this is an exciting area for many people.

One of my first work experiences at the World Health Organization had me recruiting professionals from non-health backgrounds to work in Public Health specifically from developing countries. In the beginning I thought it was going to be very difficult to motivate these professionals to work in the subject, however, it was highly sought by those who were informed about the job opportunities and areas of work. The main challenge was just to get out there and to deliver the message effectively for public health to be known within some target groups.

The fields of work in Public Health are broad as well. You can work for local, regional, national or world offices, governmental or non-governmental, private and educational institutions. Next is an example of a job description for a non-health professional to work in Public Heath:

Example: Sample Job Description: Performance Improvement Manager
Position Overview: Manages and coordinates organization-wide efforts to ensure that performance management (PM) and quality improvement (QI) programs are developed and managed using a data driven focus that sets priorities for improvements aligned to ongoing strategic imperatives.
Minimum Requirements: Master's degree in public health or MBA and 10 or more years of experience in public health management, planning or public policy development. Experience in Performance Improvement Management and Quality is desired [7].

In the beginning of my public health career, I quickly learned that Public Health needs the work and support of different disciplines and backgrounds. To analyze and act upon a health issue you need the participation of a health professional who knows the theory behind the health issue, people with some knowledge in administration and finances, people that know about policy development, statistics and so on, if you really want to target properly the matter of study and have some impact.

You are able to find all the levels of training in Public Health, while in developing countries, you can mainly find graduate programs such as Masters or PhDs. Perhaps, developing countries are just now entering the world of policy development in public health issues and training programs are just starting to grow.

There are many different degree programs for those interested in studying public health. Some of the programs include:

BA = Bachelor's in public health: Designed to give students a basic grounding in public health issues and methods. [8]

- MPH = Master of Public Health: include coursework in a number of public health disciplines, such as administration, epidemiology, environmental health, and behavioral health. Specialized degrees such as a Master of Health Administration will be more focused on a specific topic.

- MHA = Master of Health Administration: People with experience in public health but often don't have MPH degrees

- MHSA = Master of Health Services Administration: For people interested in administration of Public Health.

- MSPH = Master of Science in Public Health

- DrPH = Doctor of Public Health: It is for people with an interest in public health leadership, or a desire for deeper knowledge than an MPH program can provide.

- PhD = Doctor of Philosophy

The MPH, DrPH, and MHA are example of degrees which are geared towards those who want careers as practitioners of public health in traditional health departments, managed care organizations, community-based organizations, hospitals, consulting firms, international agencies, state and federal agencies, among others.

MS, PhD, and ScD are examples of academic degrees. They are more oriented toward students wishing to seek a career in academics and research rather than public health practice.

However, each school of public health can tailor their degree programs significantly. Students interested in getting a degree in public health should check with individual schools for more information on specific degree programs.

In your classroom, you will have you have an array of backgrounds that represent an opportunity to make your class exciting and fulfilling. Know your students, who they are, what they do, what their expectations are, and more importantly, identify how can they contribute to the public health world.

Exercise 2	Exercise 2 Characteristics
Greet your students and ask them the following information 1. What is your name? 2. What is your background? 3. What do you expect from the class? 4. What previous experiences in public health have you had? 5. Is there a particular career path or job you seek?	**Type of exercise:** Getting acquainted **Setting:** Classroom **Number of students recommended:** From 5 to 30 **Materials:** - **Duration:** 15 to 30 minutes. **Expected outcome:** Knowing your students, identifying what they expect and what they could give to the class.

Figure 4. Exercise 2 – Getting acquainted

Public health is a rewarding field. The field of public health offers great personal fulfillment - working towards improving people's health and well-being is a rewarding day's work. Health status indicators or health outcomes, can tell you whether you've got a clean bill of health or if you and your community are in need of some regular public health attention [9].

4. What skills and competences are needed in a public health practitioner?

An array of skills and competences become the tools of good performance in the field. Those skills and competences need to be developed during public health training. The teacher is directly responsible for assuring that the students get what is needed to execute impeccably the plans and goals delineated for taking action in the community or research fields.

Competency is defined as the ability to apply particular knowledge, skills, attitudes, and values to the standard of performance required in specified contexts. The Core Competencies can serve as a starting point for public health practice and academic organizations as they create workforce development plans, identify training and workforce needs, prepare for accreditation, and more [10]. Generic competencies are the minimum baseline set of competencies that are common to all public health roles across all public health sectors and disciplines and that are necessary for the delivery of essential public health services [11].

The competencies are organized into twelve topic areas. Each topic comprises a set of competency statements as follows (Table 1):

Topic	Generic Competency statement
1. Health systems	• Demonstrates knowledge of the health systems and structures • Demonstrates knowledge of key international agreements.
2. Public Health Science	• Demonstrates knowledge of what constitutes public health and how it relates to public health practice in specific contexts. • Demonstrates knowledge of the determinant factors that affect health and health inequalities. • Demonstrates knowledge of the basic concepts of health. • Demonstrates knowledge of the basic epidemiological concepts.
3. Policy, Legislation and Regulation	• Demonstrates knowledge of the use of policy in a public health context. • Demonstrates knowledge of how legislation and regulations are applied in public health contexts.
4. Research and evaluation	• Demonstrates understanding of the principles of research and its applications in public health. • Demonstrates understanding of the principles of evaluation and its applications in public health.
5. Community health development	• Demonstrates knowledge of community development in a public health context.
6. Public Health Practice	• Demonstrates knowledge and understanding of the intent of public health interventions. • Analyses public health issues.

Topic	Generic Competency statement
	• Uses culturally appropriate values processes and protocols when working in teams.
7. Working across and understanding cultures	• Demonstrates knowledge of the nature of culture. • Demonstrates knowledge of the principles of cultural • safety and takes responsibility for maintaining safety in • regards to cultural values, norms, and practices.
8. Communication	• Listens actively. • Uses different communication styles to facilitate understanding accommodate. • Uses oral communication effectively in a range of contexts. • Communicates clearly in writing for the given context. • Consults with others in a range of settings.
9. Leadership, Teamwork, and professional liaison	• Positively influences the way teams work together. • Demonstrates understanding of the many aspects of leadership. • Instigates, coordinates and facilitates groups. • Establishes and maintains effective professional relationships to improve health outcomes.
10. Advocacy	• Demonstrates the ability to advocate in achieving public health outcomes. • Demonstrates the ability to negotiate to achieve public health outcomes.
11. Professional Development and Self- Management	• Manages self to improve performance and professional development.
12. Planning and Administration	• Accesses a range of organizational information. • Describes how work plan fits with organizational and wider public health priorities. • Completes appropriate administration record keeping and allocated financial responsibilities according to contractual and legal frameworks and organizational policies as they apply. • Demonstrates understanding of the public heath role in an emergency response.

Source: Keating, Gay et al. Generic Competencies for Public Health in Aotearoa-New Zealand. New Zealand: The Public Health Association of New Zealand.

Table 1. Topic areas with their generic competencies in Public Health

A skill is the ability to do something well; to have the expertise. Some of the most important skills for a public health professional to have are: Analytic Assessment Skills, Policy Development/Programa Planning Skills, Communication Skills, Cultural Competency Skills, Community Dimensions of Practice Skills, Basic Public Health Sciences Skills, Financial Planning and Management Skills and Leadership and Systems Thinking Skills [12]

For each domain of skills there are a group of specific competences that apply as shown in table 2.

Skill	Specific Competence
Analytic Assessment Skills	• Defines a problem
	• Determines appropriate uses and limitations of both quantitative and qualitative data
	• Selects and defines variables relevant to defined public health problems
	• Identifies relevant and appropriate data and information sources
	• Evaluates the integrity and comparability of data and identifies gaps in data sources
	• Applies ethical principles to the collection, maintenance, use, and dissemination of data and information
	• Partners with communities to attach meaning to collected quantitative and qualitative data
	• Makes relevant inferences from quantitative and qualitative data
	• Obtains and interprets information regarding risks and benefits to the community
	• Applies data collection processes, information technology applications, and computer systems storage/retrieval strategies
	• Recognizes how the data illuminates ethical, political, scientific, economic, and overall public health issues
Policy Development/Program Planning Skills	• Collects, summarizes, and interprets information relevant to an issue
	• States policy options and writes clear and concise policy statements
	• Identifies, interprets, and implements public health laws, regulations, and policies related to specific programs
	• Articulates the health, fiscal, administrative, legal, social, and political implications of each policy option
	• States the feasibility and expected outcomes of each policy option
	• Utilizes current techniques in decision analysis and health planning
	• Decides on the appropriate course of action
	• Develops a plan to implement policy, including goals, outcome and process objectives, and implementation steps
	• Translates policy into organizational plans, structures, and programs
	• Prepares and implements emergency response plans
	• Develops mechanisms to monitor and evaluate programs for their
	• effectiveness and quality
Communication Skills	• Communicates effectively both in writing and orally, or in other ways
	• Solicits input from individuals and organizations
	• Advocates for public health programs and resources
	• Leads and participates in groups to address specific issues
	• Uses the media, advanced technologies, and community networks to communicate information
	• Effectively presents accurate demographic, statistical, programmatic, and scientific information for professional and lay audiences
Cultural Competency Skills	• Utilizes appropriate methods for interacting sensitively, effectively,

Skill	Specific Competence
	• and professionally with persons from diverse cultural, socioeconomic, educational, racial, ethnic and professional
	• backgrounds, and persons of all ages and lifestyle preferences
	• Identifies the role of cultural, social, and behavioral factors in
	• determining the delivery of public health services
	• Develops and adapts approaches to problems that take into
	• account cultural differences
Community Dimensions of Practice Skills	• Establishes and maintains linkages with key stakeholders
	• Utilizes leadership, team building, negotiation, and conflict
	• resolution skills to build community partnerships
	• Collaborates with community partners to promote the health of
	• the population
	• Identifies how public and private organizations operate within a community
	• Accomplishes effective community engagements
	• Identifies community assets and available resources
	• Develops, implements, and evaluates a community public health assessment,
	• Describes the role of government in the delivery of community
	• health services
Basic Public Health Sciences Skills	• Identifies the individual's and organization's responsibilities within the context of the Essential Public Health Services and core functions
	• Defines, assesses, and understands the health status of populations, determinants of health and illness, factors contributing
	• to health promotion and disease prevention, and factors influencing the use of health services
	• Understands the historical development, structure, and interaction of public health and health care systems
	• Identifies and applies basic research methods used in public health
	• Applies the basic public health sciences including behavioral and social sciences, biostatistics, epidemiology, environmental public
	• health, and prevention of chronic and infectious diseases and injuries
	• Identifies and retrieves current relevant scientific evidence
	• Identifies the limitations of research and the importance of observations and interrelationships
Financial Planning and Management Skills	• Develops and presents a budget
	• Manages programs within budget constraints
	• Applies budget processes
	• Develops strategies for determining budget priorities
	• Monitors program performance
	• Prepares proposals for funding from external sources

Skill	Specific Competence
	• Applies basic human relations skills to the management of organizations, motivation of personnel, and resolution of conflicts
	• Manages information systems for collection, retrieval, and use of data for decision-making
	• Negotiates and develops contracts and other documents for
	• the provision of population-based services
	• Conducts cost effectiveness, cost benefit, and cost utility analyses
Leadership and Systems Thinking Skills	• Creates a culture of ethical standards within organizations and communities
	• Helps create key values and shared vision and uses these principles to guide action
	• Identifies internal and external issues that may impact delivery of
	• essential public health services (i.e. strategic planning)
	• Facilitates collaboration with internal and external groups to
	• ensure participation of key stakeholders
	• Promotes team and organizational learning
	• Contributes to development, implementation, and monitoring of organizational performance standards
	• Uses the legal and political system to effect change
	• Applies theory of organizational structures to professional practice

Source: PHF. Core Competencies for Public Health Professionals. Washington: Public Health Foundation; 2012.

Table 2. Skills and specific competences in Public Health.

You can observe in tables 1 and 2, public health professional needs to develop: a series of skills and competences that will make s/he a professional that will be able to perform different duties in several areas and to have a broader understanding of the health problems in his community and the world.

According to the discipline, profiles are outlined to meet the requirement of the tasks as it is presented in the following example:

> **Example: Sample Job Description: Performance Improvement Manager**
> *Position Overview*: Lecturer / Senior Lecturer in Public Health
> *Essential Factors and Skills*: Master's degree or equivalent, Ability to inspire and collaborate, Establishes writing skills, Specialist expertise and experience in public health, Previous experience in coordinating public health research, writing and submitting proposals and bids and mentoring and supervising staff. Excellent verbal and communication skills, presentation skills and IT skills. Organized, with an ability to work methodically, accurately and to deadlines. [13].

Exercise 3	Exercise 3 Characteristics
Invite a guest speaker to your class, who's profile is an experienced Public Health Professional. Ask him to talk about his experience in the field; how he has done it, what skills and competences he has developed. Finish the session with questions and answers from your students.	**Type of exercise:** Guest speaker **Setting:** Classroom or auditorium **Number of students recommended:** From 15 to 100 **Materials:** Audiovisual, video beam, computer **Duration:** 30 to 60 minutes. **Expected outcome:** Students motivated about Public Health

Figure 5. Exercise 3 – Guest speaker

5. Importance of knowing your students and identifying their particular skills

This is a special section with some strategies to identify the potential of your students in the classroom, how to explore and encourage their development and applicability towards public health practice.

It doesn't matter how good a professional can be if s/he doesn't care for who s/he is teaching. A success factor for any one's learning experience is having a teacher that can actively search and find the talents of his/her students.

I always recommend to anyone who works in education, more so in health education, to devote a good amount of time to get to know their students well. I say especially in health education because health sciences tend to depersonalize learning experiences; leaving the themes as just science to be learned no matter the individual makes learning sterile.

From the first encounter with your students take some time getting acquainted, for example, use icebreakers, ask about your student's family, habits, hobbies and why not get into some of the public health subjects you are going to be teaching them utilizing their own health risk factors or determinants of health. That way you will know how much resonance you will have in your lectures. This will also give you the opportunity to select examples that will reach your students in a deeper level that will touch them, that will make them remember!

Learners can be classified according to their learning style or preference as visual, auditory or tactile/kinesthetic [14].

For visual learners it is important to use pictures, diagrams, photographs, graphs, videos, illustrations, flipcharts or any other visual aid that will accompany the main message. Body language it is also important with these types of students. It can become a powerful tool for keeping their interest in the class and the subject.

Auditory learners are those who learn best by listening. Be prepared to use a decisive tone of voice, make changes in volume, intensity, accentuation and speed. Learners get the most out of discussions in small groups, short lectures and interesting subjects. Sometimes you can also use music to emphasize parts of the lecture or discussion.

Tactile or kinesthetic learners learn better by doing, moving or touching. In teaching public health, any type of community work, such as data collection, surveying, prevention activities in the community, education, etc. it is a very used method to motivate and train your students in a particular subject.

Example: Learning Styles

AUDITORY LEARNERS

Like to be read to
Like to read at loud
Like to use mnemonics to help learn material
Like to talk with others about their ideas

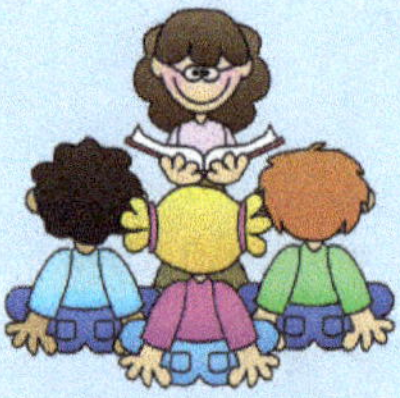

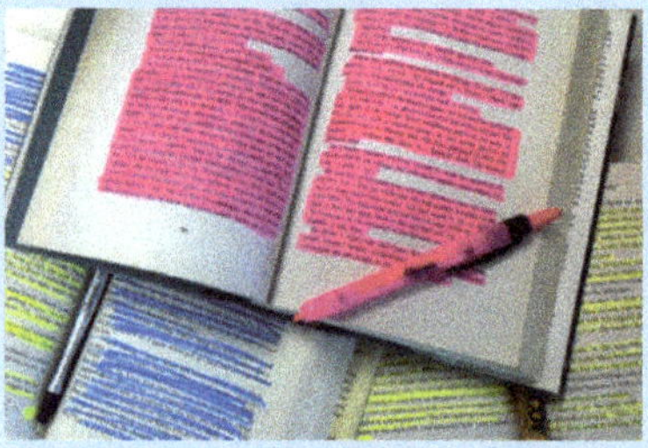

VISUAL LEARNERS

Like to learn from reading, taking notes,
and using worksheets
Like to use highlighters to outline
important facts
Like to see a visual representation of the
information
Like to use multimedia materials such as
computers and transparencies

KINESTHETIC LEARNERS

Like to move around to learn new information
Like to take frequent breaks
Like to use rhythms or music to learn
Like to learn in different settings

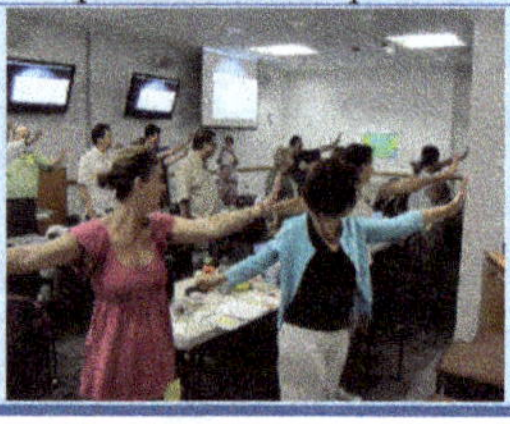

Figure 6. Example of learning styles. Source: BENSLEY, Robert and BROOKINS-FISHER, Jodi. Community Health education and methods. A practical guide. United States: Jones and Barlett Publishers, LLC; 2009.

You can use either or all the methods whenever you feel you need them. Public Health teaching is not limited to the classroom, but can be done in all kinds of settings. Where ever you are, try to use it for your convenience and apply your skills to achieve your main goal: capture your student's interest [15]. You can do this by stimulating research on the theory and practice of health education; supporting high quality performance standards for the practice of health education and health promotion; and finally, advocating policy and legislation affecting health education.

In the next table there are several methods that can be used in the exercise of teaching public health by developing three types of objectives: cognitive objectives, affective objectives and psychomotor objectives.

Method	Cognitive	Affective	Psychomotor	Time required
Getting acquainted (icebrakers)	X	P	P	15+
Audio	X	P	P	15+
Audiovisual materials	X	P	P	15+
Case studies	X	X		30+
Computer-assisted instruction	X	P		30+
Cooperative learning	P	P	P	30+
Debates	P	P		30+
Educational games	X			20+
Field trips		P		60+
Guest speakers	X	P		30+
Lecture	X			5+
Panels	P	X		30+
Peer education	P	X		120+
Problem solving		X	P	30+
Self-appraisals		X		10+
Service learning	X	X	P	120+
Simulations	X	X	X	30+
Storytelling	P	X		10+

Legend: X = Yes, common use; P = possible

Table 3. Methods for teaching public health and their objectives

Some of the methods described above have been used as examples in this chapter.

> **Example: Selecting team members**
> After a getting acquainted section, you noticed you have at least 5 students that know very well SPSS, 3 more that are great speakers, 2 that have field experiences in public health interventions, 4 students with grant writing experiences, and 2 students with managerial and financial skills. You need to put to put together a team of 5 people that can manage and run an intervention in the community. You are able know to select the individuals for your team after knowing the skills your students have.

In order to have a good point of departure in a modern public health course, I recommend choosing an authoritative book on the main concepts of Public Health to be used as course text. Depending on the focus of the class, that book can have only public health theory or more specific information on any of the public health areas.

Prepare your class using at least one of the methods that have been explained or more than one depending on the content of the lecture, number of students, available resources and time.

Create a course syllabus. Schedule topics in advance and inform your students about the materials to be used in the class. Assign some readings so the students have a previous review of the information to be discussed in the class and make sure to make a round of questions (Q&A) about the assigned reading.

This will help you and your students to trace a baseline from which your class will start with generated expectations and a basic knowledge to be developed.

Exercise 4	Exercise 4 Characteristics
Prepare an outline for a lecture using at least 3 methods described in table 3. Input the time dedicated to each activity, materials used and bibliography. Make sure to include exercises for your students.	**Type of exercise:** Lecture **Setting:** Classroom or auditorium **Number of students recommended:** From 5 to 30 **Materials:** Audiovisual, video beam, computer **Duration:** 45 to 90 minutes. **Expected outcome:** Objectives of the lecture met.

Figure 7. Exercise 4 – Lecture

Again, using either one or several of those methods, you should be able to include the students and make them full participant in your class activity. Once you have identified what the student can do and what it that makes her/him special in the classroom, reinforce it and promote it.

6. Guiding your students to generate actions in public health

Public health is a field that offers an abundance of job opportunities to suit a variety of interests and skills. Whether you are more interested in crunching numbers, conducting research, or working with people, there is a place for you. Recent college graduates and those that have been in the field for years have something to offer and to gain in this field. Public health is ideal for those that gain satisfaction knowing that they are working to improve the lives of others.

It is very important for a student to understand the public health priorities that surround her/him, and in that way, should be able to propose solutions that can be taken to actions. Some of the key public health priorities which have become achievements for the world and the United States of America are listed in table 4.

No.	Worldwide 2001-2010	United States 2001-2010
1	Reductions in child mortality	Vaccine-Preventable Diseases
2	Vaccine-Preventable Diseases	Prevention and control of Infectious Diseases
3	Access to Safe Water and Sanitation	Tobacco Control
4	Malaria Prevention and Control	Maternal and Infant Health
5	Prevention and control of HIV/AIDS	Motor Vehicle Safety
6	Tuberculosis Control	Cardiovascular Disease Prevention
7	Control of Neglected Tropical Diseases	Occupational Safety
8	Tobacco Control	Cancer Prevention
9	Increased Awareness and Response for Improving Global Road Safety	Childhood Lead Poisoning Prevention
10	Improved Preparedness and Response to Global Health Threats	Public Health Preparedness and Response

Source: CDC. Ten Great Public Health Achievements

Table 4. Ten great Public Health Achievements

Public Health needs to transcend the assessment of health issues and professionals should be able to propose and deliver interventions in the field that make changes in communities and hopefully in public policies.

Many public health practitioners find the problems, analyze them and give plausible explanations of the causes to health issues. Less come out with ideas for interventions and activities to be made, and even less are able to conjugate the results of those interventions to proposing political exits to public health problems.

Exercise 5	Exercise 5 Characteristics
Take your students on a field trip to visit a vulnerable community to a health problem, example, a community with water problems. Have them talk to the people, look for the water sources, identify the problems, propose solutions and implement intervention activities if already outlined. Wrap up the session with lessons learned. Take pictures and write a field trip report.	**Type of exercise:** Field trip **Setting:** Field **Number of students recommended:** 5 to 15 **Materials:** Transportation mean, identifications for students, camera **Duration:** 90 to 180+ minutes. **Expected outcome:** Students motivation, intervention goals reviewed and measured.

Figure 8. Exercise 5 – Field trip

7. Use of technology in the teaching and practicing of public health

Globalization has changed the way in which we work, especially as a scientific community. Networking and technology are quintessential tools for teaching public health now.

Teaching and assessing public health has changed within a century, and now, we face an age in which the Information and communication technologies (ITCs) are the gold standard. ITCs are the integration of telecommunications, computers, audio-visual systems, wired and wireless signals, software, storage and others in order to transmit, store, manipulate and share information efficiently between users.

The ITCs join what used to be telephone networks with computer networks, and has facilitated the delivery of messages to public health practitioners and community.

Dr. Mirta Roses Periago, former Director of the Panamerican Health Organization said in 2003 the following words that I consider relevant: "This century will be the century of networks, connectivity and interdependence, and this will allow us to overcome the barriers of time and space, opening possibilities that we never imagined to improve the life conditions of our people..." [18]

Health services are complex in the way they are built, based upon scientific research and evidence based medicine. In order to do this, it is necessary the collaboration and participation of multiple actors with different profiles, knowledge and skills.

Communication between parties that work in public health has significantly improved through ITCs and social networks. There are other technologies that include digital content and video streaming that also facilitate the interaction of interdisciplinary groups.

The source of knowledge and their spread has evolved as follows (figure 3):

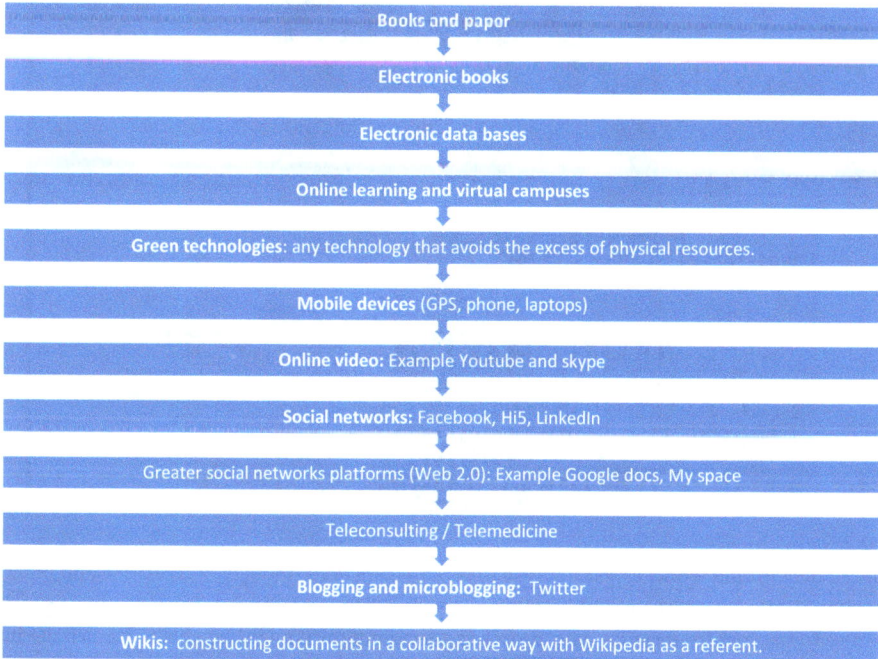

Figure 9. Evolution of knowledge sources and their communication resources

With the use of ITCs you can interact with others, share information and resources efficiently, however, one has to be very cautious when protecting the security and privacy of the health information that is being managed, because of its efficiency and ease of use, sharing this type of knowledge through ITCs can put people at risk.

This is why users, roles and privileges in accessing any type of ITC resource has to be well defined. Computer accounts need to be secure, data storage and back up has to be warranted. [19]

I have personally used all of the tools named in figure 3 for both clinical and public health practice. I believe ITCs and social networking are a powerful tool to access the community and generate highly impacting interventions. However, I also believe the management of the messages being distributed, the discussions created and the rising questions need a careful treatment in order not to allow the transformation or deviation of the core messages that were intended to be delivered.

Example: Blog: U.S Strategy to prevent and respond to gender-based violence globally [20]

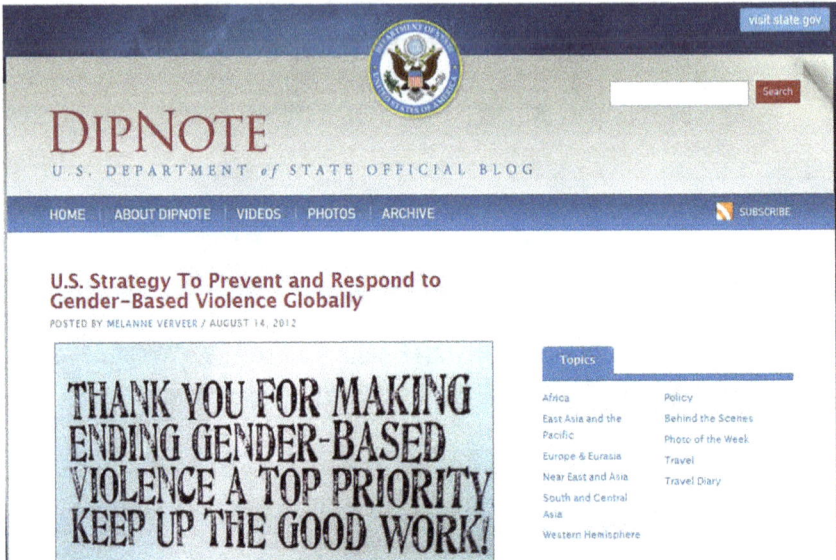

Social networking works especially well in settings where technology is accessible and other communication practices might be more expensive. Some developing countries have good access to internet for instance, and people in the community might be able to participate in activities and discussions, read messages, post queries or getting actively involved in a public health strategy without having to spend a lot or resources.

Exercise 6	Exercise 6 Characteristics
At the computer lab give your students a public health topic to research. Provide them with a list of health databases to be used. Ask them to look for at least 5 scientific articles that discuss the topic selected. Students should write a report and send it to the instructor by e-mail at the end of the class.	**Type of exercise:** Computer-assisted instruction **Setting:** Computer lab **Number of students recommended:** 5 to 30 **Materials:** Computer, video beam **Duration:** 60 to 120 minutes **Expected outcome:** Data bases management

Figure 10. Exercise 6 – Computer-assisted instruction

8. Results expected in the learning process of public health

One of the key messages to be taught is to keep in mind that partnering with the community is the key to success of Public Health practice.

Community diversity and culture must be recognized and respected. Community engagement can only be sustained by identifying and mobilizing community assets, and by developing capacities and resources for community health decisions and action.

The concerns of society are always in the forefront of public health. These concerns keep changing and the methods for addressing keep expanding. New technologies and global, local, and national interventions are becoming a necessary part of public health. [21]

The impact of any public health initiative is proportional to the amount of community involvement and collaboration. They are who, in the end, will acquire long-term commitments with their own health and we as public health practitioners, are the ones who will partner with them and other organizations to make those relationships long lasting and productive.

The final outcome of a public health learning process involves:

• Basic knowledge in public health generalities

• Acute sense of research

• Highly committed and sensible professionals with the community

• Community involvement

• Setting realistic goals that should progress to highly impact the social setting to be applied.

• Setting performance indicators

Goals, objectives, and performance indicators function very much like the elements of an archer and his or her target, in that, they clarify the purpose of the health education intervention.

9. Conclusion

Teaching public health means training individuals to assess effectively health issues, assure the maintenance of health in a community and develop policies, strategies and interventions to improve health.

Public health is an exciting and growing field of study that challenges its professionals to confront complex health issues, such as improving access to health care, controlling infectious disease, and reducing environmental hazards, violence, substance abuse, and injury. The field is dynamic and diverse, and Public Health professionals come from varying educational backgrounds and can specialize in an array of fields. A host of specialists, including teachers, journalists, researchers, administrators, environmentalists, demographers, social workers, laboratory scientists, and attorneys, work to protect the health of the public.

Public health is also a field geared toward serving others. Public health professionals serve local, national, and international communities. They are leaders who meet the many exciting challenges in protecting the public's health today and in the future.

As public health trainers we have the obligation to educate our students develop their skills and make them competent in the areas they select as their preference. A well trained professional should be capable of taking on challenges with confidence, effectiveness and assertiveness.

During training, students need to explore all three dimensions of the core functions of public health: assessment, assurance and policy development. In this way, they would be able to choose which direction to go once they are practicing.

A public health trainer needs to be proficient in the use of ICTs and apply them not only during the academic exercise of teaching public health but during his practice. ICTs facilitate public health intervention outcomes and are an efficient and cost-effective way to promote health.

Author details

Claudia Marin-Kelso[1,2]

Address all correspondence to: claudiamarin@utp.edu.co

1 School of Medicine, Faculty of Health Sciences (Colombian Associated Center for the Iberoamerican Cochrane Network), Universidad Tecnológica de Pereira (UTP), Pereira, Colombia

2 Faculty of Health Sciences (Colombian Associated Center for the Iberoamerican Cochrane Network), Universidad Tecnológica de Pereira (UTP), Pereira, Risaralda, Colombia

References

[1] Winslow, Charles-Edward Amory. The cost of sickness and the price of health. In: Bulletin of the World Health Organization. Geneva: World Health Organization; 2006. Available from http://www.ncbi.nlm.nih.gov/pmc/articles/PMC2626527/pdf/16501735.pdf (accessed August 31, 2012).

[2] Gilbert, Glen; Sawyer, Robin and McNeill, Lisa Beth. Health Education: Creating strategies for school & Community Health. United States: Jones and Barlett Publishers, LLC; 2011.

[3] Saracci, Rodolfo. Introducing the history of epidemiology. In: teaching epidemiology. A guide for teachers in epidemiology, public health and clinical medicine. Third Edition. Oxford: Oxford University Press, 2010.

[4] Novick, Lloyd and Morrow, Cynthia. Defining Public health: Historial and contemporary developments. In: Public Health Administration: Principles for Population-Based Management, Second Edition. Burlington: Jones & Barlett Learning; 2008.

[5] WHO. Closing the gap in a generation. Health equity through action on the social determinants of health. In: commission on social determinants of health. Final Report. Geneva: WHO;   2008.   Available   from   http://whqlibdoc.who.int/hq/2008/ WHO_IER_CSDH_08.1_eng.pdf (accessed August 10, 2012).

[6] HSS. Framework. Healthy People 2020. Washington D.C: U.S Department of Health and Human Services (HSS); 2012. Available from http://www.healthypeople.gov/ 2020/Consortium/HP2020Framework.pdf (accessed August 15, 2012).

[7] CDC. Sample Job Description. Sample Job Description: Performance Improvement Manager. Atlanta: Center for Disease Control and Prevention; 2010. Available from http://www.cdc.gov/stltpublichealth/docs/PHF%20-%20PIM%20Sample%20Job %20Description.pdf (accessed August 1, 2012).

[8] Seltzer, Beth. 101 Careers in Public Health. New York: Springer Publishing Company, LLC; 2011.

[9] Carney, Jan. Public Health in Action: Practicing in the Real world. United States: Jones and Barlett Learning; 2006.

[10] PHF. About the core competencies for public health professionals. Washington: Public Health Foundation; 2012. Available from: http://www.phf.org/programs/corecompetencies/Pages/ About_the_Core_Competencies_for_Public_Health_Professionals.aspx (accessed August 25, 2012)

[11] Keating, Gay et al. Generic Competencies for Public Health in Aotearoa-New Zealand. New Zealand: The Public Health Association of New Zealand. Available from http://www.pha.org.nz/documents/GenericCompetenciesforPublicHealth-March2007.pdf (accessed August 28, 2012)

[12] PHF. Core Competencies for Public Health Professionals. Washington: Public Health Foundation;   2012.   Available   from: https://www.train.org/competencies/corecomp.pdf (accessed August 25, 2012)

[13] WHO. Vacancy: Lecturer / Senior Lecturer in Public Health. Liverpool John Moores University. Liverpool: Collaborating Centre for Violence Prevention, World Health Organization.   Available   from   http://www.nwph.net/JD%20Senior%20Lecturer %20Public%20Health%20IC.pdf (accessed August 20, 2012)

[14] Bensley, Robert and Brookins-Fisher, Jodi. Community Health education and methods. A practical guide. United States: Jones and Barlett Publishers, LLC; 2009.

[15] Barnes, Louis, Roland, Christensen and Hansen, Abby. Teaching and the case method: Text, Cases and Readings. United States: Harvard Business School Press, 1994.

[16] CDC. Ten Great Public Health Achievements – United States, 2001 – 2010. In: Morbidity and Mortality Weekly Report. Vol 19. Atlanta: CDC; 2011. http://www.cdc.gov/mmwr/pdf/wk/mm6019.pdf

[17] CDC. Ten Great Public Health Achievements – Worldwide, 2001 – 2010. In: Morbidity and Mortality Weekly Report. Vol 24. Atlanta: CDC; 2011. http://www.cdc.gov/mmwr/pdf/wk/mm6024.pdf

[18] PAHO. Herramientas y metodologias TIC para mejorar la salud pública en la Región de las Américas. Washington: eSalud OPS. Pan American Health Organization; 2003. Available from http://www.cepal.org/elac/noticias/paginas/7/40837/jorge-walters.pdf (accessed August 30, 2012).

[19] Minelli, Mark and Breckon, Donald. Community Health Education: Settings, Roles, and Skills. 5th edition. United States: Jones and Barlett Publishers; 2009.

[20] USA. U.S. Strategy To Prevent and Respond to Gender-Based Violence Globally. Washingon: U.S Department of State; 2012. Available from http://blogs.state.gov/index.php/site/entry/us_strategy_gbv (accessed August 5, 2012)

[21] Riegelman, Richard. Public Health 101. Healthy people-Healthy populations. United States: Jones and Barlett Publishers, LLC; 2010.

Permissions

The contributors of this book come from diverse backgrounds, making this book a truly international effort. This book will bring forth new frontiers with its revolutionizing research information and detailed analysis of the nascent developments around the world.

We would like to thank Alfonso J. Rodriguez-Morales, for lending his expertise to make the book truly unique. He has played a crucial role in the development of this book. Without his invaluable contribution this book wouldn't have been possible. He has made vital efforts to compile up to date information on the varied aspects of this subject to make this book a valuable addition to the collection of many professionals and students.

This book was conceptualized with the vision of imparting up-to-date information and advanced data in this field. To ensure the same, a matchless editorial board was set up. Every individual on the board went through rigorous rounds of assessment to prove their worth. After which they invested a large part of their time researching and compiling the most relevant data for our readers. Conferences and sessions were held from time to time between the editorial board and the contributing authors to present the data in the most comprehensible form. The editorial team has worked tirelessly to provide valuable and valid information to help people across the globe.

Every chapter published in this book has been scrutinized by our experts. Their significance has been extensively debated. The topics covered herein carry significant findings which will fuel the growth of the discipline. They may even be implemented as practical applications or may be referred to as a beginning point for another development. Chapters in this book were first published by InTech; hereby published with permission under the Creative Commons Attribution License or equivalent.

The editorial board has been involved in producing this book since its inception. They have spent rigorous hours researching and exploring the diverse topics which have resulted in the successful publishing of this book. They have passed on their knowledge of decades through this book. To expedite this challenging task, the publisher supported the team at every step. A small team of assistant editors was also appointed to further simplify the editing procedure and attain best results for the readers.

Our editorial team has been hand-picked from every corner of the world. Their multi-ethnicity adds dynamic inputs to the discussions which result in innovative outcomes. These outcomes are then further discussed with the researchers and contributors who give their valuable feedback and opinion regarding the same. The feedback is then collaborated with the researches and they are edited in a comprehensive manner to aid the understanding of the subject.

Apart from the editorial board, the designing team has also invested a significant amount of their time in understanding the subject and creating the most relevant covers. They scrutinized every image to scout for the most suitable representation of the subject and create an appropriate cover for the book.

The publishing team has been involved in this book since its early stages. They were actively engaged in every process, be it collecting the data, connecting with the contributors or procuring relevant information. The team has been an ardent support to the editorial, designing and production team. Their endless efforts to recruit the best for this project, has resulted in the accomplishment of this book. They are a veteran in the field of academics and their pool of knowledge is as vast as their experience in printing. Their expertise and guidance has proved useful at every step. Their uncompromising quality standards have made this book an exceptional effort. Their encouragement from time to time has been an inspiration for everyone.

The publisher and the editorial board hope that this book will prove to be a valuable piece of knowledge for researchers, students, practitioners and scholars across the globe.

List of Contributors

Leonardo Sosa Valencia and Erika Rodriguez-Wulff
CITE (National Center of Ecoendoscopia), Caracas, Venezuela

Adrián Bolívar-Mejía
Medical School, Faculty of Health, Universidad Industrial de Santander, Bucaramanga, Santander, Colombia

Boris E. Vesga-Angarita
Instituto del Corazón de Bucaramanga, Internal Medicine Department, Universidad Industrial de Santander, Bucaramanga, Santander, Colombia

Maria de Lourdes Pereira
Departament of Biology & CICECO, Aveiro University, Aveiro, Portugal

Fernando Garcia e Costa
Departament of Morphology & Function, CIISA, Faculty of Veterinary Medicine, Technical University of Lisbon, Portugal

Irvathur Krishnananda Pai
Department of Zoology, Goa University, Goa, India

Matthew R. Hipsey
School of Earth and Environment, The University of Western Australia, Nedlands, Australia

Justin D. Brookes
School of Earth and Environmental Science, The University of Adelaide, Adelaide, Australia

John Berry
Department of Chemistry and Biochemistry, Florida International University, USA

Klara Slezakova
LEPAE, Departamento de Engenharia Química, Faculdade de Engenharia, Universidade do Porto, Portugal
REQUIMTE, Instituto Superior de Engenharia do Porto, Instituto Politécnico do Porto, Portugal

Maria do Carmo Pereira
LEPAE, Departamento de Engenharia Química, Faculdade de Engenharia, Universidade do Porto, Portugal

Simone Morais
REQUIMTE, Instituto Superior de Engenharia do Porto, Instituto Politécnico do Porto, Portugal

Naser Al-Jaser, M. Cli. Epi and Niyi Awofeso
School of Population Health, University of Western Australia, Australia

J. Ateudjieu
Faculty of Medicine and Biomedical Sciences, University of Yaounde 1, Centre Region, Cameroon
Faculty of Sciences, University of Dschang; Division of Health Operations Research, Ministry of Public Health Cameroon, Cameroon

E. A. Tembe-Fokunang and O. M. T. Abena
Faculty of Medicine and Biomedical Sciences, University of Yaounde 1, Centre Region, Cameroon

P. C. Chi and Lazare Kaptue
Cameroon National Ethics Committee (CNEC), Yaoundé, Cameroon

P. Awah
Faculty of Arts and Modern Letters, University of Yaoundé 1, Ipas, Chapel Hill, North Carolina, United States

R. Langsi
Health Division, University of Bamenda, Cameroon

C. N. Fokunang
Faculty of Medicine and Biomedical Sciences, University of Yaounde 1, Centre Region, Cameroon
Cameroon National Ethics Committee (CNEC), Yaoundé, Cameroon

M. Djuidje Ngounoue
Cameroon National Ethics Committee (CNEC), Yaoundé, Cameroon
Faculty of Sciences, University of Yaoundé 1, Centre Region, Cameroon

CN Fokunang
Faculty of Medicine and Biomedical Sciences, University of Yaoundé 1, Cameroon
Cameroon National Ethics Committee (CNEC), Yaoundé, Cameroon
Faculty of Health Sciences, University of Bamenda, Bambili, Cameroon

EA Tembe-Fokunang and O.M.T. Abena
Faculty of Medicine and Biomedical Sciences, University of Yaoundé 1, Cameroon

M. Djuidje Ngounoue, P.C. Chi, J Ateudjieu, G. Magne, N.M. Ndje and Kaptue Lazare
Cameroon National Ethics Committee (CNEC), Yaoundé, Cameroon

Awah Pascal
Department of Philosophy, Faculty of Arts and Social Sciences, University of Yaoundé 1, Cameroon

D. Sprumont
Chaire de Droit de la Santé, University of Neuchatel, Switzerland

Emma Bassett and Spencer Moore
School of Kinesiology and Health Studies, Queen's University, Kingston Ontario, Canada

Claudia Marin-Kelso
School of Medicine, Faculty of Health Sciences (Colombian Associated Center for the Iberoamerican Cochrane Network), Universidad Tecnológica de Pereira (UTP), Pereira, Colombia
Faculty of Health Sciences (Colombian Associated Center for the Iberoamerican Cochrane Network), Universidad Tecnológica de Pereira (UTP), Pereira, Risaralda, Colombia